Fifth Edition

Lifetime Physical Fitness and Wellness
A Personalized Program

Werner W. K. Hoeger

Boise State University

Sharon A. Hoeger

Morton Publishing Company
925 W. Kenyon, Unit 12
Englewood, Colorado 80110

Interior Design: Joanne R. Saliger
Cover Design: Bob Schram, Bookends
Cover Photo: Amber Lee Hoeger
Illustrator: Jennifer Johnson
Copy Editor: Carolyn Acheson
Typography: Ash Street Typecrafters, Inc.

Printed in the United States of America

10   9   8   7   6   5   4   3   2   1

ISBN: 0–89582–390–X

Preface

The current American way of life does not provide the human body with sufficient physical activity to enhance or maintain adequate health. Further, many present lifestyle patterns are such a serious threat to our health that they actually increase the deterioration rate of the human body and often lead to premature illness and mortality.

Although people in the United States are firm believers in the benefits of physical activity and positive lifestyle habits as a means to promote better health, most do not reap these benefits because they simply do not know how to implement a sound physical fitness and wellness program that will indeed yield the desired results. According to the Surgeon General, more than 60% of U.S. adults do not achieve the recommended amount of physical activity, and 25% are not physically active at all.

Scientific evidence has clearly shown that improving the quality and most likely the longevity of our lives is a matter of personal choice. The biggest challenge that we are faced with as we approach the 21st century is to teach individuals how to take control of their personal health habits to insure a better, healthier, happier, and more productive life. The information presented in this book has been written with this objective in mind, providing you with the opportunity to initiate your own healthy lifestyle program.

As you work through the different chapters in this book, you will be able to develop and regularly update your own lifetime program to improve the various components of physical fitness and wellness. The emphasis is on teaching you how to take control of your personal health and lifestyle habits, so that you can make a constant and deliberate effort to stay healthy and realize your highest potential for well-being.

What's New in the Fifth Edition

All chapters in this edition of Lifetime Physical Fitness and Wellness have been revised and updated to conform with advances and recommendations made since the publication of the fourth edition. The most significant changes in this new edition are:

- Key terms appear in boldface type and, together with their definitions, appear in boxes within the text. The terms are also combined in a glossary at the end of the book.
- The 1996 U.S. Surgeon General's Report on Physical Activity and Health has been reviewed and information from this report has been included in this fifth edition.
- Chapter 1 has been extensively revised and now includes a much broader discussion on wellness and its dimensions, an update on the association between fitness and mortality, the relevance of initiating and adhering to a fitness/wellness program during youth, and the effects of a healthy lifestyle on quality of life and longevity. The new definitions of physical activity and exercise are also provided in this chapter. Further, new and essential information on motivation and behavior modification to help students implement a lifetime wellness program are included. As a result of the latter addition, tips for behavior modification are provided throughout chapters in the book.
- New information on the effectiveness of Aerobelt exercise has been included under mode of exercise in the cardiorespiratory exercise prescription chapter. This chapter now also emphasizes the importance of strength conditioning prior to starting an aerobic exercise program to

minimize the risk of exercise-related injuries. Guidelines for exercise during pregnancy have been updated and additional information on exercise clothing is provided.

- Due to several reports regarding the validity and reliability of the abdominal crunch test and the large number of requests and concerns expressed by instructors throughout the country, the Bent-leg Curl-up test has again been incorporated into the Muscular Strength and Endurance and the Muscular Endurance Tests in Chapter 3. The Abdominal Crunch Test has been left as an alternate test item recommended for use by individuals who are at risk for low back injury.

- The nutrition chapter has also been extensively revised and contains an update on recent information released on antioxidant nutrients, phytochemicals, and the recent 1995 Dietary Guidelines for North Americans. The list of nutrients in Appendix A has also been expanded to 514 food items. Most of the new additions to this list are commercially prepared meals.

- Based on the latest research reports, the importance of physical activity as a major factor, if not the most important one, in the prevention of obesity and maintenance of recommended body weight has been enhanced in the weight control chapter. Further, evidence showing that lack of physical activity, and not excessive weight itself, as the cause of premature death rates associated with obesity is presented in this chapter. This finding is of significance because it appears that aerobically fit/overweight men have a lower risk of death than unfit men of normal weight and as low a risk of death as fit men of normal weight.

- The prescription of flexibility exercise conforms with the new 1995 guidelines for exercise testing and prescription by the American College of Sports Medicine (ACSM). Also, because of multiple requests, the tables containing flexibility test data now provide these data in both inches and in centimeters (cm).

- The cardiovascular disease prevention chapter has been updated to conform with recent developments in this area.

- Information on nicotine substitution products has been added to the Smoking Cessation chapter.

- Chapter 14 contains an update on health/fitness club membership and issues related to the selection, purchase, and maintenance of exercise equipment.

- New color photography and many new graphs have been added throughout the book.

● Ancillaries

The following ancillaries are provided free of charge to all qualified Lifetime Physical Fitness & Wellness adopters:

- Profile Plus for Windows: The most comprehensive computer software packages available with any fitness/wellness textbook. This software is custom-designed for this textbook and it includes a Fitness and Wellness Profile, a Personalized Cardiorespiratory Exercise Prescription, a Nutrient Analysis, and a weekly and monthly Exercise Log. This software package helps provide a more meaningful experience to all participants and greatly decreases the workload of course instructors.

- A video containing a detailed explanation of many of the fitness assessment test items used in the book. Instructors can use this video to help familiarize themselves with the proper test protocols for each fitness test. This audio-visual aid contains the following test items: 1.5-Mile Run Test, Step Test, Astrand-Ryhming Test, Muscular Strength and Endurance Test, Muscular Endurance Test, Strength-to-Body Weight Ratio Test, Modified Sit-and-Reach Test, Body Rotation Test, Shoulder Rotation Test, Skinfold Thickness Test, and Girth Measurements Test.

- Microtest, edited by Allan S. Cohen Consulting Services, a Fitness and Wellness Computerized Testbank contains the following options: (a) over 800 multiple choice questions, (b) capability to add/or edit test questions, (c) previously generated tests can be recalled — creating new exam versions because multiple choice answers can be rotated with each new test generated, and (d) capability to generate tests using a LaserJet printer.

- Over 60 color overhead transparency acetates of the book's most important illustrations and figures to facilitate class instruction and help explain key fitness and wellness concepts.

● An instructor's manual to aid with the implementation of your physical fitness and wellness course.

● Student Supplement for the World Wide Web

The World Wide Web has emerged as a valuable educational resource, and visiting cyberspace can make for a unique teaching and learning experience. The problem is: How do students identify sites that are academically appropriate and begin to use WWW sites in an educational context?

To make use of the resources of the World Wide Web in a practical way, JumpStart with WebLinks: A Guidebook for Fitness/Wellness/Personal Health is a suggested supplement. Edited by Professor Eileen L. Daniel, Ph.D., this spiral-bound guidebook (168 pages) contains 36 topics on fitness, wellness, and personal health. For each topic (e.g., cardiorespiratory endurance, eating disorders), a topic introduction orients students to the topic and concludes with a mix of personal assessment and content-related questions.

Following the topic introduction is a directory of WebLinks: the addresses (URLs) of four to six relevant WWW sites and a brief description of each site. These sites are appropriate for students and faculty alike. Each site has been fully verified and approved by a WebAdvisory Board made up of academics from colleges and universities throughout the United States and Canada. A brief Instructor's Resource Guide provides general information on how to incorporate JumpStart with WebLinks into any classroom setting.

Morton Publishing Company
1-800-348-3777
Web Site
http://www.morton-pub.com

Acknowledgments

We wish to express our gratitude to colleagues throughout the country who evaluated the fourth edition of *Lifetime Physical Fitness and Wellness*. The feedback received greatly enhanced the preparation of this edition.

Special thanks to Kaselah Crockett and Debbie Thompson who helped with the new photography in this fifth edition.

Contents

4 Muscular Strength Assessment and Prescription 87

6 Body Composition Assessment 141

5 Muscular Flexibility Assessment and Prescription 121

7 Nutrition for Wellness 159

8 Principles of Weight Management 195

9 Preventing Cardiovascular Disease 221

10 Cancer Risk Management 243

11 Stress Assessment and Management Techniques 267

Introduction to Lifetime Physical Fitness and Wellness

*M*ovement and physical activity are basic functions for which the human organism was created. Advances in modern technology have almost completely eliminated the need for physical activity in daily living. Physical activity is no longer a natural part of our existence. We now live in an automated society, in which most of the activities that used to require strenuous physical exertion can be accomplished by machines with the simple pull of a handle or push of a button.

The available scientific evidence shows that physical inactivity and a sedentary lifestyle seriously threaten our health and rapidly increase the deterioration rate of the human body. Physically active people live longer than their inactive counterparts, even if activity is started later in life. Estimates indicate that more than 250,000 deaths yearly in the United States are attributed to lack of regular physical activity.[1] Similar trends are found in most industrialized nations throughout the world.

Objectives

- Define wellness, list its dimensions, and identify components of wellness.
- Define physical fitness and list health-related and skill-related fitness components.
- Learn the differences between physical fitness and wellness.
- Distinguish between health standards and physical fitness standards.
- Identify the major health problems in the United States.
- Understand the benefits and the significance of participating in a lifetime fitness and wellness program.
- Identify lifestyle factors that help improve health and longevity.
- Learn motivation and behavior modification techniques to enhance compliance with a fitness and wellness program.
- Identify risk factors that may interfere with safe participation in exercise.

1

At the beginning of the 20th century, the most common health problems in the Western world were infectious diseases such as tuberculosis, diphtheria, influenza, kidney disease, polio, and other diseases of infancy. Progress in the field of medicine has largely eliminated these diseases. As the North American people started to enjoy the so-called good life (sedentary living, alcohol, fatty foods, excessive sweets, tobacco, drugs), we saw a parallel increase in the incidence of **chronic diseases** such as hypertension, coronary heart disease, atherosclerosis, strokes, diabetes, cancer, emphysema, and cirrhosis of the liver (see Figure 1.1).

As the incidence of chronic diseases climbed, we came to recognize prevention as the best medicine. Consequently, a new fitness and wellness movement developed gradually over the last three decades. People began to realize that good health is mostly self-controlled and that the leading causes of premature death and illness in North America could be prevented by adhering to positive lifestyle habits.

● Physical Activity Versus Exercise

Based on the abundance of scientific research on physical activity and exercise over the last three

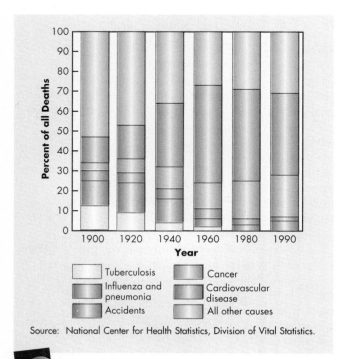

Source: National Center for Health Statistics, Division of Vital Statistics.

Figure 1.1 ● *Causes of death in the United States for selected years.*

decades, a clear distinction has been established between physical activity and exercise. **Physical activity** is defined as bodily movement produced by skeletal muscles that requires energy expenditure and produces progressive health benefits.[2] Examples of physical activity are walking to and from work and the store, taking stairs (instead of elevators and escalators), gardening, doing household chores, dancing, and washing the car by hand. Physical inactivity, on the other hand, implies a level of activity that is lower than that required to maintain good health.

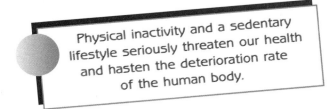

Physical inactivity and a sedentary lifestyle seriously threaten our health and hasten the deterioration rate of the human body.

Exercise is considered a type of physical activity that requires "planned, structured, and repetitive bodily movement done to improve or maintain one or more components of physical fitness."[3] A regular weekly program of walking, jogging, cycling, aerobics, swimming, strength training, or stretching exercises are all examples of exercise.

● Surgeon General's Report on Physical Activity and Health

A landmark report on the influence of regular physical activity on health was released in July of 1996 by the U.S. Surgeon General.[4] The significance of this historic document cannot be underestimated. Until 1996, only two previous reports had been released by the Surgeon General: one on smoking and health in 1964 and a second one on nutrition and health in 1988. More than 1,000 scientific studies from the fields of epidemiology, exercise physiology, medicine, and the behavioral sciences are summarized in this document on physical activity and health.

The report states that regular moderate physical activity provides substantial benefits in health and well-being for the vast majority of Americans who are not physically active. Among these benefits are a significant reduction in the risk of developing or dying from heart disease, diabetes, colon cancer, and high blood pressure. Regular physical activity is important for health of muscles, bones, and joints. It seems to reduce symptoms of depression and anxiety, improve mood, and enhance the ability to

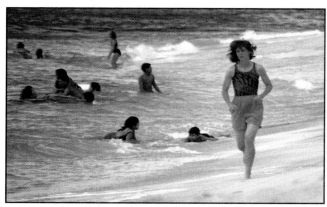

Exercise and an active lifestyle help increase health, quality of life, and longevity.

perform daily tasks throughout life. For individuals who are moderately active already, greater health benefits can be achieved by increasing the amount of physical activity.

According to the Surgeon General, improving health through physical activity is a serious public health issue that we must meet head-on at once. More than 60% of adults do not achieve the recommended amount of physical activity, and 25% are not physically active at all. Further, almost half of all people between age 12 and 21 are not vigorously active on a regular basis. This report has become a call to nationwide action.

Regular moderate physical activity can prevent premature death, unnecessary illness, and disability. It can also help control health care costs and help to maintain a high quality of life into old age. In the report, **moderate physical activity** has been defined as physical activity that uses 150 calories of energy per day, or 1,000 calories per week. People should strive to achieve at least 30 minutes of physical activity per day most days of the week. Examples of moderate physical activity include walking, cycling, playing basketball or volleyball, swimming, water aerobics, dancing fast, pushing a stroller, raking leaves, shoveling snow, washing or waxing a car, washing windows or floors, and gardening.

Most people recognize that participating in fitness programs improves their quality of life. In recent years, however, we came to realize that improving physical fitness alone was not always sufficient to lower the risk for disease and ensure better health. For example, individuals who run 3 miles (about 5 km) a day, lift weights regularly, participate in stretching exercises, and watch their body weight can be classified as having good or excellent fitness.

If these same people, however, have high blood pressure, smoke, are under constant stress, consume alcohol excessively, and eat too many fatty foods, they are at risk for cardiovascular disease and may not be aware of it. These characteristics that predict which people may develop a certain disease are called **risk factors**.

One of the best examples that good fitness does not always provide a risk-free guarantee of a healthy and productive life was the tragic death in 1984 of Jim Fixx, author of the best selling book *The Complete Book of Running*. At the time of his death by heart attack, Fixx was 52 years old. He had been running between 60 and 80 miles a week and had believed that people at his high level of fitness could not die from heart disease.

At age 36, Jim Fixx smoked two packs of cigarettes per day, weighed about 215 pounds, did not participate in regular physical activity, and had a family history of heart disease. His father, having had a first heart attack at age 35, later died at age 43.

Perhaps in an effort to lessen his risk for heart disease, Fixx began to raise his level of fitness. He started to jog, lost 50 pounds, and quit cigarette smoking. On several occasions, though, Fixx declined to have an exercise electrocardiogram (ECG) test, which most likely would have revealed his cardiovascular problem. His unfortunate death is a tragic example that exercise programs by themselves will not make high-risk people immune to heart disease, though they may delay the onset of a serious or fatal problem.

Good health, therefore, no longer is viewed as simply the absence of illness. The notion of good health has evolved notably in the last few years and

TERMS

Chronic diseases Illnesses that develop and last over a long time.

Physical activity Bodily movement produced by skeletal muscles that requires energy expenditure and produces progressive health benefits.

Exercise A type of physical activity that requires planned, structured, and repetitive bodily movement done to improve or maintain one or more components of physical fitness.

Moderate physical activity Physical activity that uses 150 calories of energy per day, or 1,000 calories per week.

Risk factors Characteristics that predict which people may develop a certain disease.

continues to change as scientists learn more about lifestyle factors that bring on illness and affect wellness. Once the idea took hold that fitness by itself would not always decrease the risk for disease and ensure better health, a new wellness concept developed in the 1980s.

● Wellness

Wellness is defined as the constant and deliberate effort to stay healthy and achieve the highest potential for well-being. Wellness is an all-inclusive umbrella covering a variety of activities aimed at helping individuals recognize components of lifestyle that are detrimental to their health. Wellness living requires implementing positive programs to change behavior to improve health and quality of life, prolong life, and achieve total well-being.

To enjoy a wellness lifestyle, a person needs to practice behaviors that will lead to positive outcomes in the five dimensions of wellness: physical, emotional, intellectual, social, and spiritual (see Figure 1.2). These dimensions are interrelated, and one dimension frequently affects the others. For example, a person who is emotionally down often has no desire to exercise, study, socialize with friends, or attend church.

In looking at the five dimensions of wellness, high-level wellness clearly goes beyond the absence of disease and optimal fitness. Wellness incorporates factors such as adequate fitness, proper nutrition, stress management, disease prevention, spirituality, smoking cessation, personal safety, substance abuse control, regular physical examinations, health education, and environmental support (see Figure 1.3).

Figure 1.2 ● *Dimensions of wellness.*

Figure 1.3 ● *Components of wellness.*

For a wellness way of life, not only must individuals be physically fit and manifest no signs of disease, but they also must have no risk factors for disease (such as hypertension, cigarette smoking, negative stress, faulty nutrition, careless sex). The relationship between adequate fitness and wellness is illustrated in the wellness continuum in Figure 1.4 Even though an individual tested in a fitness center may demonstrate adequate or even excellent fitness, indulgence in unhealthy lifestyle behaviors still will increase the risk for chronic diseases and decrease the person's well-being.

● Leading Health Problems in North America

The most prominent causes of death in North America today are largely lifestyle-related (see Figure 1.5). Current statistics indicate that about 65% of all deaths in the United States are caused by cardiovascular disease and cancer.[5] Nearly 80% of these deaths could be prevented through a healthy lifestyle program. The third cause of death, chronic and obstructive pulmonary disease, is related mostly to tobacco use. Accidents comprise the fourth leading cause of death. Even though not all accidents are preventable, many are. Fatal accidents are often related to abusing drugs and not wearing seat belts.

In looking at the underlying causes of death in the United States, estimates (see Figure 1.6) indicate that 9 of the 10 causes are related to lifestyle and lack of common sense. The "big three" — tobacco use, poor diet and inactivity, and alcohol abuse — are responsible for more than 800,000 deaths annually.

As the incidence of chronic diseases increased, it became obvious that prevention was the best medicine. Estimates indicate that more than half of disease is lifestyle-related, a fifth is attributed to the environment, and a tenth is influenced by the health care the individual receives. Only 16% is related to genetic factors.[6] Thus, the individual controls 84% of

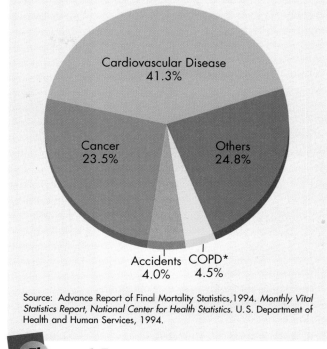

Source: Advance Report of Final Mortality Statistics,1994. *Monthly Vital Statistics Report, National Center for Health Statistics.* U.S. Department of Health and Human Services, 1994.

Figure 1.5 ● *Leading causes of death in the United States: 1991.*

disease and quality of life (see Figure 1.7). Further, according to estimates, 83% of deaths before age 65 are preventable. In essence, most North Americans are threatened by the very lives they lead today.

Ideally, healthy lifestyle habits should be taught and reinforced in early youth. Unfortunately, many young people are in such poor physical condition that they will add to national health concerns in years to come. Surveys conducted during the past decade have raised public concern regarding the fitness level of American youth. As compared to the

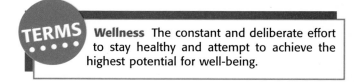

TERMS **Wellness** The constant and deliberate effort to stay healthy and attempt to achieve the highest potential for well-being.

Figure 1.4 ● *Wellness continuum.*

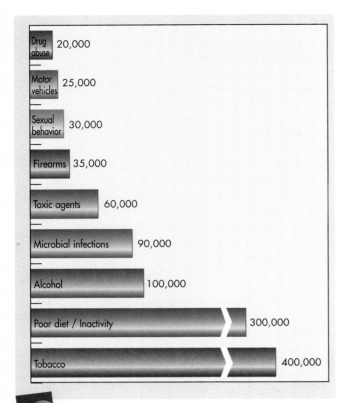

Figure 1.6 ● *Underlying causes of death in the United States.*

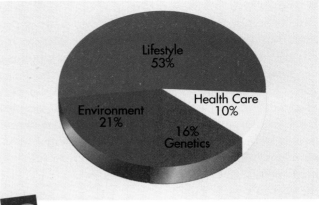

Figure 1.7 ● *Factors that affect health and well-being.*

1960s and 1970s, cardiorespiratory endurance and upper body strength have decreased and body fat has increased. These findings suggest that current physical education programs are not promoting lifetime fitness and wellness adequately.

Although the incidence of cardiovascular disease has declined remarkably in the last two decades, concern over youth fitness led Dr. Kenneth Cooper, Director of the Aerobics Research Institute in Dallas, Texas, to state: "It's discouraging and I'm afraid that as these kids grow up, we will see all the gains made against heart disease in the last twenty years wiped out in the next twenty years."[7] Even 5- and 6-year-old children already have coronary heart disease risk factors such as high blood pressure, excessive body fat, and low fitness.[8]

Because of the unhealthy lifestyles that many young adults lead, physically they may be middle-aged or older! Healthy choices made today influence health a decade or two later. Many physical education programs do not emphasize the skills necessary for our youth to maintain a high level of fitness and health throughout life. That is the intent of this book: to provide the skills and help to prepare you for a

lifetime of physical fitness and wellness. A healthy lifestyle is self-controlled, and people need to be taught how to be responsible for their own health and fitness.

Cardiovascular Disease

The most prevalent degenerative diseases in the United States are those of the cardiovascular system (see Figures 1.1 and 1.5). Almost half of all deaths in this country are attributed to diseases of the heart and blood vessel.

In 1997, according to estimates by the American Heart Association,[9] more than 57 million people in the United States were afflicted with diseases of the cardiovascular system, including 50 million with hypertension (high blood pressure) and 13.6 million with coronary heart disease. Many of these people have more than one type of cardiovascular disease.

In addition, the 1997 estimated cost of heart and blood vessel disease in the U.S. was expected to be around 259 billion dollars. Heart attacks alone cost American industry approximately 132 million workdays annually, including 24.6 billion dollars in lost productivity because of physical and emotional disability. About 38% of the people who die are in their most productive years, below age 75.

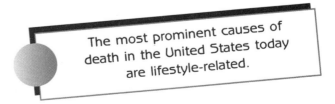

The most prominent causes of death in the United States today are lifestyle-related.

The American Heart Association estimates that more than $700 million a year in the United States is spent in replacing employees who have had heart attacks. About a million and a half people in the United States have heart attacks each year. Half a million of those people die as a consequence. About half the time, the first symptom of coronary heart disease is the heart attack itself, and 40% of those who have a first heart attack die within the first 24 hours. In one of every five cardiovascular deaths, sudden death is the initial symptom.

Most coronary heart disease risk factors are reversible and preventable. They can be controlled by modifying the lifestyle. A complete cardiovascular disease prevention program is outlined in Chapter 9.

Cancer

The second leading cause of death in the United States is cancer. The mortality rate for cancer had increased steadily over the last few decades (see Figure 1.1), but in 1996 the cancer rate decreased slightly for the first time. Even though cancer is not the number-one killer, it certainly is the number-one health fear of the American people.

Cancer is an uncontrolled growth and spread of abnormal cells in the body. Some cells grow into a mass of tissue called a tumor, which can be either benign or malignant. Benign tumors do not invade other tissues and rarely cause death. They may, however, interfere with normal body functions. A malignant tumor is considered a cancer. If the spread of cells is not controlled or checked, death is the inevitable result.

Approximately 24% of all deaths in the United States are attributable to cancer.[10] About 555,000 people died from this disease in 1996, and an estimated 1.4 million new cases were reported the same year. The major cause of increased cancer deaths the last four decades has been lung cancer. Without lung cancer, cancer mortality rates would have decreased by 14% between 1950 and 1990.

Testing procedures for early detection of cancer, as well as treatment modalities, are changing and improving continuously. More than 8 million Americans with a history of cancer now are alive, and close to 5 million of them can be considered cured. The American Cancer Society maintains that the most influential factor in fighting cancer today is prevention through health education programs. Evidence indicates that as much as 80% of all human cancer can be prevented through positive lifestyle behaviors.

The basic recommendations for preventing cancer include a diet high in fruits and vegetables, fiber, vitamins A and C, and low in fat. Alcohol, as well as salt-cured, smoked, and nitrite-cured foods, should be consumed in moderation. Cigarette smoking and tobacco use in general should be eliminated, and obesity should be avoided. A comprehensive cancer prevention program is presented in Chapter 10.

Wellness, Fitness, and Longevity

During the late 1960s and in the 1970s, we began to realize that good fitness is important in the fight against chronic diseases, particularly those of the cardiovascular system. Because of more participation in fitness programs in the last few years, cardiovascular mortality rates have dropped. The rate started to decline in about 1963, and between 1970 and 1988 heart disease dropped by 34%. This decrease is credited to higher levels of wellness and better health care in the United States. More than half of the decline is attributed to improvements in diet and fewer people smoking.

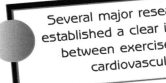

Several major research studies have established a clear inverse relationship between exercise and premature cardiovascular mortality.

Furthermore, several studies have shown an inverse relationship between physical activity and premature cardiovascular mortality rates. In a study conducted among 16,936 Harvard alumni linking physical activity habits and mortality rates, as the amount of weekly physical activity increased, the risk of cardiovascular deaths decreased.[11] The largest decrease in cardiovascular deaths was observed among alumni who used up more than 2000 calories per week through physical activity. Figure 1.8 graphically illustrates the study results.

A major study published in the *Journal of the American Medical Association*, based on data from 13,344 people followed over an average of 8 years, upheld the findings of the Harvard alumni study.[12] The results confirmed that the level of cardiorespiratory fitness is related to mortality from all causes.

TERMS

Cancer Uncontrolled growth and spread of abnormal cells in the body; a malignancy.

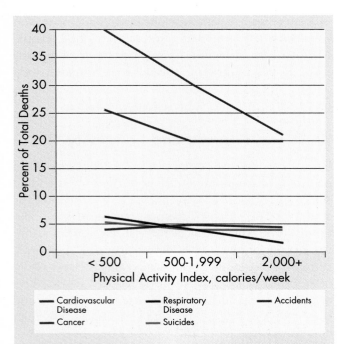

NOTE: The graph represents cause-specific death rates per 10,000 man-years of observation among 16,936 Harvard alumni, 1962–1978, by physical activity index; adjusted for differences in age, cigarette smoking, and hypertension.

Source: "A Natural History of Athleticism on Cardiovascular Health," by R. S. Paffenbarger, R. T. Hyde, A. L. Wing,. and C. H. Steinmetz, *Journal of the American Medical Association*, 252 (1989), 491–495. Used by permission.

Figure 1.8 ● *Death rates by physical activity index.*

The study revealed a graded and consistent inverse relationship between cardiorespiratory fitness and mortality, regardless of age and other risk factors. As illustrated in Figure 1.9, the higher the level of cardiorespiratory fitness, the lower the mortality rate. Death rates from all causes for the least fit (group 1) men were 3.4 times higher than the most fit (group 5) men. For the least fit women, the death rates were 4.6 times higher than the most fit women.

This study also reported a greatly reduced rate of premature death, even at moderate fitness levels that most adults can achieve easily. Even greater protection is attained when increased fitness levels are combined with reduction in other risk factors such as hypertension, serum cholesterol, cigarette smoking, and excessive body fat.

In another major research study conducted in the 1980s, a healthy lifestyle was shown to contribute to some of the lowest mortality rates ever reported in the literature.[13] As illustrated in Figure 1.10, compared with the general White population, this group of 5,231 men and 4,631 women (wives) had much lower cancer, cardiovascular, and overall death rates.

Healthy lifestyle habits include abstaining from tobacco, alcohol, caffeine, and drugs, and adhering to a well-balanced diet, based on grains, fruits, and vegetables, and moderate consumption of poultry

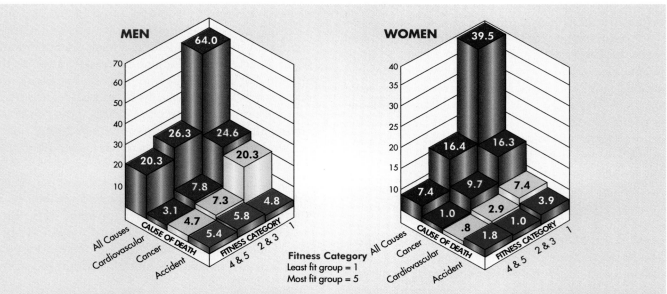

Based on data from "Physical Fitness and All-Cause Mortality: A Prospective Study of Healthy Men and Women," by S. N. Blair, H. W. Kohl III, R. S. Paffenbarger, Jr., D. G. Clark, K. H. Cooper, and L. W. Gibbons. *Journal of the American Medical Association*, 262 (1989), 2395–2401.

Figure 1.9 ● *Death rates by physical fitness groups.*

and red meat. The investigators in this study looked at three general health habits among the participants: lifetime abstinence from smoking, regular physical activity, and sleep.

Men in this study had one-third the death rate from cancer, one-seventh the death rate from cardiovascular disease, and one-fifth the rate of overall mortality. The wives had about half the rate of cancer and overall mortality and a third the death rate from cardiovascular disease. Life expectancies for 25-year-olds who adhered to the three health habits were 85 and 86 years, respectively, as compared to 74 and 80 for the average U.S. White man and woman (see Figure 1.11).

From this study we can conclude that people who adhere to a lifetime healthy lifestyle indeed will reap healthy rewards. Better health leads to improvements in quality of life. The additional 6 to 11 years of "golden" life are precious to those who maintain a lifetime wellness program.

Additional research that looked at changes in fitness and mortality found a substantial (44%) reduction in mortality risk when people abandon a sedentary lifestyle and become moderately fit.[14] The lowest death rate was found in people who were fit and remained fit, and the highest rate was found in men who remained unfit (see Figure 1.12).

Subsequent research published in 1995 in the *Journal of the American Medical Association* substantiated the previous findings but also indicated that primarily vigorous activities are associated with

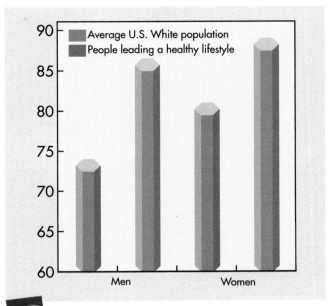

Figure 1.11 ● *Life expectancy for 25-year-olds who adhere to a lifetime healthy lifestyle program as compared to the average U.S. White population.*

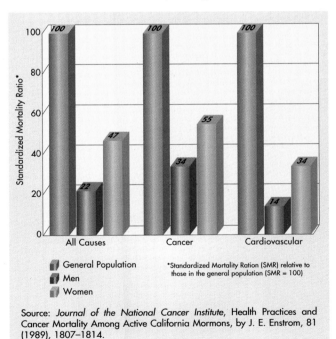

Source: *Journal of the National Cancer Institute*, Health Practices and Cancer Mortality Among Active California Mormons, by J. E. Enstrom, 81 (1989), 1807–1814.

Figure 1.10 ● *Effects of a healthy lifestyle on all causes, cancer, and cardiovascular death rates in White men and women.*

* Death rate per 10,000 man-years observation. Based on data from "Changes in Physical Fitness and All-Cause Mortality: A Prospective Study of Healthy Men," Journal of the American Medical Association, 273 (1995), 1193–1198.

Source: J. E. Enstrom, "Health Practices and Cancer Mortality Among Active California Mormons," Journal of the National Cancer Institute, 81 (1989), 1807–1814.

Figure 1.12 ● *Five-year follow-up in mortality rates associated with maintenance and improvements in fitness.*

greater longevity.[15] **Vigorous activity** was defined as any activity that requires a MET level equal to or greater than 6 METs (21 ml/kg/min — see Health Fitness Standards, below). One **MET** is the body's energy expenditure at rest, or approximately 3.5 ml/kg/min. Six or more METs represents exercising at an oxygen uptake (VO_2) equal to or greater than 6 times the resting energy requirement.

Examples of vigorous activities used in the previous study include brisk walking, jogging, swimming laps, squash, racquetball, tennis, and shoveling snow. Results also indicated that vigorous exercise is as important as not smoking and maintaining recommended weight.

The results of these studies clearly indicate that fitness improves wellness, quality of life, and longevity. If people are able to do vigorous exercise, it is preferable because it is most clearly associated with longer life.

● Physical Fitness

The most comprehensive definition of physical fitness is that of the American Medical Association, which has defined **physical fitness** as the general capacity to adapt and respond favorably to physical effort. As the fitness concept grew during the 1970s, it became clear that no single test was sufficient to assess overall fitness. A battery of tests was necessary because several specific components have to be established to determine an individual's overall level of fitness.

Physical fitness can be classified into health-related and motor skill-related fitness. As shown in Figure 1.13, the four health-related fitness components are: cardiorespiratory (aerobic) endurance, muscular strength and endurance, muscular flexibility, and body composition. Skill-related fitness components consist of agility, balance, coordination, power, reaction time, and speed (Figure 1.14). The latter are aimed primarily at succeeding in athletics and may not be as crucial in developing better health. In terms of preventive medicine, the main emphasis of fitness programs should be on the health-related components. That is the focus of this book.

Fitness Standards: Health Versus Physical Fitness

Throughout the discussion of health-related fitness assessment in Chapters 2, 4, 5, and 6, several tests are identified to assess fitness. A meaningful debate regarding age- and gender-related fitness standards for the general population has resulted in the two standards: a health fitness standard (criterion-referenced) and a physical fitness standard.

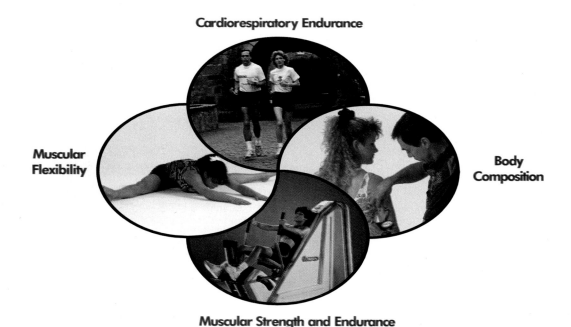

Figure 1.13 ● *Health-related components of physical fitness.*

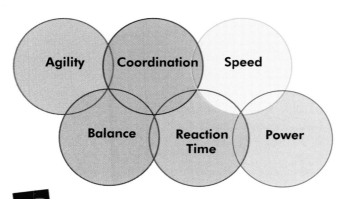

Figure 1.14 • *Motor skill-related components of physical fitness.*

Health Fitness Standards

As illustrated in Figure 1.15, although fitness (VO_{2max} — see discussion below) improvements with a moderate aerobic activity program are not as notable, significant health benefits are reaped with such a program. These improvements are quite striking, and only slightly greater health benefits are obtained with a more intense exercise program. These benefits include a reduction in blood lipids, lower blood pressure, decreased risk for diabetes, weight loss, stress release, and lower risk for disease and premature mortality. More specifically, improvements in the **metabolic profile** (better insulin sensitivity and glucose tolerance and improved plasma lipid and lipoprotein levels) can be notable in spite of little or no improvement in aerobic capacity or weight loss. These improvements in the metabolic profile through an active lifestyle and exercise are referred to as **metabolic fitness**.

The **health fitness** (or criterion-referenced) **standards** used in this book are based on epidemiological data linking minimum fitness values to disease prevention and health. Attaining the health fitness standards requires only moderate amounts of physical activity. For example, a 2-mile walk in less than 30 minutes, five to six times per week, seems to be sufficient to achieve the health-fitness standard for cardiorespiratory endurance.

Cardiorespiratory endurance is measured in terms of the maximal amount of oxygen the body is able to utilize per minute of physical activity (maximal oxygen uptake or VO_{2max}). VO_{2max} commonly is

TERMS

Vigorous activity Any activity that requires a MET level equal to or greater than 6 METs.

MET The body's energy expenditure at rest.

Physical fitness General capacity to adapt and respond favorably to physical effort.

Metabolic profile Used to assess risk for diabetes and cardiovascular disease through plasma insulin, glucose, lipid, and lipoprotein levels.

Metabolic fitness Denotes improvements in the metabolic profile through a moderate-intensity exercise program in spite of little or no improvements in health-related fitness.

Health fitness standards The lowest fitness requirements for maintaining good health, decreasing the risk for chronic diseases, and lowering the incidence of muscular-skeletal injuries.

Cardiorespiratory endurance The ability of the lungs, heart, and blood vessels to deliver adequate amounts of oxygen to the cells to meet the demands of prolonged physical activity.

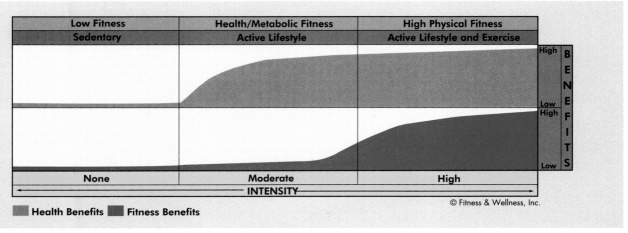

Figure 1.15 • *Health and fitness benefits based on the type of lifestyle and physical activity program.*

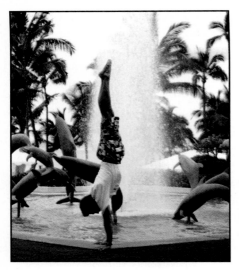

Good health- and skill-related fitness are required to participate in highly skilled activities.

expressed in milliliters of oxygen per kilogram of body weight per minute (ml/kg/min). Individual values can range from about 10 ml/kg/min in cardiac patients to approximately 80 to 90 ml/kg/min in world-class runners and cross-country skiers.

Data from the research study presented in Figure 1.9 indicate that VO_{2max} values of 35 and 32.5 ml/kg/min for men and women, respectively, may be sufficient to lower the risk for all-cause mortality significantly. Although greater improvements in fitness yield a slightly lower risk for premature death, the largest drop is seen between the least fit (group 1) and the moderately fit (groups 2 and 3). Therefore, the 35 and 32.5 ml/kg/min values could be selected as the health fitness standards.

Physical Fitness Standards

Physical fitness standards are set higher than the health fitness norms and require a more vigorous exercise program. Many experts believe that people who meet the criteria of "good" physical fitness should be able to do moderate to vigorous physical activity without undue fatigue and to maintain this capability throughout life. In this context, physically fit people of all ages will have the freedom to enjoy most of life's daily and recreational activities to their fullest potential. Current health fitness standards may not be enough to achieve these objectives.

Sound physical fitness gives the individual a degree of independence throughout life that many people in North America no longer enjoy. Most older people should be able to carry out activities similar to those conducted in their youth, though

not with the same intensity. Although a person does not have to be an elite athlete, activities such as changing a tire, chopping wood, climbing several flights of stairs, playing a vigorous game of basketball, mountain biking, playing soccer with grandchildren, walking several miles around a lake, and hiking through a national park require more than the current "average fitness" level of the American people.

If the main objective of the fitness program is to lower the risk for disease, attaining the health fitness standards may be enough to ensure better health. On the other hand, if the individual wants to participate in moderate to vigorous fitness activities, achieving a high physical fitness standard is recommended. For the purposes of this book, therefore, both health fitness and physical fitness standards are given for each fitness test. The individual then needs to decide the personal objectives for the fitness program.

● Benefits of a Comprehensive Wellness Program

A most inspiring story illustrating what fitness can do for a person's health and well-being is that of George Snell from Sandy, Utah. At age 45, Snell weighed approximately 400 pounds, his blood pressure was 220/180, he was blind because of diabetes he did not know he had, and his blood glucose level was 487.

Snell had determined to do something about his physical and medical condition, so he started a walking/jogging program. After about 8 months of conditioning, Snell had lost almost 200 pounds, his eyesight had returned, his glucose level was down to 67, and he was taken off medication. Two months later, less than 10 months after beginning his personal exercise program, he completed a marathon, a running course of 26.2 miles.

Health Benefits

Most people exercise because it improves their personal appearance and makes them feel good about themselves. Although many benefits accrue from participating in a regular fitness and wellness program and active people generally live longer, the greatest benefit of all is that physically fit individuals enjoy a better quality of life. These people live life to its fullest, with fewer health problems than inactive individuals who also may indulge in negative lifestyle patterns. Although compiling an all-inclusive list of the benefits reaped from participating in a fitness and wellness program is difficult, the following list summarizes many of these benefits.

1. Improves and strengthens the cardiorespiratory system (by facilitating oxygen supply to all parts of the body, including the heart, muscles, and brain).
2. Maintains better muscle tone, muscular strength, and endurance.
3. Improves muscular flexibility.
4. Helps maintain recommended body weight.
5. Improves posture and physical appearance.
6. Lowers the risk for chronic diseases (such as diseases of the cardiovascular system and cancer).
7. Decreases the mortality rate from chronic diseases.
8. Thins the blood so it is less likely to clot (decreasing the risk for coronary heart disease and strokes).
9. Prevents or delays the development of high blood pressure and lowers blood pressure in people with hypertension.
10. Lowers the risk of developing non-insulin-dependent-diabetes.
11. Helps achieve peak bone mass in young adults and maintain bone mass later in life.
12. Helps people sleep better.
13. Helps prevent chronic back pain.
14. Relieves tension and helps in coping with life stresses.
15. Raises levels of energy and job productivity.
16. Extends longevity and slows down the aging process.
17. Improves self-image and morale and helps fight depression and anxiety.
18. Motivates toward positive changes in lifestyle (better nutrition, quitting smoking, alcohol and drug abuse control).
19. Speeds recovery time following physical exertion.
20. Speeds recovery following injury and disease.
21. Regulates and improves overall body functions.
22. Improves physical stamina and counteracts chronic fatigue.
23. Improves quality of life; makes people feel better and live a healthier and happier life.

Economic Benefits

The economic impact of sedentary living can leave a strong impression on a nation's economy. As the need for physical exertion in Western countries decreased steadily during the last century, health-care expenditures have increased dramatically. Health-care costs in the United States rose from $12 billion in 1950 to approximately $1 trillion in 1995 (Figure 1.16). At the present rate of escalation, health-care expenditures will reach $1.6 trillion by the year 2002. The 1995 figure represents about 14% of the gross national product (GNP). It is projected to reach about 18% by the year 2002 and 37% by 2030.

Unhealthy behaviors are contributing to the staggering U.S. health-care costs. Risk factors for disease carry a heavy price tag (see Figure 1.17). According to estimates, 1% of Americans account

Figure 1.16 ● *U.S. health care cost increments since 1950.*

TERMS

Physical fitness standards A fitness level that allows a person to sustain moderate to vigorous physical activity without undue fatigue and the ability to closely maintain this level throughout life.

for 30% of these costs.[16] Half of the people use up about 97% of the health-care dollars. Furthermore, and as illustrated in Figure 1.18, the 1989 average health-care cost per person in the United States ($2,354) was almost twice as high as for most other industrialized nations.

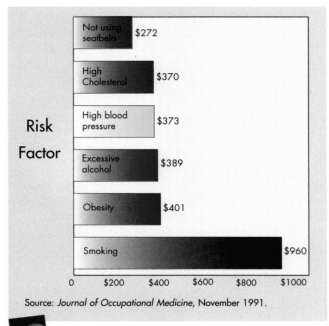

Source: *Journal of Occupational Medicine*, November 1991.

Figure 1.17 ● *Average annual health care costs for leading risk factors.*

Strong scientific evidence now links participation in fitness and wellness programs not only to better health but also to lower medical costs and higher job productivity. Most of this research is being conducted and reported by organizations that already have implemented fitness or wellness programs. Approximately half of the health-care expenditures in the United States are being absorbed by American business and industry. In 1989, business spending on health insurance premiums and health care for employees and former employees was more than 100% of after-tax profits by all U. S. companies combined.

As a result of the staggering rise in medical costs, many organizations are beginning to realize that keeping employees healthy costs less than treating them once they are sick. A 1991 survey by the American Institute for Preventive Medicine found that large corporations are finding health-cost savings by implementing health promotion programs.[17] A sample return on investment per dollar spent is provided in Figure 1.19. Containing the costs of health care through fitness and wellness programs has become a major issue for many organizations around North America. Let's examine the evidence.

The Prudential Insurance Company of Houston, Texas, conducted a study on its 1,386 employees and found that those who participated for at least

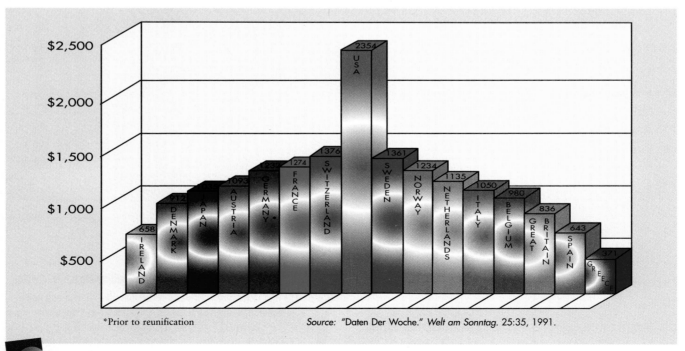

Prior to reunification　　　　　　Source: "Daten Der Woche." Welt am Sonntag. 25:35, 1991.

Figure 1.18 ● *1989 average health care costs per person for selected countries.*

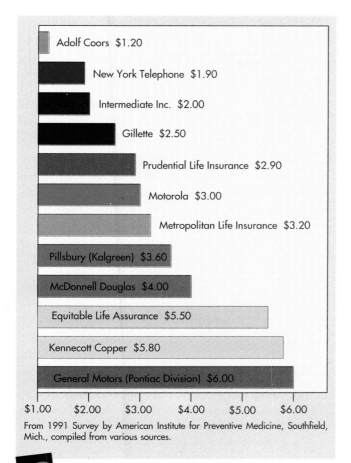

Adolf Coors	$1.20
New York Telephone	$1.90
Intermediate Inc.	$2.00
Gillette	$2.50
Prudential Life Insurance	$2.90
Motorola	$3.00
Metropolitan Life Insurance	$3.20
Pillsbury (Kalgreen)	$3.60
McDonnell Douglas	$4.00
Equitable Life Assurance	$5.50
Kennecott Copper	$5.80
General Motors (Pontiac Division)	$6.00

$1.00 $2.00 $3.00 $4.00 $5.00 $6.00

From 1991 Survey by American Institute for Preventive Medicine, Southfield, Mich., compiled from various sources.

Figure 1.19 • *Health care cost savings by selected corporations per dollar spent on health promotion programs.*

one year in the company's fitness program averaged 3.5 days of disability, compared to 8.6 days for nonparticipants. A further breakdown by level of fitness showed no disability days for those in the high-fitness group, 1.6 days for the good-fitness group, and 4.1 days for the fair-fitness group.

Since 1979, the Mesa Petroleum Company in Amarillo, Texas, has offered an on-site fitness program to its employees and their family members. Data analysis showed the average medical costs per person to be 150% higher for the nonparticipating group than for the fitness-participating group. Sick leave time also was significantly less for the physically active group — 27 hours per year, compared to 44 for the inactive group.

A similar study, conducted by Tenneco Incorporated in Houston, also showed a significant reduction in medical-care costs for men and women who participated in an exercise program. Annual medical care costs for male and female nonexercisers were 79% and 140% higher than those of the exercisers. Sick leave also was reduced in the men and women participants.

Furthermore, a survey of the more than 3,000 employees at Tenneco found that job productivity is related to fitness. The company reported that individuals with high job performance ratings also rated high in exercise participation.

Strong data also are coming in from Europe. Research in Germany reported 68.6% less absenteeism among workers with cardiovascular symptoms who participated in a fitness program. The law mandates that corporations employing workers for sedentary jobs must provide an in-house facility for physical exercise.

The Goodyear Company in Norrkoping, Sweden, indicated a 50% reduction in absenteeism following implementation of a fitness program. Studies in the former Soviet Union report expanded physical work capacity and motor coordination, lower incidence of disease, shorter duration of illness, and fewer relapses among individuals participating in industrial fitness programs.

Another reason some organizations are offering wellness programs to their employees — overlooked by many because it does not seem to affect the bottom line directly — is simply concern by top management for the physical well-being of employees. Whether the program lowers medical costs is not the main issue. The only reason that really matters to top management is that wellness programs help individuals feel better about themselves and improve their quality of life.

Such is the case of Mannington Mills Corporation, which invested $1.8 million in an on-site fitness center. The return on investment is secondary to the company's interest in happier and healthier employees. The center also is open to dependents and retirees. As a result of this program, Mannington Mills believes the participants — about half of the 1,600 people who are eligible — can enjoy life to its fullest potential, and the employees most likely will be more productive simply because of the company's caring attitude.

In addition to the financial and physical benefits, some corporations are offering health promotion programs as an incentive to attract, hire, and retain employees. Many companies are taking a hard look at the fitness and health level of potential employees and are using this information in their screening process. Some organizations refuse to hire smokers or overweight individuals.

Other executives believe that an on-site health promotion program is the best fringe benefit they can offer at their company. Young executives are looking for organizations such as these, not only for the added health benefits but also because the head corporate officers are showing an attitude of concern and care.

● The Wellness Challenge for the 21st Century

Because a better and healthier life is something every person should strive for, our biggest challenge as we look to the turn of the century is to teach people how to take control of their personal health habits and adhere to a positive lifestyle. Considering the wealth of information available on the benefits of fitness and wellness programs, improving the quality and possible length of our lives is a matter of personal choice.

Research indicates that to significantly improve health and extend life, a person should:

1. *Participate in a lifetime physical activity program.* Exercise regularly at least three times per week and try to accumulate a minimum of 30 minutes of physical activity each day of your life. The exercise program should consist of 20 to 60 minutes of aerobic exercise, along with some strengthening and stretching exercises.

2. *Do not smoke cigarettes.* Cigarette smoking is the largest preventable cause of illness and premature death in the United States. When considering all related deaths, smoking is responsible for more than 400,000 unnecessary deaths each year.

3. *Eat right.* Eat a good breakfast and two additional well-balanced meals every day. Unless snacks consist of healthy foods, refrain from snacking between meals. Avoid eating too many calories and foods with a lot of sugar, fat, and sodium (salt). Increase your daily consumption of fruits, vegetables, and whole-grain products.

4. *Maintain recommended body weight.* Maintain proper body weight through adequate nutrition and exercise. This is important in preventing chronic diseases and in developing a higher level of fitness.

5. *Get enough rest.* Sleep 7 to 8 hours each night.

6. *Lower stress levels.* Reduce your vulnerability to stress, and practice stress management techniques as needed.

7. *Be wary of alcohol.* Drink alcohol moderately or not at all. Alcohol abuse leads to mental, emotional, physical, and social problems.

8. *Surround yourself with healthy friendships.* Unhealthy friendships contribute to destructive behaviors and low self-esteem. Associating with people who strive to maintain good fitness and health reinforces a positive outlook in life and encourages positive behaviors. Constructive social interactions enhance well-being.

9. *Be informed about the environment.* Seek clean air, clean water, and a clean environment. Be aware of pollutants and occupational hazards: asbestos fibers, nickel dust, chromate, uranium dust, and so on. Take precautions when using pesticides and insecticides.

10. Take personal safety measures. Although not all accidents are preventable, many are. Taking simple precautionary measures, such as using seat belts and keeping electrical appliances away from water (see Appendix C), lessens the risk for avoidable accidents.

Thanks to current scientific data and the fitness and wellness movement of the past three decades, most Americans now see a need to participate in programs that improve and maintain health. The typical American, however, is not a good role model when cardiorespiratory fitness is concerned. Almost 60% of U.S. adults engage in little or no leisure-time physical activity. In 1996, only 40% of the adults in the United States exercised strenuously three or more days per week.[18]

Aerobic activities are the most popular form of exercise, so even a lower percentage of the population probably engages in and derives benefits from strength and flexibility programs. In addition, an estimated half or more of the adult population in the United States has a weight problem, and a third of all adults is considered obese (20% or more above recommended weight).

Even though people in the United States believe a positive lifestyle has a great impact on health and longevity, most do not reap the benefits because they don't know how to implement a safe and effective fitness and wellness program. Others are exercising incorrectly and therefore are not reaping the full benefits of their program.

● U.S. Health Objectives for the Year 2000

Every 10 years the U.S. Department of Health and Human Services releases a list of objectives for preventing disease and promoting health. From its onset in 1980, this 10-year plan has helped instill a new sense of purpose and focus for public health and preventive medicine. The Year 2000 objectives, published in the document *Healthy People 2000*,[19] address three important points:

1. *Personal responsibility:* The need for individuals to become ever more health-conscious. Responsible and informed behaviors are the key to good health.

2. *Health benefits for all people:* Lower socio-economic conditions and poor health often are interrelated. Extending the benefits of good health to all people is crucial to the health of the nation.

3. *Health promotion and disease prevention:* A shift from treatment to preventive techniques will drastically cut health-care costs and help all Americans achieve a higher quality of life.

Development of the Year 2000 health objectives involved more than 10,000 people representing 300 national organizations, including the Institute of Medicine of the National Academy of Sciences, all state health departments, and the federal Office of Disease Prevention and Health Promotion. A summary of key objectives is provided in Figure 1.20. Living the fitness and wellness principles provided in this book not only will enhance the quality of your life but also will allow you to be an active participant in achieving the Healthy People 2000 objectives.

● Motivation and Behavior Modification

Scientific evidence of the benefits derived from living a healthy lifestyle continues to mount each day. Although the data are impressive, most people still don't adhere to a healthy lifestyle. Understanding why people do not live a healthy lifestyle may help increase your readiness and motivation to do so.

To answer this question, one has to examine what motivates people and what actions are required to make permanent changes in behavior.

Motivation is often set forth as an explanation for why some people succeed and others don't. Although motivation comes from within, external factors trigger the inner desire to accomplish a given task. These external factors, then, control behavior.

When studying motivation, understanding **locus of control** is helpful. People who believe they have control over events in their lives are said to have an internal locus of control. People with an external locus of control believe that what happens to them is a result of chance — the environment — and is unrelated to their behavior.

People with an internal locus of control are healthier and have an easier time initiating and adhering to a wellness program. In contrast, those who perceive that they have no control think of themselves as powerless and vulnerable. Becoming motivated is often a challenge. These people are also at greater risk for illness. When illness strikes, restoring a sense of control is vital to regain health.

Few people have either a completely external or a completely internal locus of control. They fall somewhere along a continuum. Where a person is along the continuum relates to his or her health. Also, the more external, the greater is the challenge in adhering to exercise and other healthy lifestyle behaviors. Fortunately, developing a more internal locus of control can be accomplished. Understanding that most events in life are not controlled genetically or environmentally helps people pursue goals and gain control over their lives. Three impediments, however, can keep people from taking action: lack of competence, confidence, and motivation.[20]

1. *Problems of competence.* Lacking the skills to get a given task done leads to decreased competence. If your friends play basketball regularly but you don't know how to play, you might not be inclined to participate. The solution to the problem of competence is to master the skills needed to participate. Most people are not born

---

TERMS

Motivation   The desire and will to do something.

Locus of control   The extent to which a person believes he or she can influence the external environment.

HEALTHY PEOPLE 2000:
SELECTED HEALTH OBJECTIVES FOR THE YEAR 2000

I. Physical Activity and Fitness

1. Increase the proportion of people who engage regularly, preferably daily, in *light* to *moderate* physical activity for at least 30 minutes per day.
2. Increase the proportion of people who engage in *vigorous* physical activity that promotes the development and maintenance of cardio-respiratory fitness 3 or more days per week for 20 or more minutes per occasion.
3. Increase the proportion of people who regularly perform physical activities that enhance and maintain muscular strength, muscular endurance, and flexibility.
4. Reduce the proportion of people who engage in no leisure-time physical activity.
5. Reduce overweight to a prevalence of no more than 20% among people aged 20 and older and no more than 15% among adolescents aged 12 through 19.
6. Increase to at least 50% the proportion of overweight people aged 12 and older who have adopted sound dietary practices combined with regular physical activity to attain an appropriate body weight.

II. Nutrition

1. Reduce dietary fat intake to an average of 30% of calories or less and average saturated fat intake to less than 10% of calories among people aged 2 and older.
2. Increase complex carbohydrate and fiber-containing foods in the diets of adults to 5 or more daily servings for vegetables and fruits, and to 6 or more daily servings for grain products.
3. Increase calcium consumption in the diet.
4. Reduce iron deficiency among children ages 1 through 4 and women of childbearing age.
5. Decrease salt and sodium intake in the diet.
6. Increase to at least 85% the proportion of people aged 18 and older who use food labels to make nutritious selections.

III. Chronic Diseases

1. Increase years of healthy life to at least 65 years.
2. Reduce coronary heart disease deaths.
3. Reduce the mean serum cholesterol level among adults to no more than 200 mg/dL.
4. Increase the proportion of adults with high blood cholesterol who are aware of their condition and are taking action to reduce their blood cholesterol to recommended levels.
5. Increase the proportion of people with high blood pressure whose blood pressure is under control.
6. Increase the proportion of people with high blood pressure who are taking action to help control their blood pressure.
7. Reverse the rise in cancer deaths.
8. Slow the rise in lung cancer deaths.
9. Reduce the rate of breast cancer deaths.
10. Reduce colorectal cancer deaths.
11. Reduce diabetes-related deaths.
12. Reduce the proportion of people with asthma who experience limitation in activity.
13. Reduce deaths from cirrhosis of the liver.
14. Reduce hip fractures among older adults.
15. Reduce limitation in activity because of chronic back conditions.
16. Reduce the proportion of people who experience a limitation in major activity because of chronic conditions.

IV. Mental Health and Disorders

1. Reduce the prevalence of mental disorders.
2. Reduce the suicide rate.
3. Reduce the proportion of people who experience adverse health effects from stress.
4. Decrease the proportion of people who experience stress who do not take steps to reduce or control their stress.

V. Tobacco

1. Reduce the incidence of cigarette smoking.
2. Reduce the initiation of cigarette smoking by children and youth.
3. Reduce the proportion of children who are exposed regularly to tobacco smoke at home.
4. Reduce use of smokeless tobacco.
5. Increase the proportion of worksites with a formal smoking policy that prohibits or severely restricts smoking at the workplace.

VI. Alcohol and Other Drugs

1. Reduce the proportion of young people who have used alcohol, marijuana, and cocaine.
2. Reduce the proportion of high school seniors and college students engaging in recent occasions of heavy drinking of alcoholic beverages.
3. Reduce alcohol consumption by people aged 14 and older to an annual average of no more than 2 gallons of ethanol per person.
4. Increase the proportion of high school seniors who associate risk of physical or psychological harm with the heavy use of alcohol, occasional use of marijuana, and experimentation with cocaine.
5. Reduce the proportion of male high school seniors who use anabolic steroids.
6. Reduce deaths caused by alcohol-related motor vehicle crashes.
7. Reduce drug-related deaths.
8. Increase the proportion of all intravenous drug abusers who are in drug abuse treatment programs.
9. Increase the proportion of intravenous drug abusers not in treatment who use only uncontaminated drug paraphernalia ("works").

VII. AIDS, HIV Infection, and Sexually Transmitted Diseases

1. Confine annual incidence of diagnosed AIDS cases to no more than 98,000 cases.
2. Confine the prevalence of HIV infection to no more than 800 per 100,000 people.
3. Increase the proportion of sexually active, unmarried people who used a condom at last sexual intercourse.
4. Reduce the incidence of gonorrhea.
5. Reduce the incidence of chlamydia.
6. Reduce the incidence of primary and secondary syphilis.
7. Reduce the incidence of genital herpes and genital warts.
8. Reduce the incidence of pelvic inflammatory disease.
9. Reduce the incidence of sexually transmitted hepatitis B infection.

VIII. Family Planning

1. Reduce the number of pregnancies that are unintended.
2. Reduce the proportion of adolescents who have engaged in sexual intercourse.
3. Increase the proportion of sexually active, unmarried people aged 19 and younger who use contraception, especially combined-method contraception that both effectively prevents pregnancy and provides barrier protection against disease.

IX. Unintentional Injuries

1. Reduce deaths caused by unintentional injuries.
2. Increase use of occupant protection systems, such as safety belts, inflatable safety restraints, and child safety seats among motor vehicle occupants.
3. Increase use of helmets among motorcyclists and bicyclists.

Excerpted from *Healthy People 2000: National Health Promotion and Disease Prevention Objectives*, U.S. Department of Health and Human Services, Public Health Service, (Boston: Jones and Bartlett Publishers, 1992). Refer to this publication for further information on these objectives.

Figure 1.20 •

with all-inclusive natural abilities, including playing sports.

A college professor continuously watched a group of students play an entertaining game of basketball every Friday at noon. Having no basketball skills, he was reluctant to play. The desire to join in the fun was strong enough that he enrolled in a beginning course at the college so he would learn to play the game. To his surprise, most students were impressed that he was willing to do this. Now, with greater competence, he is able to join in on Friday's "pick-up" games.

Another alternative is to select an activity in which you are skilled. It may not be basketball, but it could well be aerobics. Don't be afraid to try new activities. Similarly, if your body weight is a problem, you could learn to cook low-fat meals. Try different recipes until you find dishes you like.

Fear and feelings of inadequacy often interfere with the ability to perform a task.

2. *Problems of confidence.* When the skills are there but you don't believe you can get it done, problems with confidence arise. Fear and feelings of inadequacy often interfere with the ability to perform the task.

You never should talk yourself out of something until you have given it a fair try. If the skills are there, the sky is the limit. Initially, try to visualize yourself doing the task and getting it done. Repeat this several times, then give it a try. You will surprise yourself.

Sometimes lack of confidence develops when the task appears insurmountable. In these situations, dividing a goal into smaller realistic objectives helps to accomplish the task. You may know how to swim, but to swim a continuous mile may take several weeks to accomplish. Set up your training program so that each day you swim a little farther until you are able to swim the entire mile. If on a given day you don't meet your objective, try it again, reevaluate, cut back a little, and, most important, don't give up.

3. *Problems of motivation.* In problems of motivation, both the competence and the confidence

are there, but the individual is unwilling to change because the reasons for change are not important to him or her. For example, people begin contemplating a smoking cessation program when the reasons for quitting outweigh the reasons for smoking.

When it comes to quality of life, lack of knowledge and lack of goals are the primary causes of unwillingness to change. Knowledge often determines goals, and goals determine motivation. How badly you want it dictates how hard you'll work at it. Many people are unaware of the magnitude of the benefits of a wellness program. Unfortunately, when it comes to a healthy lifestyle, there may not be a second chance. A stroke, a heart attack, or cancer can lead to irreparable or fatal consequences. Greater understanding of what leads to disease may be all that is needed to initiate change.

Also, feeling physically fit is difficult to explain unless you have experienced it yourself. Feelings of fitness, self-esteem, confidence, health, and quality of life cannot be conveyed to someone who is confined to sedentary living. In a way, wellness is like reaching the top of a mountain. The quietness, the clean air, the lush vegetation, the flowing water in the river, the wildlife, and the majestic valley below are difficult to explain to someone who has spent a lifetime within city limits.

Behavior Modification

Over the course of many years, we all develop habits that at some point in time we would like to change. Old habits die hard. **Behavior modification** requires continual effort. The sooner we implement a healthy lifestyle program, the greater are the health benefits and quality of life that lie ahead. The following principles can be adopted to help change behavior.

1. *Self-analysis.* The first step in behavior modification is a decisive desire to do so. If you have no interest in changing a behavior, you won't do it. A person who has no intention of quitting smoking will not quit, regardless of what anyone may

TERMS **Behavior modification** The process of replacing destructive or negative behaviors permanently with positive behaviors that will lead to better health and well-being.

say or how strong the evidence is against it. In your self-analysis, you may want to prepare a list of reasons for continuing or discontinuing a certain behavior. When the reasons for change outweigh the reasons for not changing, you are ready for the next step.

2. *Behavior analysis.* Determine the frequency, circumstances, and consequences of the behavior to be altered or implemented. If the desired outcome is to decrease your consumption of fat, you first must find out what foods in your diet are high in fat, when you eat them, and when you don't eat them. Knowing when you don't eat them points to circumstances under which you exert control of your diet and will help as you set goals.

3. *Goal setting.* Goals motivate change in behavior. The stronger the goal (desire), the more motivated you'll be to either change unwanted behaviors or implement new, healthy behaviors. The discussion on goal setting that follows will help you write goals and prepare an action plan to achieve those goals. The process will aid with behavior modification.

4. *Social support.* Surround yourself by people who either will work toward a common goal with you or will encourage you along the way. When attempting to quit smoking, it helps to do so with others who are trying to quit. You also may get help from friends who already have done so. Peer support is a strong incentive for behavioral change.

During this process, it's important also to avoid people who will not support you. Friends who have no desire to quit smoking actually may tempt you to smoke and encourage relapse of unwanted behaviors. People who are beyond the goal you are trying to reach may not be supportive either. For instance, someone may say: "I can do six consecutive miles." Your response should be: "I'm proud that I can jog three consecutive miles."

5. *Monitoring.* Continuous behavior monitoring increases awareness of the desired outcome. Sometimes this principle by itself is sufficient to cause change. For example, keeping track of daily food intake reveals sources of fat in the diet. It can help you cut down gradually or completely eliminate high-fat foods before consuming them. If the goal is to increase daily fruit and vegetable intake, keeping track of the number of servings you eat each day will raise awareness and may help increase their intake.

6. *Positive outlook.* You should take a positive approach from the beginning and believe in yourself. Following the guidelines set out in this chapter will help you pace yourself so you can work toward change. Also look at the outcomes — how much healthier you will be, how much better you will look, or being able to jog a certain distance, for instance.

7. *Reinforcement.* People tend to repeat behaviors that are rewarded and disregard those that are not rewarded or are punished. If you have been successful in cutting down your fat intake during the week, reward yourself by going to a show or buying a new pair of shoes. Do not reinforce yourself with destructive behaviors such as eating a high-fat dinner. If you fail to change a desired behavior (or to implement a new one), you may want to put off buying those new shoes you planned for that week. When a positive behavior becomes habitual, give yourself an even better reward. Treat yourself to a vacation weekend or go on a short trip.

Goal Setting

Goals are critical to initiate change. Goals motivate behavioral change and provide a plan of action. Goals are most effective when they are:

● *Well planned.* Only a well conceived action plan will help you attain your goal. The items below, as well as others discussed in different chapters, will help you design your plan of action. You also should write specific objectives to help you reach each goal. Examples of specific objectives are provided in Chapter 14, under "Behavioral Objectives for the Future," page 340.

● *Personalized.* Goals that you set for yourself are more motivational than goals someone else sets for you.

● *Written.* An unwritten goal is simply a wish. A written goal, in essence, becomes a contract with yourself. Show this goal to a friend or an instructor and have him or her witness, by way of a signature, the contract you made with yourself.

● *Realistic.* Goals should be within reach. If you have not exercised regularly, it would be unrealistic to start a daily exercise program consisting of 45 minutes of step aerobics at a vigorous intensity level. Unattainable goals lead to discouragement and loss of interest. Setting smaller, attainable goals is better.

At times, even with realistic goals, problems arise. Try to anticipate potential difficulties as much as possible, and plan for ways to deal with them. If your goal is to jog 30 minutes on six consecutive days, what are the alternatives if the weather turns bad? Possible solutions are to jog in the rain, find an indoor track, jog at a different time of day when the weather improves, or participate in a different aerobic activity, such as stationary cycling, swimming, or step aerobics.

- *Measurable.* Write your goals so they are clear, and state specifically the objective to accomplish. "I will lose weight" is not clear enough and is not measurable. A better example is: "I will decrease my body fat to 17%."

- *Time-specific.* A goal always should have a specific date set for completion. This date should be realistic but not too distant in the future.

- *Monitored.* Monitoring your progress as you move toward a goal reinforces behavior. Keeping a physical activity log or doing a body composition assessment periodically determines where you are at at any given time.

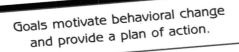

Goals motivate behavioral change and provide a plan of action.

- *Evaluated.* Periodic reevaluations are vital for success. You may find that a given goal is unreachable. If so, reassess the goal. On the other hand, if a goal is too easy, you will lose interest and may stop working toward it. Once you achieve a goal, set a new one to improve or maintain what you have achieved. Goals keep you motivated.

In addition to these guidelines, throughout this book you will find additional information on behavioral change. Examples are the tips for behavior modification and adherence to a lifetime weight management program on page 212, the Exercise Readiness Questionnaire on page 49, getting started and adhering to a lifetime exercise program on page 77, tips for a healthy cancer-fighting diet on page 249, stress management techniques on page 267, tips for smoking cessation on page 311, and behavioral objectives for the future and tips for behavioral change on page 340.

● General Objectives

Because fitness and wellness needs vary significantly from one individual to another, all exercise and wellness prescriptions must be personalized to obtain best results. The information in the following chapters and the worksheets within these chapters set forth the necessary guidelines to develop a personal lifetime program to improve fitness and promote preventive health care and personal wellness.

The worksheets have been prepared on tear-out sheets so they can be turned in to class instructors. As you study this book and complete the respective worksheets, you will learn to:

- Determine whether medical clearance is needed for your safe participation in exercise.
- Conduct nutritional analyses and follow the recommendations for adequate nutrition.
- Write sound diet and weight-control programs.
- Assess the health-related components of fitness (cardiorespiratory endurance, muscular strength and endurance, muscular flexibility, and body composition).
- Write exercise prescriptions for cardiorespiratory endurance, muscular strength and endurance, and muscular flexibility.
- Determine your potential risk for cardiovascular disease, and implement a risk-reduction program.
- Follow a cancer risk-reduction program.
- Determine your levels of tension and stress, lessen your vulnerability to stress, and implement a stress management program if necessary.
- Implement a smoking cessation program, if applicable.
- Avoid chemical dependency, and know where to find assistance if needed.
- Learn the health consequences of sexually transmitted diseases, including AIDS, and guidelines for preventing STDs.
- Discover the relationship between fitness and aging.

- Write objectives to improve your fitness and wellness, and learn how to chart a wellness program for the future.
- Discern between myths and facts of exercise and health-related concepts.
- Learn behavioral modification techniques to help you adhere to a lifetime fitness and wellness program.

● Wellness Lifestyle Questionnaire

Most people go to college to learn how to make a living, but a fitness and wellness course will teach you how to live — how to truly live life to its fullest potential. Some people seem to think that success in life is measured by how much money they make. Making a good living will not help you unless you live a wellness lifestyle that will allow you to enjoy what you have.

Lifestyle choices that you make now will have an impact on how well you live the rest of your life.

Everyone would like to enjoy good health and wellness, but most people don't know how to reach this objective. Lifestyle is the most important factor affecting our personal well-being. Although some people live long because of genetic factors, the quality of life during middle age and the "golden years" is related more often to wise choices initiated during youth and continued throughout life.

In a few short years, lack of wellness leads to a loss of vitality and gusto for life, as well as premature morbidity and mortality. The Wellness Lifestyle Questionnaire, given in Figure 1.21 at the end of this chapter, will provide an initial rating of your current efforts to stay healthy and well. The components of a wellness lifestyle are discussed in subsequent chapters of this book.

Upon completing the questionnaire, select the areas in which you think you will need the most improvement. Even though you need to pay attention to all aspects of wellness, initially work on the lifestyle factors in which definite improvements are required. Lifestyle choices that you make now will have an impact on how well you live the rest of your life.

● A Word of Caution

Even though exercise testing and participation is relatively safe for most apparently healthy individuals under age 45, the reaction of the cardiovascular system to higher levels of physical activity cannot be totally predicted. Consequently, a small but real risk exists for exercise-induced abnormalities in people with a history of cardiovascular problems and those who are at higher risk for disease.[21] These include abnormal blood pressure, irregular heart rhythm, fainting, and, in rare instances, a heart attack or cardiac arrest.

Before you start to engage in an exercise program or participate in any exercise testing, you should fill out the questionnaire in Figure 1.22. If your answer to any of the questions is yes, you should see a physician before participating in a fitness program. Exercise testing and participation is not wise under some of the conditions listed in this questionnaire and may require a stress electrocardiogram (ECG) test. If you have any questions regarding your current health status, consult your doctor before initiating, continuing, or increasing your level of physical activity.

● Evaluation of Wellness Dimensions

Now that you are about to embark in a wellness lifestyle program, sit down and subjectively determine where you are at on each of the five dimensions of wellness. Use Figure 1.23 to help you with this exercise. The following scale should be used to determine your wellness rating for each dimension: poor = 5, fair = 4, average = 3, good = 2, and excellent = 1. Record the date and at the top of the respective column. Next, write a general objective (goal) for each wellness dimension to be accomplish prior to the end of this course. Also list three specific objectives that will help you accomplish each goal. As you continue to study the content of this book, use this same figure to monitor your progress. At least once a month make adjustments in your specific objectives so that you may reach the desired goals. Modifying unhealthy behaviors and developing new positive habits take time. The plan of action that you are about to develop will help you achieve the desired outcomes.

Notes

1. U.S. Centers for Disease Control and Prevention and American College of Sports Medicine, Summary Statement: Workshop on Physical Activity and Public Health, *Sports Medicine Bulletin*, 28(4), 7.

2. National Institutes of Health, *Consensus Development Conference Statement: Physical Activity and Cardiovascular Health*, Washington, DC, December 18–20, 1995.

3. National Institutes of Health.

4. U. S. Department of Health and Human Services, "Physical Activity and Health: A Report of the Surgeon General," Atlanta, GA: U.S. Department of Health and Human Services, Centers for Disease Control and Prevention, National Center for Chronic Disease Prevention and Health Promotion, 1996.

5. U. S. Department of Health and Human Services, National Center for Health Statistics, *Monthly Vital Statistics Report: Advance Report of Final Mortality Statistics*, 45:3, Supplement (1994), September 30, 1996.

6. T. A. Murphy and D. Murphy, *The Wellness for Life Workbook* (San Diego: Fitness Publications, 1987).

7. P. E. Allsen, J. M. Harrison, and B. Vance, *Fitness for Life* (Madison, WI: Brown & Benchmark, 1993), p. 3.

8. B. Gutin et al., "Blood Pressure, Fitness, and Fitness in 5- and 6-Year-Old Children," *Journal of the American Medical Association*, 264 (1990), 1123–1127.

9. American Heart Association, *Heart and Stroke Statistical Update: 1997 Statistical Supplement*. Dallas: AHA, 1996.

10. American Cancer Society, *1997 Cancer Facts and Figures* (New York: ACS, 1997).

11. R. S. Paffenbarger, Jr., R. T. Hyde, A. L. Wing, and C. H. Steinmetz, "A Natural History of Athleticism and Cardiovascular Health," *Journal of the American Medical Association*, 252 (1984), 491–495.

12. S. N. Blair, H. W. Kohl III, R. S. Paffenbarger, Jr., D. G. Clark, K. H. Cooper, and L. W. Gibbons, "Physical Fitness and All-Cause Mortality: A Prospective Study of Healthy Men and Women," *Journal of the American Medical Association*, 262 (1989), 2395–2401.

13. J. E. Enstrom, "Health Practices and Cancer Mortality Among Active California Mormons," *Journal of the National Cancer Institute*, 81 (1989), 1807–1814.

14. S. N. Blair, H. W. Kohl III, C. E. Barlow, R. S. Paffenbarger, Jr., L. W. Gibbons, and C. A. Macera, "Changes in Physical Fitness and All-Cause Mortality: A Prospective Study of Healthy and Unhealthy Men," *Journal of the American Medical Association*, 273 (1995), 1193–1198.

15. I. Lee, C. Hsieh, and R. S. Paffenbarger, Jr., "Exercise Intensity and Longevity in Men: The Harvard Alumni Health Study," *Journal of the American Medical Association*, 273 (1995), 1179–1184.

16. "Wellness Facts," University of California at Berkeley *Wellness Letter* (Palm Coast, FL: The Editors, April, 1995).

17. Robert C. Chadbourne, "Fit for Hire," *Fitness Management*, 12:2 (1996), 28–30.

18. Editors of *Prevention* Magazine, *The Prevention Index 1996: A Report Card on the Nation's Health* (Emmaus, PA: Rodale Press, 1996).

19. U. S. Department of Health and Human Services, Public Health Service, *Healthy People 2000: National Health Promotion and Disease Prevention Objectives* (Boston: Jones and Bartlett Publishers, 1992).

20. G. S. Howard, D. W. Nance, and P. Myers, *Adaptive Counseling and Therapy* (San Francisco: Jossey-Bass Publishers, 1987).

21. American College of Sports Medicine, *Guidelines for Exercise Testing and Prescription* (Baltimore: Williams & Wilkins, 1995).

Suggested Readings

American College of Sports Medicine. "The Recommended Quantity and Quality of Exercise for Developing and Maintaining Cardiorespiratory and Muscular Fitness in Healthy Adults." *Medicine and Science in Sports and Exercise*, 22 (1990), 265–274.

Davies, N. E., and L. H. Felder. "Applying Brakes to the Runaway American Health Care System." *Journal of the American Medical Association*, 263 (1990) 73–76.

Gettman, L. R. "Cost/Benefit Analysis of a Corporate Fitness Program." *Fitness in Business*, 1:1 (1986), 11–17.

Hatziandreu, E. L., J. P. Koplan, M. C. Weinstein, C. J. Caspersen, and K. E. Warner. "A Cost-Effectiveness Analysis of Exercise as a Health Promotion Activity." *American Journal of Public Health*, 78 (1988), 1417–1421.

Hoeger, W. W. K., and S. A. Hoeger. *Principles & Labs for Fitness & Wellness*. Englewood, CO: Morton Publishing, 1997.

Koplan, J. P., C. J. Caspersen, and K. E. Powell. "Physical Activity, Physical Fitness, and Health: Time to Act." *Journal of the American Medical Association* 262 (1989) 2437.

Smith, L. K. "Cost-Effectiveness of Health Promotion Programs." *Fitness Management*, 2:3 (1986), 12–15.

"New Fitness Data Verifies: Employees Who Exercise Are Also More Productive." *Athletic Business*, 8:12 (1984), 24–30.

Van Camp, S. P. "The Fixx Tragedy: A Cardiologist's Perspective." *Physician and Sportsmedicine*, 12:9 (1984), 153–155.

Wilmore, J. H. "Design Issues and Alternatives in Assessing Physical Fitness Among Apparently Healthy Adults in a Health Examination Survey of the General Population." In *Assessing Physical Fitness and Activity in General Population Studies* (F. Drury, Editor).Washington, DC: U.S. Public Health Service, National Center for Health Statistics, 1988.

WELLNESS LIFESTYLE QUESTIONNAIRE

Please circle the appropriate answer to each question and total your points as indicated at the end of the questionnaire. Circle 5 if the statement is ALWAYS true, 4 if the statement is FREQUENTLY true, 3 if the statement is OCCASIONALLY true, 2 if the statement is SELDOM true, 1 if the statement is NEVER true.

1. I am able to identify the situations and factors that overstress me.   5 4 3 2 1
2. I eat only when I am hungry.   5 4 3 2 1
3. I don't take tranquilizers or other drugs to relax.   5 4 3 2 1
4. I support efforts in my community to reduce environmental pollution.   5 4 3 2 1
5. I avoid buying foods with artificial colorings.   5 4 3 2 1
6. I rarely have problems concentrating on what I'm doing because of worrying about other things.   5 4 3 2 1
7. My employer (school) takes measures to ensure that my work (study) place is safe.   5 4 3 2 1
8. I try not to use medications when I feel unwell.   5 4 3 2 1
9. I am able to identify certain bodily responses and illnesses as my reactions to stress.   5 4 3 2 1
10. I question the use of diagnostic x-rays.   5 4 3 2 1
11. I try to alter personal living habits that are risk factors for heart disease, cancer, and other lifestyle diseases.   5 4 3 2 1
12. I avoid taking sleeping pills to help me sleep.   5 4 3 2 1
13. I try not to eat foods with refined sugar or corn sugar ingredients.   5 4 3 2 1
14. I accomplish goals I set for myself.   5 4 3 2 1
15. I stretch or bend for several minutes each day to keep my body flexible.   5 4 3 2 1
16. I support immunization of all children for common childhood diseases.   5 4 3 2 1
17. I try to prevent friends from driving after they drink alcohol.   5 4 3 2 1
18. I minimize extra salt intake.   5 4 3 2 1
19. I don't mind when other people and situations make me wait or lose time.   5 4 3 2 1
20. I walk four or fewer flights of stairs rather than take the elevator.   5 4 3 2 1
21. I eat fresh fruits and vegetables.   5 4 3 2 1
22. I use dental floss at least once a day.   5 4 3 2 1
23. I read product labels on foods to determine their ingredients.   5 4 3 2 1
24. I try to maintain a normal body weight.   5 4 3 2 1
25. I record my feelings and thoughts in a journal or diary.   5 4 3 2 1
26. I have no difficulty falling asleep.   5 4 3 2 1
27. I engage in some form of vigorous physical activity at least three times a week.   5 4 3 2 1
28. I take time each day to quiet my mind and relax.   5 4 3 2 1
29. I am willing to make and sustain close friendships and intimate relationships.   5 4 3 2 1
30. I obtain an adequate daily supply of vitamins from my food or vitamin supplements.   5 4 3 2 1
31. I rarely have tension or migraine headaches, or pain in the neck or shoulders.   5 4 3 2 1
32. I wear a safety belt when driving.   5 4 3 2 1
33. I am aware of the emotional and situational factors that lead me to overeat.   5 4 3 2 1
34. I avoid driving my car after drinking any alcohol.   5 4 3 2 1
35. I am aware of the side effects of the medicines I take.   5 4 3 2 1
36. I am able to accept feelings of sadness, depression, and anxiety, knowing that they are almost always transient.   5 4 3 2 1
37. I would seek several additional professional opinions if my doctor were to recommend surgery for me.   5 4 3 2 1
38. I agree that nonsmokers should not have to breathe the smoke from cigarettes in public places.   5 4 3 2 1
39. I agree that pregnant women who smoke harm their babies.   5 4 3 2 1

(Continued)

Edlin: *Health and Wellness,* © 1992, Boston: Jones and Bartlett Publishers. Reprinted with permission.

Figure 1.21 •

40. I think I get enough sleep. 5 4 3 2 1
41. I ask my doctor why a certain medication is being prescribed and inquire about alternatives. 5 4 3 2 1
42. I am aware of the calories expended in my activities. 5 4 3 2 1
43. I am willing to give priority to my own needs for time and psychological space by saying "no" to others' requests of me. 5 4 3 2 1
44. I walk instead of drive whenever feasible. 5 4 3 2 1
45. I eat a breakfast that contains about one-third of my daily need for calories, proteins, and vitamins. 5 4 3 2 1
46. I prohibit smoking in my home. 5 4 3 2 1
47. I remember and think about my dreams. 5 4 3 2 1
48. I seek medical attention only when I have symptoms or believe that some (potential) condition needs checking, rather than have routine yearly checkups. 5 4 3 2 1
49. I endeavor to make my home accident-free. 5 4 3 2 1
50. I ask my doctor to explain the diagnosis of my problem until I understand all that I care to. 5 4 3 2 1

51. I try to include fiber or roughage (whole grains, fresh fruits and vegetables, or bran) in my daily diet. 5 4 3 2 1
52. I can deal with my emotional problems without alcohol or other mood-altering drugs. 5 4 3 2 1
53. I am satisfied with my school/work. 5 4 3 2 1
54. I require children riding in my car to be in infant seats or in shoulder harnesses. 5 4 3 2 1
55. I try to associate with people who have a positive attitude about life. 5 4 3 2 1
56. I try not to eat snacks of candy, pastries, and other "junk" foods. 5 4 3 2 1
57. I avoid people who are "down" all the time and bring down those around them. 5 4 3 2 1
58. I am aware of the calorie content of the foods I eat. 5 4 3 2 1
59. I brush my teeth after meals. 5 4 3 2 1
60. (for women only) I routinely examine my breasts. 5 4 3 2 1
(for men only) I am aware of the signs of testicular cancer. 5 4 3 2 1

How to Score

Enter the numbers you've circled next to the question number and total your score for each category. Then determine your degree of wellness for each category using the wellness status key.

Emotional health	Fitness and body care	Environmental health	Stress	Nutrition	Medical self-responsibility
6___	15___	4___	1___	2___	8___
12___	20___	7___	3___	5___	10___
25___	22___	17___	9___	13___	11___
26___	24___	32___	14___	18___	16___
36___	27___	34___	19___	21___	35___
40___	33___	38___	28___	23___	37___
47___	42___	39___	29___	30___	41___
52___	44___	46___	31___	45___	48___
55___	58___	49___	43___	51___	59___
57___	59___	54___	53___	56___	60___
Total___	Total___	Total___	Total___	Total___	Total___

Wellness Status

To assess your status in each of the six categories, compare your total score in each to the following key:

0–34 Need improvement   35–44 Good   45–50 Excellent

Figure 1.21 • *Continued.*

HEALTH HISTORY QUESTIONNAIRE

Although exercise testing and exercise participation are relatively safe for most apparently healthy individuals, the reaction of the cardiovascular system to increased physical activity cannot always be totally predicted. Consequently, a person takes a small but real risk of certain changes occurring during exercise testing or participation. These changes may include abnormal blood pressure, irregular heart rhythm, fainting, and, in rare instances, a heart attack or cardiac arrest.

Therefore, it is imperative that you provide honest answers to this questionnaire. Exercise may be ill-advised under some of the conditions listed below; others simply may require special consideration. **If any of the conditions apply, consult your physician before you participate in an exercise program.** Also, promptly report to your instructor any exercise-related abnormalities that you may experience during exercise participation.

A. Have you ever had or do you now have any of the following conditions?

☐   1. Myocardial infarction
☐   2. Coronary artery disease
☐   3. Congestive heart failure
☐   4. Elevated blood lipids (cholesterol and triglycerides)
☐   5. Chest pain at rest or during exertion
☐   6. Shortness of breath
☐   7. Abnormal resting or stress electrocardiogram
☐   8. Uneven, irregular, or skipped heartbeats (including racing or fluttering heart)
☐   9. Blood embolism
☐   10. Thrombophlebitis
☐   11. Rheumatic heart fever
☐   12. Elevated blood pressure
☐   13. Stroke
☐   14. Diabetes
☐   15. Family history of coronary heart disease, syncope, or sudden death before age 60
☐   16. Any other heart problem that makes exercise unsafe

B. Do you have any of the following conditions?

☐   1. Arthritis, rheumatism, or gout
☐   2. Chronic low back pain
☐   3. Any other joint, bone, or muscle problems
☐   4. Any respiratory problems
☐   5. Obesity (more than 30% overweight)
☐   6. Anorexia
☐   7. Bulimia
☐   8. Mononucleosis
☐   9. Any physical disability that could interfere with safe participation in exercise

C. Do any of the following conditions apply?

☐   1. Do you smoke cigarettes?
☐   2. Are you taking any prescription drug?
☐   3. Men: Are you 40 or older?
☐   3. Women: Are you 50 or older?

D. Do you have any other concern regarding your ability to safely participate in an exercise program? If so, explain?

_____

_____

Student's Signature: _____ Date: _____

Figure 1.22 •

Name:_____ Course: _____ Section:_____

Date: Wellness Dimension										
Physical										
Emotional										
Social										
Intellectual										
Spiritual										

Goals and Objectives

Physical Goal: _____
Specific Objectives
1. _____
2. _____
3. _____

Emotional Goal: _____
Specific Objectives
1. _____
2. _____
3. _____

Social Goal: _____
Specific Objectives
1. _____
2. _____
3. _____

Intellectual Goal: _____
Specific Objectives
1. _____
2. _____
3. _____

Spiritual Goal: _____
Specific Objectives
1. _____
2. _____
3. _____

Figure 1.23 ● *Wellness scale.*

Cardiorespiratory Endurance Assessment

2

*T*he most important component of physical fitness and best indicator of overall health is cardiorespiratory endurance. Physical activity is no longer a natural part of our existence. Current technological developments have driven most people in developed countries into sedentary lifestyles. For instance, if there is a need to go to a store only a couple of blocks away, most people drive their automobiles and then spend a couple of minutes driving around the parking lot to find a spot 10 to 20 yards closer to the store's entrance. They do not even have to carry out the groceries any more. A youngster working at the store usually takes them out in a cart and places them in the vehicle.

Similarly, during a visit to a multi-level shopping mall, almost everyone chooses to ride the escalators instead of taking the stairs. Automobiles, elevators, escalators, telephones, intercoms, remote controls, electric garage door openers — all are modern-day commodities that minimize the amount of movement and effort required of the human body.

Photo Courtesy of Quinton Instrument Co., 2121 Terry Ave., Seattle, WA 98121-2791.

Objectives

- Define cardiorespiratory endurance and the benefits of cardiorespiratory endurance training.
- Understand the importance of adequate cardiorespiratory endurance in maintaining good health and well-being.
- Define aerobic and anaerobic exercise.
- Be able to assess cardiorespiratory fitness through six different test protocols (1.5-Mile Run Test, 1.0-Mile Walk Test, Step Test, Astrand-Ryhming Test, and 12-Minute Swim Test).
- Learn to interpret cardiorespiratory endurance assessment test results according to health fitness and physical fitness standards.

One of the most harmful effects of modern-day technology is an increase in chronic conditions related to a lack of physical activity. These include hypertension, heart disease, chronic low-back pain, and obesity. They are referred to as **hypokinetic diseases.** The term "hypo" means low or little, and "kinetic" implies motion. Lack of adequate physical activity is a fact of modern life that most people can avoid no longer. To enjoy modern-day commodities and still expect to live life to its fullest, however, a personalized lifetime exercise program must become a part of daily living.

> To enjoy modern-day commodities and still expect to live life to its fullest, a personalized lifetime exercise program must become a part of daily living.

For most people around the world, modern-day technology has led to a lower level of **cardiorespiratory endurance.** As a person breathes, part of the oxygen in the air is taken up in the lungs and transported in the blood to the heart. The heart then is responsible for pumping the oxygenated blood through the circulatory system to all organs and tissues of the body. At the cellular level, oxygen is used to convert food substrates, primarily carbohydrates and fats, into energy necessary to conduct body functions and maintain constant internal equilibrium. During physical exertion, more energy is needed to perform the activity. As a result, the heart, lungs, and blood vessels have to deliver more oxygen to the cells to supply the required energy.

During prolonged exercise, an individual with a high level of cardiorespiratory endurance is able to deliver the required amount of oxygen to the tissues

Advances in modern technology have almost completely eliminated the need for physical activity, significantly contributing to deterioration of the human body.

with relative ease. The cardiorespiratory system of a person with a low level of endurance has to work much harder, as the heart has to pump more often to supply the same amount of oxygen to the tissues and, consequently, fatigues faster. Hence, a higher capacity to deliver and utilize oxygen (oxygen uptake or VO_2) indicates a more efficient cardiorespiratory system.

● Aerobic and Anaerobic Exercise

Cardiorespiratory endurance activities often are called **aerobic** exercises. Examples of cardiorespiratory or aerobic exercises are walking, jogging, swimming,

The epitome of physical inactivity is to drive around a parking lot for several minutes in search of a parking spot 10 to 20 yards closer to the store's entrance.

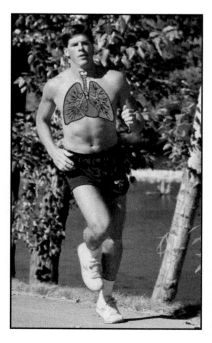

Cardiorespiratory endurance is the ability of the lungs, heart, and blood vessels to deliver adequate amounts of oxygen to the cells to meet the demands of prolonged physical activity.

cycling, cross-country skiing, water aerobics, rope skipping, and aerobics.

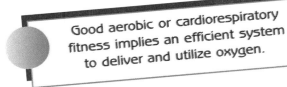

Good aerobic or cardiorespiratory fitness implies an efficient system to deliver and utilize oxygen.

The intensity of **anaerobic** exercise is so high that oxygen cannot be delivered and utilized to produce energy. Because energy production is limited in the absence of oxygen, these activities can be carried out for only short periods — 2 to 3 minutes. The higher the intensity of the activity, the shorter the duration.

Activities such as the 100, 200, and 400 meters in track and field, the 100 meters in swimming, gymnastics routines, and strength training are good examples of anaerobic activities. Anaerobic activities do not contribute much to development of the cardiorespiratory system. Only aerobic activities will help increase cardiorespiratory endurance. The basic guidelines for cardiorespiratory exercise prescription are set forth in Chapter 3.

TERMS

Hypokinetic diseases Diseases associated with a lack of physical activity.

Cardiorespiratory endurance The ability of the lungs, heart, and blood vessels to deliver adequate amounts of oxygen to the cells to meet the demands of prolonged physical activity.

Aerobic Exercise that requires oxygen to produce the necessary energy to carry out the activity.

Anaerobic Exercise that does not require oxygen to produce the necessary energy to carry out the activity.

Sample Aerobic Activities

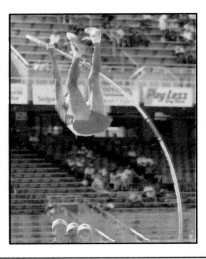

Sample Anaerobic Activities

● Benefits of Aerobic Training

Everyone who participates in a cardiorespiratory or aerobic exercise program can expect a number of physiological adaptations from training. Among these benefits are:

1. *A higher maximal oxygen uptake. The amount of oxygen the body is able to use du*ring physical activity increases significantly. This allows the individual to exercise longer and at a higher rate before becoming fatigued. Depending on the initial fitness level, maximal oxygen uptake may increase as much as 30%, although higher increases have been reported in people with very low initial levels of fitness.

2. *An increase in the oxygen-carrying capacity of the blood.* As a result of training, the red blood cell count goes up. Red blood cells contain hemoglobin, which transports oxygen in the blood.

3. *A decrease in resting heart rate and an increase in cardiac muscle strength.* During resting conditions, the heart ejects between 5 and 6 liters of blood per minute (a liter is slightly larger than a quart). This amount of blood, also referred to as **cardiac output**, meets the body's energy demands in the resting state.

    Like any other muscle, the heart responds to training by increasing in strength and size. As the heart gets stronger, the muscle can produce a more forceful contraction, which causes the heart to eject more blood with each beat. This **stroke volume** yields a lower heart rate. The lower heart rate also allows the heart to rest longer between beats. Average resting and maximal cardiac outputs, stroke volumes, and heart rates for sedentary, trained, and highly trained (elite) individuals are shown in Table 2.1.

    Resting heart rates frequently decrease by 10 to 20 beats per minute (bpm) after only 6 to 8 weeks of training. A reduction of 20 bpm saves the heart about 10,483,200 beats per year. The average heart beats between 70 and 80 bpm. As seen in Table 2.1, resting heart rates in highly trained athletes are often around 45 bpm.

4. *A lower heart rate at given **workloads**.* When compared with untrained individuals, a trained person has a lower heart rate response to a given task. This is because of the greater efficiency of the cardiorespiratory system. Individuals also are surprised to find that, following several weeks of

Table 2.1	*Average Resting and Maximal Cardiac Output, Stroke Volume, and Heart Rate, for Sedentary, Trained, and Highly Trained Males*					
	RESTING			**MAXIMAL**		
	$\dot{Q}$ (l/min)	SV (ml)	HR (bpm)	$\dot{Q}$ (l/min)	SV (ml)	HR (bpm)
Sedentary	5	68	74	20	100	200
Trained	5	90	56	30	150	200
Highly Trained	5	110	45	35	175	200

$\dot{Q}$ = cardiac output
SV = stroke volume
HR = heart rate

training, a given workload (let's say a 10-minute mile) elicits a much lower heart rate response as compared to the response when training first started.

5. *An increase in the number and size of the **mitochondria**.* All energy necessary for cell function is produced in the mitochondria. As the size and number increase, so does the potential to produce energy for muscular work.

6. *An increase in the number of functional **capillaries**.* These smaller vessels allow for the exchange of oxygen and carbon dioxide between the blood and the cells. As more vessels open up, more gas exchange can take place, delaying the onset of fatigue during prolonged exercise. This increase in capillaries also speeds up the rate at which waste products of cell metabolism can be removed. Increased capillarization also is seen in the heart, which enhances the oxygen delivery capacity to the heart muscle itself.

7. *Faster recovery time.* Trained individuals recover more rapidly after exercising. A fit system is able to restore more quickly any internal equilibrium disrupted during exercise.

8. *Lower blood pressure and blood lipids.* A regular aerobic exercise program leads to lower blood pressure and fats such as cholesterol and triglycerides, all of which have been linked to the formation of atherosclerotic plaque, which obstructs the arteries. This decreases the risk of coronary heart disease (see Chapter 9). High blood pressure also is a leading risk factor for strokes.

9. *An increase in fat-burning enzymes.* The role of fat-burning enzymes is significant because fat is

lost primarily by burning it in muscle. As the concentration of the enzymes increases, so does the ability to burn fat.

● Assessment of Cardiorespiratory Endurance

The level of cardiorespiratory endurance, cardiorespiratory fitness, or aerobic capacity is determined by the maximal amount of oxygen the human body is able to utilize per minute of physical activity. This value can be expressed in liters per minute (l/min) or milliliters per kilogram per minute (ml/kg/min). The relative value in ml/kg/min is used most often because it considers total body mass (weight). When comparing two individuals with the same absolute value, the one with the lesser body mass will have a higher relative value, indicating that more oxygen is available to each kilogram (2.2 pounds) of body weight. Because all tissues and organs of the body need oxygen to function, higher oxygen consumption indicates a more efficient cardiorespiratory system.

The most precise way to determine **maximal oxygen uptake** (VO_{2max}) is through gas analysis. This is done by using a metabolic cart through which the amount of oxygen consumption can be measured directly. This type of equipment is not available in most health/fitness centers. Therefore, several alternative methods of estimating maximal oxygen uptake have been developed using limited equipment.

Even though most cardiorespiratory endurance tests probably are safe to administer to apparently healthy individuals (those with no major coronary risk factors or symptoms), the American College of Sports Medicine recommends that a physician be present for all maximal exercise tests on apparently healthy men over age 40 and women over age 50. A maximal test is any test that requires the participant's all-out or nearly all-out effort. For submaximal exercise tests, a physician should be present when testing higher risk/symptomatic individuals or diseased people, regardless of the participant's current age.

Five exercise tests used to assess cardiorespiratory fitness are introduced in this chapter: the 1.5-Mile Run Test, 1.0-Mile Walk Test, Step Test, Astrand-Ryhming Test, and 12-Minute Swim Test. The test procedures are explained in detail in Figures 2.1, 2.2, 2.3, 2.4, and 2.5, respectively.

Depending on time, equipment, and individual physical limitations, you may perform one or more of these tests. For example, people who can't jog or walk could take the bike or swim test. Because these are different tests, they will not necessarily yield the exact same results. Therefore, to make valid comparisons, you should take the same test when doing pre- and post-assessments.

● 1.5-Mile Run Test

This test is used most frequently to predict cardiorespiratory fitness according to the time the person takes to run or walk a 1.5-mile course (see Figure 2.1). Maximal oxygen uptake is estimated based on the time the person takes to cover the distance (see Table 2.2).

The only equipment necessary to conduct this test is a stopwatch and a track or premeasured

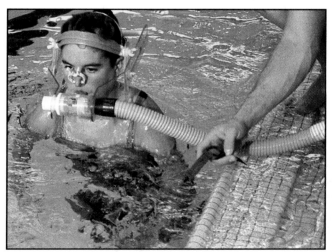

Oxygen uptake (cardiorespiratory fitness) is assessed during a water aerobics exercise test.

1.5 MILE RUN TEST

1. Make sure you qualify for this test. This test is contraindicated for unconditioned beginners, individuals with symptoms of heart disease, and those with known heart disease or risk factors.

2. Select the testing site. Find a school track (each lap is one-fourth of a mile) or a premeasured 1.5-mile course.

3. Have a stopwatch available to determine your time.

4. Conduct a few warm-up exercises prior to the test. Do some mild stretching exercises, some walking, and slow jogging.

5. Initiate the test and try to cover the distance in the fastest time possible (walking or jogging). Time yourself during the run to see how fast you have covered the distance. If any unusual symptoms arise during the test, do not continue. Stop immediately and re-take the test after another 6 weeks of aerobic training.

6. At the end of the test, cool down by walking or jogging slowly for another 3 to 5 minutes. Do not sit or lie down after the test.

7. According to your performance time, look up your estimated maximal oxygen uptake (VO_{2max}) in Table 2.2.

    Example: A 20-year-old female runs the 1.5-mile course in 12 minutes and 40 seconds. Table 2.2 shows a VO_{2max} of 39.8 ml/kg/min for a time of 12:40. According to Table 2.8, this VO_{2max} would place her in the good cardiorespiratory fitness category.

Figure 2.1 ● *Procedure for the 1.5-Mile Run Test.*

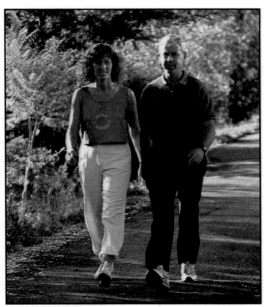

Even moderate physical activity enhances health and longevity.

Table 2.2 — *Estimated Maximal Oxygen Uptake for the 1.5-Mile Run Test*

Time	VO_{2max} (ml/kg/min)	Time	VO_{2max} (ml/kg/min)
6:10	80.0	12:40	39.8
6:20	79.0	12:50	39.2
6:30	77.9	13:00	38.6
6:40	76.7	13:10	38.1
6:50	75.5	13:20	37.8
7:00	74.0	13:30	37.2
7:10	72.6	13:40	36.8
7:20	71.3	13:50	36.3
7:30	69.9	14:00	35.9
7:40	68.3	14:10	35.5
7:50	66.8	14:20	35.1
8:00	65.2	14:30	34.7
8:10	63.9	14:40	34.3
8:20	62.5	14:50	34.0
8:30	61.2	15:00	33.6
8:40	60.2	15:10	33.1
8:50	59.1	15:20	32.7
9:00	58.1	15:30	32.2
9:10	56.9	15:40	31.8
9:20	55.9	15:50	31.4
9:30	54.7	16:00	30.9
9:40	53.5	16:10	30.5
9:50	52.3	16:20	30.2
10:00	51.1	16:30	29.8
10:10	50.4	16:40	29.5
10:20	49.5	16:50	29.1
10:30	48.6	17:00	28.9
10:40	48.0	17:10	28.5
10:50	47.4	17:20	28.3
11:00	46.6	17:30	28.0
11:10	45.8	17:40	27.7
11:20	45.1	17:50	27.4
11:30	44.4	18:00	27.1
11:40	43.7	18:10	26.8
11:50	43.2	18:20	26.6
12:00	42.3	18:30	26.3
12:10	41.7	18:40	26.0
12:20	41.0	18:50	25.7
12:30	40.4	19:00	25.4

Source: Adapted from "A Means of Assessing Maximal Oxygen Intake," by K. H. Cooper, in *Journal of the American Medical Association*, 203(1968), 201-204; *Health and Fitness Through Physical Activity*, by M. L. Pollock, J. H. Wilmore, and S. M. Fox III (New York: John Wiley & Sons, 1978); and *Training for Sport and Activity*, by J. H. Wilmore and D. L. Costill (Dubuque, IA: Wm. C. Brown Publishers, 1988).

1.5-mile course. This perhaps is the easiest test to administer, but a note of caution is in order when conducting the test. As the objective is to cover the distance in the shortest time, it is considered a maximal exercise test. The 1.5-Mile Run Test should be limited to conditioned individuals who have been cleared for exercise. The test is not recommended for unconditioned beginners, men over age 40, and women over age 50 without proper medical clearance, symptomatic individuals, and those with known disease or coronary heart disease risk factors. A program of at least 6 weeks of aerobic training is recommended before unconditioned individuals take this test.

● 1.0-Mile Walk Test

This test can be used by individuals who are unable to run because of low fitness levels or injuries. All that is required is a brisk 1-mile walk that will elicit an exercise heart rate of at least 120 beats per minute at the end of the test.

You will need to know how to take your heart rate by counting your pulse. This can be done on the wrist by placing two fingers over the radial artery (inside the wrist on the side of the thumb) or over the carotid artery in the neck just below the jaw, next to the voice box.

Maximal oxygen uptake is estimated according to a prediction equation that requires the following data: 1.0-mile walk time, exercise heart rate at the end of the walk, age, gender, and body weight in pounds. The procedure for this test and the equation are given in Figure 2.2.

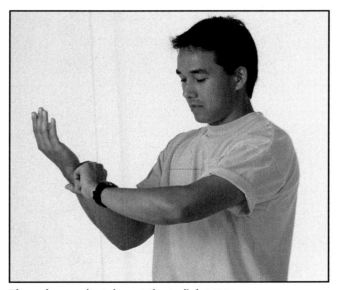

The pulse can be taken at the radial artery . . .

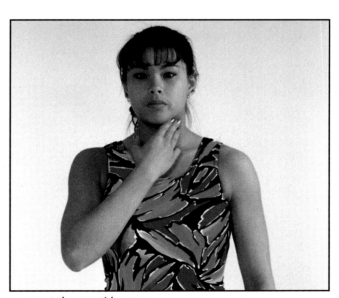

. . . or at the carotid artery.

1.0 MILE WALK TEST

1. Select the testing site. Use a 440-yard track (4 laps to a mile) or a premeasured 1.0-mile course.

2. Prior to the test, determine your body weight in pounds.

3. Have a stopwatch available to determine total walking time and exercise heart rate.

4. Walk the 1.0-mile course at a brisk pace (the exercise heart rate at the end of the test should be above 120 beats per minute).

5. At the end of the 1.0-mile walk, check your walking time and immediately count your pulse for 10 seconds. Multiply the 10-second pulse count by 6 to obtain the exercise heart rate in beats per minute.

6. Convert the walking time from minutes and seconds to minute units. Because there are 60 seconds in 1 minute, divide the seconds by 60 to obtain the fraction of a minute. For instance, a walking time of 12 minutes and 15 seconds would equal $12 + (15 \div 60)$, or 12.25 minutes.

7. To obtain the estimated maximal oxygen uptake (VO_{2max}) in ml/kg/min, plug your values in the following equation:

$$VO_{2max} = 132.853 - (.0769 \times W) - (.3877 \times A) + (6.315 \times G) - (3.2649 \times T) \times (.1565 \times HR)$$

Where:

W = Weight in pounds
A = Age in years
G = Gender (use 0 for women and 1 for men)
T = Total time for the 1-mile walk in minutes (see item 6 above)
HR = Exercise heart rate in beats per minute at the end of the 1-mile walk

Example: A 19-year-old female who weighs 140 pounds completed the 1-mile walk in 14 minutes 39 seconds and with an exercise heart rate of 148 beats per minute. The estimated VO_{2max} would be:

W = 140 lbs
A = 19
G = 0 (female gender = 0)
T = 14:39 = $14 + (39 \div 60)$ = 14.65 min
HR = 148 bpm

$$VO_{2max} = 132.853 - (.0769 \times 140) - (.3877 \times 19) + (6.315 \times 0) - (3.2649 \times 14.65) - (.1565 \times 148)$$

$$VO_{2max} = 43.7 \text{ ml/kg/min}$$

8. If you take the 1.0-Mile Walk Test, you may use the spaces below to record your data and solve the equation for your own VO_{2max}.

W = _____ lbs

A = _____

G = _____ (female gender = 0)

T = _____:_____ =   (min) + ((sec) $\div$ 60) =   min

HR = _____ bpm

$VO_{2max} = 132.853 - (.0769 \times \quad) - (.3877 \times \quad) + (6.315 \times \quad) - (3.2649 \times \quad) - (.1565 \times \quad)$

$VO_{2max} = 132.853 - (\quad) - (\quad) + (\quad) - (\quad) - (\quad)$

$VO_{2max} = \quad$ ml/kg/min

Source: "Estimation of VO_{2max} from a One-Mile Track Walk, Gender, Age, and Body Weight," by G. Kline et al., *Medicine and Science in Sports and Exercise* 19:3 (1987), 253–259. © American College of Sports Medicine. Used by permission.

Figure 2.2 • *Procedure for the 1.0-Mile Walk Test.*

● Step Test

The Step Test requires little time and equipment and can be administered to almost anyone, as a submaximal workload is used to estimate maximal oxygen uptake. Symptomatic and diseased individuals should not take this test. Significantly overweight individuals and those with joint problems in the lower extremities may have difficulty performing the test.

The actual test takes only 3 minutes. A 15-second recovery heart rate is taken between 5 and 20 seconds following the test (see Figure 2.3 and Table 2.3).

STEP TEST

1. Conduct the test with a bench or gymnasium bleacher 16¼ inches high.

2. Perform the stepping cycle to a four-step cadence (up-up-down-down). Men should perform 24 complete step-ups per minute, regulated with a metronome set at 96 beats per minute. Women perform 22 step-ups per minute, or 88 beats per minute on the metronome.

3. Allow a brief practice period of 5 to 10 seconds to familiarize yourself with the stepping cadence.

4. Begin the test and perform the step-ups for exactly 3 minutes.

5. Upon completing the 3 minutes, remain standing and take your heart rate for a 15-second interval from 5 to 20 seconds into recovery. Convert recovery heart rate to beats per minute (multiply 15-second heart rate by 4).

6. Maximal oxygen uptake (VO_{2max}) in ml/kg/min is estimated according to the following equations:

Men:
$$VO_{2max} = 111.33 - (0.42 \times \text{recovery heart rate in bpm})$$

Women:
$$VO_{2max} = 65.81 - (0.1847 \times \text{recovery heart rate in bpm})$$

Example: The recovery 15-second heart rate for a male following the 3-minute step test is found to be 39 beats. VO_{2max} is estimated as follows:

15-second heart rate = 39 beats
Minute heart rate = 39 × 4 = 156 bpm
$$VO_{2max} = 111.33 - (0.42 \times 156) = 45.81 \text{ ml/kg/min}$$

VO_{2max} also can be obtained according to recovery heart rates in Table 2.3.

From *Exercise Physiology: Energy, Nutrition, and Human Performance,* by W. D. McArdle et al. (Philadelphia: Lea & Febiger, 1996).

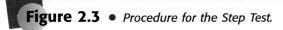

Figure 2.3 ● *Procedure for the Step Test.*

Step test.

 Table 2.3 *Predicted Maximal Oxygen Uptake for the Step Test*

15-Sec HR	HR-bpm	VO₂max Men (ml/kg/min)	VO₂max Women (ml/kg/min)
30	120	60.9	43.6
31	124	59.3	42.9
32	128	57.6	42.2
33	132	55.9	41.4
34	136	54.2	40.7
35	140	52.5	40.0
36	144	50.9	39.2
37	148	49.2	38.5
38	152	47.5	37.7
39	156	45.8	37.0
40	160	44.1	36.3
41	164	42.5	35.5
42	168	40.8	34.8
43	172	39.1	34.0
44	176	37.4	33.3
45	180	35.7	32.6
46	184	34.1	31.8
47	188	32.4	31.1
48	192	30.7	30.3
49	196	29.0	29.6
50	200	27.3	28.9

HR = heart rate
bpm = beats per minute

The equipment required is a bench or gymnasium bleacher 16¼ inches high, a stopwatch, and a metronome.

You also will need to know how to take your heart rate by counting your pulse (explained under the 1.0-Mile Walk Test). By teaching people to take their own heart rate, a large group of people can be tested at once, using gymnasium bleachers.

● Astrand-Ryhming Test

Because of its simplicity and practicality, the Astrand-Ryhming has become one of the most popular tests used to estimate maximal oxygen uptake in the laboratory setting. The test is conducted on a bicycle ergometer, and, similar to the Step Test, it requires only submaximal workloads and little time to administer.

The cautions given for the Step Test also apply to the Astrand-Ryhming Test. Nevertheless, because the participant does not have to support his or her own body weight while riding the bicycle, overweight individuals and those with limited joint problems in the lower extremities can take this test.

The bicycle ergometer to be used for this test should allow for the regulation of workloads (see the test procedure in Figure 2.4 and Tables 2.4, 2.5, and 2.6). Besides the bicycle ergometer, a stopwatch and an additional technician to monitor the heart rate are needed to conduct the test.

The heart rate is taken every minute for 6 minutes. At the end of the test, the heart rate should be in the range given for each workload in Tables 2.4, 2.5, and 2.6 (generally between 120 and 170 beats per minute).

When administering the test to older people, good judgment is essential. Low workloads should be used, because if the higher heart rates are reached (around 150 to 170 bpm), these individuals could be working near or at their maximal capacity, making it

ASTRAND-RYHMING TEST

1. Adjust the bike seat so the knees are almost completely extended as the foot goes through the bottom of the pedaling cycle.

2. During the test, keep the speed constant at 50 revolutions per minute. Test duration is 6 minutes.

3. Select the appropriate workload for the bike based on age, weight, health, and estimated fitness level. For unconditioned individuals: women, use 300 kpm (kilopounds per meter) or 450 kpm; men, 300 kpm or 600 kpm. Conditioned adults: women, 450 kpm or 600 kpm; men, 600 kpm or 900 kpm.*

4. Ride the bike for 6 minutes and check the heart rate every minute, during the last 10 seconds of each minute. Determine heart rate by recording the time it takes to count 30 pulse beats, and then converting to beats per minute using Table 2.4.

5. Average the final two heart rates (5th and 6th minutes). If these two heart rates are not within five beats per minute of each other, continue the test for another few minutes until this is accomplished. If the heart rate continues to climb significantly after the 6th minute, stop the test and rest for 15 to 20 minutes. You may then retest, preferably at a lower workload. The final average heart rate should also fall between the ranges given for each workload in Table 2.5 (men: 300 kpm = 120 to 140 beats per minute; 600 kpm = 120 to 170 beats per minute).

6. Based on the average heart rate of the final 2 minutes and your workload, look up the maximal oxygen uptake (VO_{2max}) in Table 2.5 (for example: men: 600 kpm and average heart rate = 145, VO_{2max} = 2.4 liters/minute).

7. Correct VO_{2max} using the correction factors found in Table 2.6 (if VO_{2max} = 2.4 and age 35, correction factor = .870. Multiply 2.4 × .870 and final corrected VO_{2max} = 2.09 liters/minute).

8. To obtain VO_{2max} in ml/kg/min, multiply the VO_{2max} by 1,000 (to convert liters to milliliters) and divide by body weight in kilograms (to obtain kilograms, divide your body weight in pounds by 2.2046).

Example: Corrected VO_{2max} = 2.09 liters/minute
Body weight = 132 pounds or 60 kilograms (132 ÷ 2.2046 = 60)

$$VO_{2max} \text{ in ml/kg/min} = \frac{2.09 \times 1,000}{60} = \frac{2,090}{60} = 34.8 \text{ ml/kg/min}$$

* On the Monarch bicycle ergometer, when riding at a speed of 50 revolutions per minute, a load of 1 kp = 300 kpm, 1.5 kp = 450, 2 kp = 600 kpm, and so forth, with increases of 150 kpm to each half kp.

Figure 2.4 ● *Procedure for the Astrand-Ryhming Test.*

Table 2.4 Conversion of Time for 30 Pulse Beats to Pulse Rate Per Minute

Sec.	bpm	Sec.	bpm	Sec.	bpm	Sec.	bpm	Sec.	bpm	Sec.	bpm	Sec.	bpm
22.0	82	19.9	90	17.8	101	15.7	115	13.6	132	11.5	157	9.4	191
21.9	82	19.8	91	17.7	102	15.6	115	13.5	133	11.4	158	9.3	194
21.8	83	19.7	91	17.6	102	15.5	116	13.4	134	11.3	159	9.2	196
21.7	83	19.6	92	17.5	103	15.4	117	13.3	135	11.2	161	9.1	198
21.6	83	19.5	92	17.4	103	15.3	118	13.2	136	11.1	162	9.0	200
21.5	84	19.4	93	17.3	104	15.2	118	13.1	137	11.0	164	8.9	202
21.4	84	19.3	93	17.2	105	15.1	119	13.0	138	10.9	165	8.8	205
21.3	85	19.2	94	17.1	105	15.0	120	12.9	140	10.8	167	8.7	207
21.2	85	19.1	94	17.0	106	14.9	121	12.8	141	10.7	168	8.6	209
21.1	85	19.0	95	16.9	107	14.8	122	12.7	142	10.6	170	8.5	212
21.0	86	18.9	95	16.8	107	14.7	122	12.6	143	10.5	171	8.4	214
20.9	86	18.8	96	16.7	108	14.6	123	12.5	144	10.4	173	8.3	217
20.8	87	18.7	96	16.6	108	14.5	124	12.4	145	10.3	175	8.2	220
20.7	87	18.6	97	16.5	109	14.4	125	12.3	146	10.2	176	8.1	222
20.6	87	18.5	97	16.4	110	14.3	126	12.2	148	10.1	178	8.0	225
20.5	88	18.4	98	16.3	110	14.2	127	12.1	149	10.0	180		
20.4	88	18.3	98	16.2	111	14.1	128	12.0	150	9.9	182		
20.3	89	18.2	99	16.1	112	14.0	129	11.9	151	9.8	184		
20.2	89	18.1	99	16.0	113	13.9	129	11.8	153	9.7	186		
20.1	90	18.0	100	15.9	113	13.8	130	11.7	154	9.6	188		
20.0	90	17.9	101	15.8	114	13.7	131	11.6	155	9.5	189		

The heart rate is being monitored on the carotid artery during the Astrand-Ryhming Test.

Maximal oxygen uptake improves with aerobic exercise.

Table 2.5 *Maximal Oxygen Uptake (VO$_{2max}$) Estimates for the Astrand-Ryhming Test*

Heart Rate	MEN l/min					WOMEN l/min				
	300	600	900	1200	1500	300	450	600	750	900
120	2.2	3.4	4.8			2.6	3.4	4.1	4.8	
121	2.2	3.4	4.7			2.5	3.3	4.0	4.8	
122	2.2	3.4	4.6			2.5	3.2	3.9	4.7	
123	2.1	3.4	4.6			2.4	3.1	3.9	4.6	
124	2.1	3.3	4.5	6.0		2.4	3.1	3.8	4.5	
125	2.0	3.2	4.4	5.9		2.3	3.0	3.7	4.4	
126	2.0	3.2	4.4	5.8		2.3	3.0	3.6	4.3	
127	2.0	3.1	4.3	5.7		2.2	2.9	3.5	4.2	
128	2.0	3.1	4.2	5.6		2.2	2.8	3.5	4.2	4.8
129	1.9	3.0	4.2	5.6		2.2	2.8	3.4	4.1	4.8
130	1.9	3.0	4.1	5.5		2.1	2.7	3.4	4.0	4.7
131	1.9	2.9	4.0	5.4		2.1	2.7	3.4	4.0	4.6
132	1.8	2.9	4.0	5.3		2.0	2.7	3.3	3.9	4.5
133	1.8	2.8	3.9	5.3		2.0	2.6	3.2	3.8	4.4
134	1.8	2.8	3.9	5.2		2.0	2.6	3.2	3.8	4.4
135	1.7	2.8	3.8	5.1		2.0	2.6	3.1	3.7	4.3
136	1.7	2.7	3.8	5.0		1.9	2.5	3.1	3.6	4.2
137	1.7	2.7	3.7	5.0		1.9	2.5	3.0	3.6	4.2
138	1.6	2.7	3.7	4.9		1.8	2.4	3.0	3.5	4.1
139	1.6	2.6	3.6	4.8		1.8	2.4	2.9	3.5	4.0
140	1.6	2.6	3.6	4.8	6.0	1.8	2.4	2.8	3.4	4.0
141		2.6	3.5	4.7	5.9	1.8	2.3	2.8	3.4	3.9
142		2.5	3.5	4.6	5.8	1.7	2.3	2.8	3.3	3.9
143		2.5	3.4	4.6	5.7	1.7	2.2	2.7	3.3	3.8
144		2.5	3.4	4.5	5.7	1.7	2.2	2.7	3.2	3.8
145		2.4	3.4	4.5	5.6	1.6	2.2	2.7	3.2	3.7
146		2.4	3.3	4.4	5.6	1.6	2.2	2.6	3.2	3.7
147		2.4	3.3	4.4	5.5	1.6	2.1	2.6	3.1	3.6
148		2.4	3.2	4.3	5.4	1.6	2.1	2.6	3.1	3.6
149		2.3	3.2	4.3	5.4		2.1	2.6	3.0	3.5
150		2.3	3.2	4.2	5.3		2.0	2.5	3.0	3.5
151		2.3	3.1	4.2	5.2		2.0	2.5	3.0	3.4
152		2.3	3.1	4.1	5.2		2.0	2.5	2.9	3.4
153		2.2	3.0	4.1	5.1		2.0	2.4	2.9	3.3
154		2.2	3.0	4.0	5.1		2.0	2.4	2.8	3.3
155		2.2	3.0	4.0	5.0		1.9	2.4	2.8	3.2
156		2.2	2.9	4.0	5.0		1.9	2.3	2.8	3.2
157		2.1	2.9	3.9	4.9		1.9	2.3	2.7	3.2
158		2.1	2.9	3.9	4.9		1.8	2.3	2.7	3.1
159		2.1	2.8	3.8	4.8		1.8	2.2	2.7	3.1
160		2.1	2.8	3.8	4.8		1.8	2.2	2.6	3.0
161		2.0	2.8	3.7	4.7		1.8	2.2	2.6	3.0
162		2.0	2.8	3.7	4.6		1.8	2.2	2.6	3.0
163		2.0	2.8	3.7	4.6		1.7	2.2	2.6	2.9
164		2.0	2.7	3.6	4.5		1.7	2.1	2.5	2.9
165		2.0	2.7	3.6	4.5		1.7	2.1	2.5	2.9
166		1.9	2.7	3.6	4.5		1.7	2.1	2.5	2.8
167		1.9	2.6	3.5	4.4		1.6	2.1	2.4	2.8
168		1.9	2.6	3.5	4.4		1.6	2.0	2.4	2.8
169		1.9	2.6	3.5	4.3		1.6	2.0	2.4	2.8
170		1.8	2.6	3.4	4.3		1.6	2.0	2.4	2.7

l/min = liters per minute

From Astrand, I. *Acta Physiologica Scandinavica* 49(1960). Supplementum 169:45-60.

Table 2.6　*Age-Based Correction Factors for Maximal Oxygen Uptake (VO$_{2max}$) for the Astrand-Ryhming Test*

Age	Correction Factor	Age	Correction Factor	Age	Correction Factor	Age	Correction Factor
14	1.11	27	.974	40	.830	53	.726
15	1.10	28	.961	41	.820	54	.718
16	1.09	29	.948	42	.810	55	.710
17	1.08	30	.935	43	.800	56	.704
18	1.07	31	.922	44	.790	57	.698
19	1.06	32	.909	45	.780	58	.692
20	1.05	33	.896	46	.774	59	.686
21	1.04	34	.883	47	.768	60	.680
22	1.03	35	.870	48	.762	61	.674
23	1.02	36	.862	49	.756	62	.668
24	1.01	37	.854	50	.750	63	.662
25	1.00	38	.846	51	.742	64	.656
26	.987	39	.838	52	.734	65	.650

Adapted from Astrand, I. *Acta Physiologica Scandinavica* 49(1960). Supplementum 169:45-60.

an unsafe test without adequate medical supervision. When choosing workloads for older people, final exercise heart rates should not exceed 130 to 140 bpm.

● 12-Minute Swim Test

Similar to the 1.5-Mile Run test, the 12-Minute Swim Test is considered a maximal exercise test, and the same precautions apply. The objective is to swim as far as possible during the 12-minute test.

A swimming test (Figure 2.5) is practical only for those who are planning to take part in a swimming program. Unlike land-based tests, predicting maximal oxygen uptake through a swimming test is difficult. Differences in skill level, swimming conditioning,

12-MINUTE SWIM TEST

1. Enlist a friend to time the test. The only other requisites are a stopwatch and a swimming pool. Do not attempt to do this test in an unsupervised pool.

2. Warm up by swimming slowly and doing a few mild stretching exercises before taking the test.

3. Start the test and swim as many laps as possible in 12 minutes. Pace yourself throughout the test, and do not swim to the point of complete exhaustion.

4. After completing the test, cool down by swimming another 2 or 3 minutes at a slower pace.

5. Determine the total distance you swam during the test, and look up your fitness category in Table 2.7.

Figure 2.5 ● *Procedure for the 12-Minute Swim Test.*

and body composition greatly affect the energy requirements (oxygen uptake) of swimming.

Good cardiorespiratory fitness has been linked to better health and increased longevity.

A skilled swimmer is able to swim more efficiently and expend much less energy than an unskilled swimmer. Improper breathing patterns cause premature fatigue. Overweight individuals are more buoyant in the water, and the larger surface area (body size) produces greater friction against movement in the water medium.

Lack of conditioning affects swimming test results as well. An unconditioned skilled swimmer who is in good cardiorespiratory shape because of a regular jogging program will not perform as effectively in a swimming test. Swimming conditioning is important for adequate performance on this test.

Because of these limitations, maximal oxygen uptake cannot be estimated for a swimming test and the fitness categories given in Table 2.7 are only estimated ratings. This test should be limited to people who cannot perform any of the other tests and whose primary aerobic exercise will be a swimming program. Unskilled and unconditioned swimmers can expect lower cardiorespiratory fitness ratings than those obtained with a land-based test.

Table 2.7 *12-Minute Swim Test Fitness Categories*

Distance (yards)	Fitness Category
≥700	Excellent
500–700	Good
400–500	Average
200–400	Fair
≤200	Poor

Adapted from *The Aerobics Program for Total Well-Being*, by K. H. Cooper (New York: Bantam Books, 1982).

Swimming efficiency requires skill and proper conditioning.

● Interpreting Your Maximal Oxygen Uptake Results

After obtaining your maximal oxygen uptake, you can determine your current level of cardiorespiratory fitness by consulting Table 2.8. Locate the maximal oxygen uptake in your age category, and on the top row you will find your present level of cardiorespiratory fitness. For example, a 19-year-old male with a maximal oxygen uptake of 35 ml/kg/min would be classified in the average cardiorespiratory fitness category. Once you have established your VO_{2max} and cardiorespiratory fitness category, record this information in Figure 2.6 and in your Fitness and Wellness Profile in Appendix A. After you initiate your personal cardiorespiratory exercise program (see Chapter 3), you may wish to retest yourself periodically to evaluate your progress.

● Exercise Readiness

Before proceeding to Chapter 3, on cardiorespiratory exercise prescription, and if you are not exercising now, you should ask yourself the following question: Am I willing to give exercise a try? A low percentage of the U.S. population is truly committed to exercise. Further, surveys indicate that more than half of the people who start exercising drop out during the

Table 2.8 *Cardiorespiratory Fitness Classification According to Maximal Oxygen Uptake*

Gender	Age	FITNESS CLASSIFICATION (based on VO_{2max} in ml/kg/min)				
		Poor	Fair	Average	Good	Excellent
Men	≤29	≤24.9	25–33.9	34–43.9	44–52.9	≥53
	30–39	≤22.9	23–30.9	31–41.9	42–49.9	≥50
	40–49	≤19.9	20–26.9	27–38.9	39–44.9	≥45
	50–59	≤17.9	18–24.9	25–37.9	38–42.9	≥43
	60–69	≤15.9	16–22.9	23–35.9	36–40.9	≥41
Women	≤29	≤23.9	24–30.9	31–38.9	39–48.9	≥49
	30–39	≤19.9	20–27.9	28–36.9	37–44.9	≥45
	40–49	≤16.9	17–24.9	25–34.9	35–41.9	≥42
	50–59	≤14.9	15–21.9	22–33.9	34–39.9	≥40
	60–69	≤12.9	13–20.9	21–32.9	33–36.9	≥37

▮ High physical fitness standard
▮ Health fitness standard

See Chapter 1, Fitness Standards: Health Versus Physical Fitness, page 10.

first 6 months of the program. Sports psychologists are trying to find out why some people exercise habitually and many do not. All of the benefits of exercise cannot help unless people commit to a lifetime program of physical activity.

If you are not exercising regularly, are you willing to stop contemplating and give exercise a try?

The first step is to decide positively that you will try. Using Figure 2.7, you can list the advantages and disadvantages of incorporating exercise into your lifestyle. Your list may include things such as: It will make me feel better. I will lose weight. I will have more energy. It will lower risk for chronic diseases. Your list of disadvantages might include: I don't want to take the time. I'm too out of shape. There's no good place to exercise. I don't have the willpower

to do it. When the reasons for exercise outweigh the reasons for not exercising, it will become easier to try.

The information provided in Figure 2.8 then can help you answer the question: Am I ready to start an exercise program? You are evaluated in four categories: mastery (self-control), attitude, health, and commitment. The higher you score in any category — mastery, for example — the more important that reason is for you to exercise.

Scores can vary from 4 to 16. A score of 12 and above is a strong indicator that that factor is important to you, whereas 8 and below is low. If you score 12 or more points in each category, your chances of initiating and sticking to an exercise program are good. If you do not score at least 12 points in three categories, your chances of succeeding at exercise may be slim. You need to be better informed about the benefits of exercise, and a retraining process may be helpful. More tips on how you can become committed to exercise are provided in the next chapter.

Suggested Readings

American College of Sports Medicine. *Guidelines for Exercise Testing and Prescription.* Philadelphia: Lea & Febiger, 1995.

American College of Sports Medicine. "The Recommended Quantity and Quality of Exercise for Developing and Maintaining Cardiorespiratory and Muscular Fitness in Healthy Adults." *Medicine and Science in Sports and Exercise,* 22 (1990), 265-274.

American Heart Association Committee on Exercise. *Exercise Testing and Training of Apparently Healthy Individuals: A Handbook for Physicians.* New York: AHA, 1972.

Astrand, I. *Acta Physiologica Scandinavica,* 49 (1960), Supplementum 169:45-60.

Astrand, P. O., and K. Rodahl. *Textbook of Work Physiology.* New York: McGraw-Hill, 1986.

Cooper, K. H. "A Means of Assessing Maximal Oxygen Intake." *Journal of the American Medical Association,* 203 (1968), 201-204.

Cooper, K. H. *The Aerobics Program for Total Well-Being.* New York: Mount Evans and Co., 1982.

Fox, E. L., R. W. Bowers, and H. L. Foss. *The Physiological Basis of Physical Education and Athletics.* Philadelphia: Saunders College Publishing, 1988.

Hoeger, W. W. K., and S. A. Hoeger. *Lifetime Fitness & Wellness: A Personalized Program.* Englewood, CO: Morton Publishing, 1995.

Kline, G., et al. "Estimation of VO_{2max} from a One-Mile Track Walk, Gender, Age, and Body Weight." *Medicine and Science in Sports and Exercise* 19:3 (1987), 253-259.

McArdle, W. D., F. I. Katch, and V. L. Katch. *Exercise Physiology: Energy, Nutrition and Human Performance.* Philadelphia: Lea & Febiger, 1996.

Wilmore, J. H., and D. L. Costill. *Physiology of Sport and Exercise.* Champaign, IL: Human Kinetics, 1994.

Name: _____ Age: _____

Date	Test Used	VO$_{2max}$	Fitness Classification

Figure 2.6 • *Cardiorespiratory endurance report.*

Principles of Cardiorespiratory Exercise Prescription

3

There is no drug in current or prospective use that holds as much promise for sustained health as a lifetime program of physical exercise.[1]

*W*ith the exception of older adults, cardiorespiratory endurance is the single most important component of health-related physical fitness (see Chapter 1). A person needs a certain amount of muscular strength and flexibility to engage in normal daily activities. Nevertheless, a person can get by without a lot of strength and flexibility but cannot do without a good cardiorespiratory system.

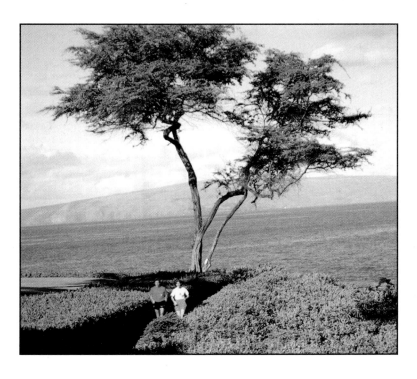

Objectives

- Determine readiness to start an exercise program.
- Learn the principles that govern cardiorespiratory exercise prescription: intensity, mode, duration, and frequency.
- Identify some popular cardiorespiratory activities and their specific benefits.
- Learn concepts for preventing and treating injuries.
- Learn some ways to enhance adherence to exercise.
- Learn to predict oxygen uptake and caloric expenditure from exercise heart rate.

Aerobic exercise is especially important in preventing coronary heart disease. A poorly conditioned heart, which has to pump more often just to keep a person alive, is subject to more wear-and-tear than a well-conditioned heart. In situations that place stren-

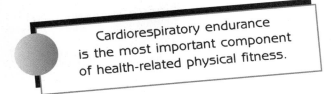

Cardiorespiratory endurance is the most important component of health-related physical fitness.

uous demands on the heart, such as doing yard work, lifting heavy objects or weights, or running to catch a bus, the unconditioned heart may not be able to sustain the strain. Regular participation in cardiorespiratory endurance activities also helps a person achieve and maintain recommended body weight, the fourth component of health-related physical fitness.

● Guidelines for Cardiorespiratory Exercise Prescription

All too often, individuals who exercise regularly and then take a cardiorespiratory endurance test are surprised to find their maximal oxygen uptake is not as good as they think it is. Although these individuals may be exercising regularly, they most likely are not following the basic principles for cardiorespiratory exercise prescription. Therefore, they do not reap significant improvements in cardiorespiratory endurance.

To develop the cardiorespiratory system, the heart muscle has to be overloaded like any other muscle in the human body. Just as the biceps muscle in the upper arm is developed through strength-training exercises, the heart muscle has to be exercised to

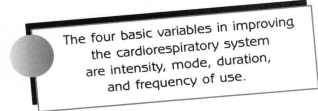

The four basic variables in improving the cardiorespiratory system are intensity, mode, duration, and frequency of use.

increase in size, strength, and efficiency. To better understand how the cardiorespiratory system can be developed, we have to be familiar with four variables: intensity, mode, duration, and frequency of exercise.

Before discussing the cardiorespiratory prescription variables, you should be aware that the American College of Sports Medicine recommends that a medical exam and a diagnostic exercise stress test be administered prior to vigorous exercise by apparently healthy men over age 40 and women over age 50.[2]

The American College of Sports Medicine has defined *vigorous exercise* as an exercise intensity above 60% of maximal oxygen uptake. This intensity is the equivalent of exercise that provides a "substantial challenge" to the participant or one that cannot be maintained for 20 continuous minutes.

Intensity of Exercise

When trying to develop the cardiorespiratory system, **intensity** of exercise is the factor that perhaps is ignored most often. For muscles to develop, they have to be overloaded to a given point. The training stimulus to develop the biceps muscle, for example, can be accomplished with arm curl-up exercises. Likewise, the cardiorespiratory system is stimulated by making the heart pump faster for a specified period of time.

Cardiorespiratory development occurs when working between 50% and 85% of heart rate reserve.[3] Working closer to 85% of heart rate reserve yields quicker results. For this reason, many experts prescribe exercise between 70% and 85% for young people. Exercise intensity can be calculated easily, and training can be monitored by checking your pulse.

Determining Training Intensity

To determine the intensity of exercise or cardiorespiratory training zone:

1. Estimate your **maximal heart rate (MHR)**. The maximal heart rate depends on the person's age and can be estimated according to the formula: MHR = 220 minus age (220 − age)

2. Check your **resting heart rate (RHR)** sometime after you have been at rest for 15 to 20 minutes. You may take your pulse for 30 seconds and multiply by 2, or take it for a full minute.

3. Determine the **heart rate reserve (HRR)**. This is done by subtracting the resting heart rate from the maximal heart rate (HRR = MHR − RHR). HRR indicates the number of beats available to go from a resting condition to an all-out maximal effort.

4. Calculate the training intensities (TI) at 50%, 70%, and 85%. Multiply the heart rate reserve by the respective 50, 70, and 85 percentages, and then add the resting heart rate to these three

figures (for example, 85% TI = HRR × .85 + RHR).

Example: The 50%, 70%, and 85% training intensities for a 20-year-old person with a resting heart rate of 68 bpm is:

MHR: 220 − 20 = 200 beats per minute (bpm)
RHR = 68 bpm
HRR: 200 − 68 = 132 beats
50% TI = (132 × .50) + 68 = 134 bpm
70% TI = (132 × .70) + 68 = 160 bpm
85% TI = (132 × .85) + 68 = 180 bpm
Cardiorespiratory training zone: 134 to 180 bpm

You can compute your own training intensity by using Figure 3.9 at the end of this chapter. The cardiorespiratory training zone indicates that whenever you exercise to improve the cardiorespiratory system, you should maintain your heart rate between the 50% and 85% training intensities to obtain adequate development (Figure 3.1). If you have been physically inactive, you should train around the 50% intensity during the first 4 to 6 weeks of the exercise program. After the first few weeks, you should exercise between 70% and 85% training intensity.

Following a few weeks of training, you may have a considerably lower resting heart rate (10 to 20 beats in 8 to 12 weeks). Therefore, you should recompute your target zone periodically. Once you have reached an ideal level of cardiorespiratory endurance, training in the 50% to 85% range will allow you to maintain your fitness level.

During the first few weeks of an exercise program, you should monitor your exercise heart rate regularly to make sure you are training in the proper zone. Wait until you are about 5 minutes into your exercise session before taking your first rate. When you check your heart rate, count your pulse for 10 seconds, and then multiply by 6 to get the per-minute pulse rate. Exercise heart rate will remain at the same level for about 15 seconds following exercise. After 15 seconds, your heart rate will drop

TERMS

Intensity In cardiorespiratory exercise, how hard a person has to exercise to improve or maintain fitness.

Maximal heart rate (MHR) Highest heart rate for a person, primarily related to age.

Resting heart rate (RHR) Heart rate after a person has been sitting quietly for 15–20 minutes.

Heart rate reserve (HRR) The difference between the maximal heart rate and the resting heart rate.

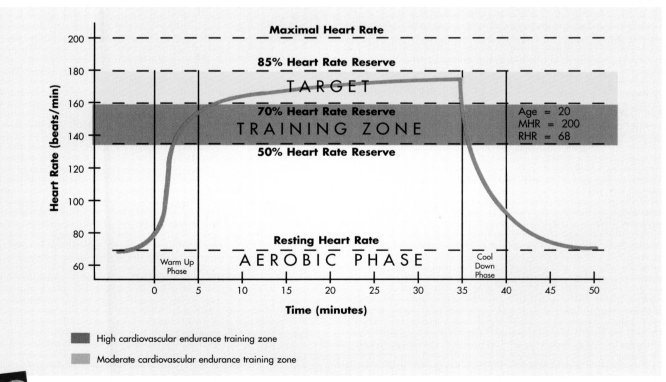

Figure 3.1 ● *Typical cardiorespiratory or aerobic training pattern.*

rapidly. Do not hesitate to stop during your exercise bout to check your pulse. If the rate is too low, increase the intensity of exercise. If the rate is too high, slow down.

To develop the cardiorespiratory system, you do not have to exercise above the 85% rate. From a fitness standpoint, training above this percentage will not produce extra benefits and actually may be unsafe for some individuals. For unconditioned people and older adults, cardiorespiratory training should be around the 50% rate. This lower rate is recommended to avoid potential problems associated with high-intensity exercise.

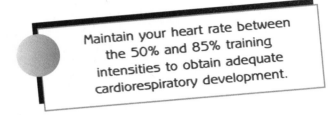

Maintain your heart rate between the 50% and 85% training intensities to obtain adequate cardiorespiratory development.

Health Fitness Versus Physical Fitness

Training benefits can be obtained by exercising at the 50% training intensity. Training at this lower percentage, however, may place a person in only an average or a "moderately fit" category (see Chapter 2, Table 2.8). As discussed later in this chapter under Specific Exercise Considerations, question 1, exercising at this lower intensity lowers the risk for cardiovascular mortality (health fitness) but does not allow the person to achieve a high cardiorespiratory fitness rating (physical fitness). The latter ratings are obtained by exercising closer to the 85% threshold.

Rate of Perceived Exertion

Because many people do not check their heart rate during exercise, an alternative method of prescribing intensity of exercise has become more popular recently. This method uses a **rate of perceived exertion (RPE)** scale developed by Gunnar Borg. Using the scale in Figure 3.2, a person subjectively rates the perceived exertion or difficulty of exercise when training in the appropriate target zone. The exercise heart rate then is associated with the corresponding RPE value.

For example, if the training intensity requires a heart rate zone between 150 and 170 bpm, the person associates this with training between "hard" and "very hard." Some individuals, however, may perceive less exertion than others when training in the

6	
7	Very, very light
8	
9	Very light
10	
11	Fairly light
12	
13	Somewhat hard
14	
15	Hard
16	
17	Very Hard
18	
19	Very, very hard
20	

From "Perceived Exertion: A Note on History and Methods," by G. Borg, *Medicine and Science in Sports and Exercise,* 5 (1983), 90–93.

Figure 3.2 ● *Rate of Perceived Exertion Scale.*

correct zone. Therefore, you have to associate your own inner perception of the task with the phrases given on the scale. You then may proceed to exercise at that rate of perceived exertion.

You must be sure to cross-check your target zone with your perceived exertion in the first weeks of your exercise program. To help you develop this association, you should keep a regular record of your activities using the form provided in Figure 3.10 at the end of this chapter. After several weeks of training, you should be able to predict your exercise heart rate just by your own perceived exertion of the exercise intensity.

Whether you monitor the intensity of exercise by checking your pulse or through rate of perceived exertion, you should be aware that changes in normal exercise conditions will affect the training zone. For example, exercising on a hot/humid day or at high altitude increases the heart rate response to a given task requiring adjustments in the intensity of your exercise.

Mode of Exercise

The **mode** of exercise that develops the cardiorespiratory system has to be aerobic in nature. Once you have established your cardiorespiratory training zone, any activity or combination of activities that will get your heart rate up to that training zone and keep it there for as long as you exercise will give you adequate development. Examples of these activities are walking, jogging, aerobics, swimming, water aerobics, cross-country skiing, rope skipping, cycling, racquetball, stair climbing, and stationary running or cycling.

The activity you choose should be based on your personal preferences, what you most enjoy doing, and your physical limitations. Choose low-impact activities, as they greatly decrease the risk for injuries. Most injuries to beginners are related to high-impact activities. General strength conditioning (see Chapter 4) is also recommended prior to initiating an aerobic exercise program for individuals who have been inactive. Strength conditioning will significantly reduce the incidence of injuries.

The amount of strength or flexibility you develop through various activities differs, but in terms of cardiorespiratory development, the heart doesn't know whether you are walking, swimming, or cycling. All the heart knows is that it has to pump at a certain rate, and as long as that rate is in the desired range, your cardiorespiratory fitness will improve.

From a health fitness point of view, training in the lower end of the cardiorespiratory zone will yield optimal health benefits. The closer the heart rate is to the higher end of the cardiorespiratory training zone, however, the greater will be the improvements in maximal oxygen uptake (high physical fitness).

Aerobic exercise has to involve the major muscle groups of the body, and it has to be rhythmic and continuous. As the amount of muscle mass involved during exercise increases, so does the effectiveness of the activity in providing cardiorespiratory development.

Cross-country skiing is regarded as the prime exercise modality for aerobic development. Several major muscle groups are used during this activity because it requires both upper and lower body work. Research has shown that, of all elite athletes, cross-country skiers have the highest maximal oxygen uptake.

Because of the greater amount of muscle mass involved, more oxygen and energy (calories) are used during cross-country skiing than with most other aerobic activities. A limitation of this activity, of course, is the lack of year-round conditions for skiing, and commercially available cross-country skiing simulating equipment is not readily available to most people.

A relatively new mode of aerobic exercise is *Aero-belt exercise*. The Aero-belt* (Aerobic Endurance Resistance Overloader) consists of a belt with an elastic band that slides freely through the belt and attaches to the wrists. The objective of using the Aero-belt is to provide resistance to the arms during lower body physical activity, thereby increasing the person's oxygen consumption, energy expenditure, and upper body strength and endurance development during aerobic exercise. As in cross-country skiing, the Aero-belt provides resistance to the arms while walking, jogging, bounding, stair stepping, riding a stationary bicycle, or doing aerobics.

Using the Aero-belt actually can provide greater upper body conditioning benefits than cross-country skiing. Depending on individual strength and fitness levels, three different tension grades for the elastic cord are available. Medium and high tension are mainly for strength conditioning, and low tension is for developing endurance.

---

*AERO-BELT is a registered trademark of Nurge Fitness Systems, P. O. Box 889, Ketchum, ID 83340 Phone: 1-800-TRY-TO-XL

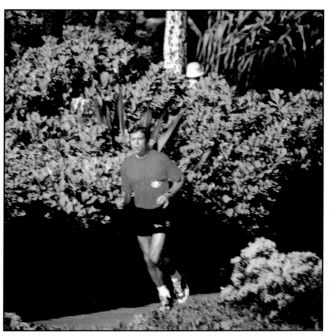

Aerobic exercise promotes cardiorespiratory development and helps decrease the risk for chronic diseases.

TERMS

Rate of perceived exertion (RPE) A perception scale to monitor or interpret the intensity of aerobic exercise.

Mode Form of exercise.

Aero-belt walking

Aero-belt step-aerobics

Aero-belt Exercise: A new exercise modality designed to provide resistance to the arms during lower body physical activity, thereby increasing the person's oxygen consumption, energy expenditure, and upper body strength development during aerobic exercise. (For more information call 1-800-TRY-TO-XL.)

The physiologic responses to Aero-belt walking (4.0 and 4.2 mph), jogging (6.0 mph), and step aerobics were investigated at Boise State University.[4,5,6] Increases in heart rate, oxygen uptake, and caloric expenditure ranged from 32% to 54% from regular walking, jogging, and step-aerobics to walking, jogging, and step-aerobics with an Aero-belt (see Figure 3.3).

Duration of Exercise

The general recommendation is that a person train between 20 and 60 minutes per session. The **duration** is based on how intensely a person trains. If the training is done around 85%, 20 minutes are sufficient. At 50% intensity, the person should train between 30 and 60 minutes. As mentioned previously, under Intensity of Exercise, unconditioned people and older adults should train at lower percentages; therefore, the activity should be carried out over a longer time.

Although most experts recommend 20 to 30 minutes of aerobic exercise per session, research indicates that three 10-minute exercise sessions per day (separated by at least 4 hours), at approximately 70% of maximal heart rate, also produce training benefits.[7]

Although the increases in maximal oxygen uptake with the latter program were not as large (57%) as those found in a group performing a continuous 30-minute bout of exercise per day, the researchers concluded that moderate-intensity exercise training,

Figure 3.3 ● *Oxygen uptake, heart rate, and energy expenditure responses to walking, jogging, and step aerobics with and without an Aero-belt.*

conducted for 10 minutes, three times per day, benefits the cardiorespiratory system significantly.

Results of this study are meaningful because people often mention lack of time as the reason for not taking part in an exercise program. Many think they have to exercise at least 20 continuous minutes to get any benefits at all. Even though 20 to 30 minutes are ideal, short, intermittent exercise bouts also are beneficial to the cardiorespiratory system.

Exercise sessions always should be preceded by a 5-minute warm-up and followed by a 5-minute cool-down period (see Figure 3.1). The **warm-up** should consist of general calisthenics, stretching exercises, or exercising at a lower intensity level than the actual target zone. The **cool-down** means decreasing the intensity of exercise *gradually*. Abruptly stopping causes blood to pool in the exercised body parts, diminishing the return of blood to the heart. Less blood return can cause dizziness and faintness or even bring on cardiac abnormalities.

Frequency of Exercise

When starting an exercise program, a **frequency** of three to five 20- to 30-minute training sessions per week are recommended to improve maximal oxygen uptake. When training is conducted more than 5 days a week, further improvements are minimal.

For individuals on a weight-loss program, 45- to 60-minute exercise sessions of low to moderate intensity, conducted five to six days per week, are recommended. Longer exercise sessions increase caloric expenditure for faster weight reduction (see Chapter 4, page 80). Three 20- to 30-minute training sessions per week, on nonconsecutive days, will maintain cardiorespiratory fitness as long as the heart rate is in the appropriate target zone. A summary of the cardiorespiratory exercise prescription guidelines according to the American College of Sports Medicine is provided in Figure 3.4.

Although three exercise sessions per week will maintain cardiorespiratory fitness, the importance of regular physical activity in preventing disease and enhancing quality of life was pointed out clearly in July 1993 at a news briefing held at the National Press Club in Washington, DC. At this briefing the American College of Sports Medicine and the U. S. Centers for Disease Control and Prevention, in conjunction with the President's Council on Physical Fitness and Sports, provided the American public with

Activity:	Aerobic (examples: walking, jogging, cycling, swimming, aerobics, racquetball, soccer, stair climbing)
Intensity:	50%–85% heart rate reserve
Duration:	20–60 minutes of continuous aerobic activity
Frequency:	3 to 5 days per week

Source: "The Recommended Quantity and Quality of Exercise for Developing and Maintaining Cardiorespiratory and Muscular Fitness in Healthy Adults by the American College of Sports Medicine," *Medicine and Science in Sports and Exercise*, 22 (1990), 265–274.

Figure 3.4 • *Cardiorespiratory exercise prescription guidelines.*

a set of recommendations on the types of physical activity needed for maintaining and promoting health.[8]

In this summary statement every American is encouraged to accumulate at least 30 minutes of moderate-intensity physical activity almost daily. This daily routine has been promoted as an effective way to improve health. The entire statement on the benefits of physical activity is given in Figure 3.5.

The previous recommendations were subsequently upheld in the 1995 Dietary Guidelines for Americans[9] and later by the U. S. Surgeon General in its 1996 Report on Physical Activity and Health.[10] In the latter report the Surgeon General states that Americans can improve their health and quality of life substantially by including moderate amounts of physical activity on most, preferably all, days of the week. Further, it states that no one, including older adults, is too old to enjoy the benefits of regular physical activity.

To enjoy better health and fitness, physical activity must be pursued on a regular basis. According to Dr. William Haskell of Stanford University: "Most of the health-related benefits of exercise are relatively short term, so people should think of exercise

TERMS

Duration How long a person exercises.
Warm-up Starting a workout slowly.
Cool-down Tapering off an exercise session slowly.
Frequency How often a person engages in an exercise session.

— SUMMARY STATEMENT —
Workshop On
Physical Activity and Public Health

Sponsored By:
U. S. Centers for Disease Control and Prevention
and
American College of Sports Medicine

In Cooperation with the President's Council on Physical Fitness and Sports

Regular physical activity is an important component of a healthy lifestyle — preventing disease and enhancing health and quality of life. A persuasive body of scientific evidence, which has accumulated over the past several decades, indicates that regular, moderate-intensity physical activity confers substantial health benefits. Because of this evidence, the U.S. Public Health Service has identified increased physical activity as a priority in Healthy People 2000, our national health objectives for the year 2000.

A primary benefit of regular physical activity is protection against coronary heart disease. In addition, physical activity appears to provide some protection against several other chronic diseases such as adult-onset diabetes, hypertension, certain cancers, osteoporosis, and depression. Furthermore, on average, physically active people outlive inactive people, even if they start their activity late in life. It is estimated that more than 250,000 deaths per year in the U.S. can be attributed to lack of regular physical activity, a number comparable to the deaths attributed to other chronic disease risk factors such as obesity, high blood pressure, and elevated blood cholesterol.

Despite the recognized value of physical activity, few Americans are regularly active. Only 22% of adults engage in leisure time physical activity at the level recommended for health benefits in Healthy People 2000. Fully 24% of adult Americans are completely sedentary and are badly in need of more physical activity. The remaining 54% are inadequately active and they too would benefit from more physical activity. Participation in regular physical activity appears to have gradually increased during the 1960s, 1970s, and early 1980s, but has plateaued in recent years. Among ethnic minority populations, older persons, and those with lower incomes or levels of education, participation in regular physical activity has remained consistently low.

Why are so few Americans physically active? Perhaps one answer is that previous public health efforts to promote physical activity have overemphasized the importance of high-intensity exercise. The current low rate of participation may be explained, in part, by the perception of many people that they must engage in vigorous, continuous exercise to reap health benefits. Actually the scientific evidence clearly demonstrates that regular, moderate-intensity physical activity provides substantial health benefits. A group of experts brought together by the U.S. Centers for Disease Control and Prevention (CDC) and the American Col-

lege of Sports Medicine (ACSM) reviewed the pertinent scientific evidence and formulated the following recommendation:

Every American adult should accumulate 30 minutes or more of moderate-intensity physical activity over the course of most days of the week. Incorporating more activity into the daily routine is an effective way to improve health. Activities that can contribute to the 30-minute total include walking up stairs (instead of taking the elevator), gardening, raking leaves, dancing, and walking part or all of the way to or from work. The recommended 30 minutes of physical activity may also come from planned exercise or recreation such as jogging, playing tennis, swimming, and cycling. One specific way to meet the standard is to walk two miles briskly.

Because most adult Americans fail to meet this recommended level of moderate-intensity physical activity, almost all should strive to increase their participation in moderate or vigorous physical activity. Persons who currently do not engage in regular physical activity should begin by incorporating a few minutes of increased activity into their day, building up gradually to 30 minutes of additional physical activity. Those who are irregularly active should strive to adopt a more consistent pattern of activity. Regular participation in physical activities that develop and maintain muscular strength and joint flexibility is also recommended.

This recommendation has been developed to emphasize the important health benefits of moderate physical activity. But recognizing the benefits of physical activity is only part of the solution to this important public health problem. Today's high-tech society entices people to be inactive. Cars, television, and labor-saving devices have profoundly changed the way many people perform their jobs, take care of their homes, and use their leisure time. Furthermore, our surroundings often present significant barriers to participation in physical activity. Walking to the corner store proves difficult if there are no sidewalks; riding a bicycle to work is not an option unless safe bike lanes or paths are available.

Many Americans will not change their lifestyles until the environmental and social barriers to physical activity are reduced or eliminated. Individuals can help to overcome these barriers by modifying their own lifestyles and by encouraging family members and friends to become more active. In addition, local, state, and federal public health agencies; recreation boards; school groups; professional organizations; and fitness and sports organizations should work together to disseminate this critical public health message and to promote national, community, worksite, and school programs that help Americans become more physically active.

The American College of Sports Medicine and the U.S. Centers for Disease Control and Prevention, in cooperation with the President's Council on Physical Fitness and Sports, released this statement July 29, 1993, at the National Press Club in Washington, D.C.

Figure 3.5 • *Summary Statement: Workshop On Physical Activity and Public Health.*

as medication and take it on a daily basis."[11] Many of the benefits of exercise and activity diminish within 2 weeks of substantially decreased physical activity. These benefits are completely lost within 2 to 8 months of inactivity.[12]

Ideally, a person should engage in physical activity six to seven times per week. Based on the above discussion, to reap both the high-fitness and health-fitness benefits of exercise, a person needs to exercise a minimum of three times per week in the appropriate target zone for high fitness maintenance and three to four additional times per week in moderate-intensity activities to enjoy the full benefits of health fitness. All exercise/activity sessions should last about 30 minutes.

● Aerobic Activity Choices

One of the fun aspects of aerobic exercise is the variety of activities that promote cardiovascular development. You may select one or a combination of activities for your program. This choice should be based on personal enjoyment, convenience, and availability.

Most people pick and adhere to a single mode of exercise, such as walking, swimming, or jogging. No single activity develops total fitness. Many activities contribute to cardiorespiratory development. The extent of their contribution to other fitness components is limited, though, and varies among the activities. For total fitness, aerobic activities should be supplemented with strength (resistance) and flexibility exercise programs. Selecting a combination of aerobic activities (cross-training) nonetheless can add enjoyment to the program and keep exercise from becoming monotonous.

As you learn about the various aerobic activities in this chapter, keep in mind that your exercise sessions must be convenient. So that you may enjoy exercise, select a time when you will not be rushed, and find a nearby location. People do not enjoy driving across town to get to the gym, health club, track, or pool. If parking is a problem, you may quickly get discouraged and use this as an excuse not to stick to your exercise program.

Walking

The most natural, easiest, safest, and least expensive form of aerobic exercise is walking. For years many fitness practitioners believed that walking was not

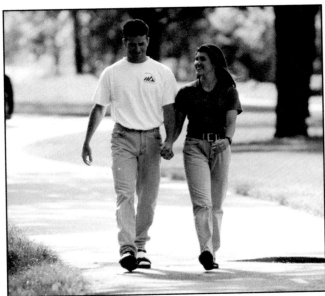

Walking is the most natural aerobic exercise.

vigorous enough to improve cardiorespiratory functioning. Studies have established, however, that brisk walking at speeds of 4 miles per hour or faster does improve cardiorespiratory fitness.

From a health-fitness viewpoint, a regular walking program can prolong life significantly. Although walking takes longer than jogging, the caloric cost of brisk walking is only about 10% lower than jogging the same distance.

Walking is perhaps the best activity to start a conditioning program for the cardiorespiratory system. Inactive people should start with 1-mile walks four to five times per week. Walk times can be increased gradually by 5 minutes each week. Following 3 to 4 weeks of conditioning, people should be able to walk 2 miles at a 4-mile-per-hour pace, five times per week. For greater aerobic benefits, walk longer and swing the arms at a faster than normal pace. A backpack (4 to 6 pounds) or an Aero-belt add to the intensity of walking. Because of the additional load to the cardiorespiratory system, extra weights are not recommended for people who have cardiovascular disease.

Walking in water (chest-deep level) is an excellent activity for people with leg and back problems. Because of water buoyancy, individuals submerged in water to armpit level weigh only about 10% to 20% of their weight outside the water. The resistance the water creates as a person walks in the pool makes the intensity quite high, providing an excellent cardiorespiratory workout.

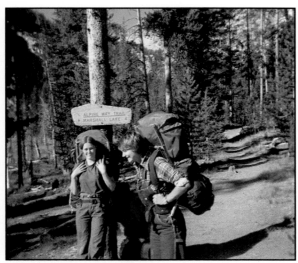

An 8-hour hike can burn as many calories as a 20-mile walk or jog.

Hiking

Many people feel guilty if they are unable to continue their exercise routine during vacations. Hiking is an excellent activity for the entire family, especially during the summer and on summer vacations. The intensity of hiking over uneven terrain is greater than walking. An 8-hour hike can burn as many calories as a 20-mile walk or jog.

Another benefit of hiking is the relaxing effects of beautiful scenery. This is an ideal activity for highly stressed people who live near woods and hills. A rough day at the office can be forgotten quickly in the peacefulness and beauty of the outdoors.

Jogging

Jogging is the most popular form of aerobic exercise. Next to walking, it is one of the most accessible and easiest forms of exercise. A person can find places to jog almost everywhere. The lone requirement to prevent injuries is a good pair of jogging shoes.

Jogging three to five times a week is one of the best ways to improve cardiorespiratory fitness. The risk of injury, however, is higher with jogging than walking, especially among beginners. For proper conditioning, jogging programs should start with 1 to 2 weeks of walking. As fitness improves, walking and jogging can be combined, gradually increasing the jogging segment until it comprises the full 20 to 30 minutes.

Unfortunately, too many people abuse this activity. People run too fast and too long. Many joggers think that if a little is good, more is better. Not so with cardiorespiratory endurance. Maximal oxygen uptake benefits of training more than five times per week are minimal. Furthermore, the risk of injury increases greatly as speed (running instead of jogging) and mileage go up.

Jogging approximately 15 miles per week near the 85% training intensity is enough to reach an excellent level of cardiorespiratory fitness. For those who want additional exercise, moderate-intensity activities (beyond the 15 miles) are recommended.

A good pair of shoes is a must for joggers. Many feet, knee, and leg problems originate from improperly fitting or worn-out shoes. A good pair of shoes should offer good lateral stability and not lean to either side when placed on a flat surface. The shoe also should bend at the ball of the foot, not at midfoot. Worn-out shoes should be replaced. After 500 miles of use, jogging shoes lose about a third of their shock absorption capabilities. If you suddenly have problems, check your shoes first. It may be time for a new pair. Guidelines for choosing the right jogging shoe are provided in Figure 3.6.

For safety reasons, joggers should stay away from high-speed roads, not wear headphones, and always run (or walk) against the traffic, so they will be able to see all oncoming traffic. At night, joggers should wear reflective clothing or fluorescent material on different parts of the body. Carrying a flashlight is even better because motorists can see the light from a distance greater than the reflective material.

An alternative form of jogging, especially for injured people, those with chronic back problems, and overweight individuals, is deep-water running (running in place while treading water). Deep-water running is almost as strenuous as jogging on land. In deep-water running, the land-running motions are accentuated by pumping the arms and legs hard through a full range of motion. The participant usually wears a floatation vest to help maintain the body in an upright position. Many elite athletes train frequently in water to lessen the wear and tear on the body caused by long-distance running. These athletes have been able to maintain high oxygen uptake values through rigorous water-running programs.

Cross-Country Skiing

Many consider cross-country skiing as the ultimate aerobic exercise because it requires vigorous lower

CHOOSING THE RIGHT SHOE

TONGUE
Should be well-padded to prevent irritation of the top of the foot.

COLLAR
About an inch rim of soft material to protect the heel cord.

ACHILLES PAD
Not too high to prevent irritation to the tendon or blistering of the skin.

UPPER
Leather, nylon mesh or other breathable materials are best for ventilation.

FIRM HEEL COUNTER
Durable plastic cup placed in the heel of the shoe to help stability.

FLARED HEEL
Added for support.

EXTERNAL STABILIZER
Supports the heel counter and offers extra stability.

TOE BOX
Allow enough space for the toes to fit comfortably.

Flexibility under forefoot.

OUTSOLE
Solid or carbon rubber outsoles are best for running, walking and cross-training traction.

MIDSOLE
Principal shock-absorbing feature of the shoe. Usually becomes worn out after 500 to 600 miles of use. Multi-density EVA or polyurethane midsoles offer best support and durability.

Figure 3.6 • *What to look for in a good pair of jogging shoes.*

and upper body movements. The large amount of muscle mass involved in cross-country skiing makes the activity intense, yet it places little strain on muscles and joints.

Research has shown that, of all elite athletes, cross-country skiers have the greatest aerobic capacity. Some of the highest maximal oxygen uptakes ever measured have been found in elite cross-country skiers. Because more muscle mass is involved, more oxygen and energy (calories) are used during cross-country skiing than with most other aerobic activities.

In addition to being an excellent aerobic activity, cross-country skiing is soothing. Skiing through the beauty of the snow-covered countryside can be highly enjoyable. Although the need for snow is an obvious limitation, cross-country skiing simulating equipment for year-round training is available at many sporting goods stores.

Some skill is necessary for proficient cross-country skiing. Poorly skilled individuals are not able to elevate the heart rate enough to cause adequate aerobic development. Individuals contemplating this activity should seek out instruction to fully enjoy and reap the rewards of cross-country skiing.

Aerobics

Aerobics, formerly known as aerobic dance, is thought to be the most common fitness activity for women in the United States. At first considered a fad, it now is a legitimate fitness activity with more than 20 million participants of all ages. Aerobics involves a series of exercise routines performed to music. Routines include a combination of stepping, walking, jogging, skipping, kicking, and arm-swinging movements. It is a fun way to exercise and promote cardiovascular development at the same time.

High-impact-aerobics (HIA), the traditional form of aerobics, involves actions in which both feet may be off the floor at the same time momentarily. These movements exert a great amount of vertical force on the feet as they contact the floor. Proper leg conditioning through other forms of weight-bearing

TERMS

High-impact aerobics (HIA) Form of aerobics in which both feet may be off the floor at the same time momentarily.

aerobic exercises (brisk walking and jogging), as well as strength training, are recommended prior to participating in high-impact aerobics.

High-impact aerobics is an intense activity, and it also produces the highest rate of aerobics injuries. Shin splints, stress fractures, low back pain, and tendinitis are all too common among high-impact aerobics enthusiasts. These injuries are caused by the constant impact of the feet on firm surfaces. As a result, several alternative forms of aerobics have been developed.

In **low-impact-aerobics (LIA)** at least one foot is in contact with the floor or ground at all times, reducing the impact as each foot contacts the surface. The recommended exercise intensity is more difficult to maintain with low-impact aerobics, though. To help elevate the exercise heart rate, all arm movements and weight-bearing actions that lower the center of gravity should be accentuated. Sustained movement throughout the program also is crucial to keep the heart rate in the target cardiovascular zone.

A relatively new form of aerobics is **step aerobics (SA)**. Using a combination of stepping and arm movements, participants step up and down benches that range in height from 2 to 10 inches. Step aerobics adds another dimension to the aerobics movement and the exercise program. As noted previously, variety adds enjoyment to aerobic workouts.

Step aerobics is viewed as a high-intensity, but low-impact activity. The intensity of the activity can

Aerobics is the most popular fitness activity for women in the United States.

be controlled easily by changing the height of the steps. Aerobic benches or plates are available commercially. The plates can be stacked together safely to adjust the height of the steps. Beginners are encouraged to use the lowest stepping height available and then advance gradually to a higher bench. This will lessen the risk of injury. Even though one foot is always in contact with the floor or bench during step aerobics, this activity is not recommended for individuals with ankle, knee, or hip problems.

Other forms of aerobics include a combination of HIA and LIA, as well as **moderate-impact aerobics (MIA)**. The latter incorporates **plyometric training**. Plyometric aerobics requires forceful jumps or springing off the ground immediately after landing from a previous jump. This type of training is used frequently by jumpers (high, long, and triple jumpers) and athletes in sports that require quick jumping ability, such as in basketball and gymnastics.

With moderate-impact aerobics, one foot is in contact with the ground most of the time. Participants, however, continually try to recover from all lower body flexion actions. This is done by quickly extending the hip, knee, and ankle joints without allowing the foot (or feet) to leave the ground. These quick movements make the exercise intensity of moderate-impact aerobics quite high.

Swimming

Swimming is another excellent form of aerobic exercise. It calls into play almost all major muscle groups in the body, providing a good training stimulus for the heart and lungs. Swimming is an excellent exercise option for individuals who cannot jog or walk for extended periods. Compared to other activities, the risk of injuries from swimming is low. The aquatic medium helps to support the body, taking pressure off bones and joints in the lower extremities and the back.

Maximal heart rates during swimming are approximately 13 beats per minute (bpm) lower than during running. The horizontal position of the body is thought to aid blood flow distribution throughout the body, decreasing the demand on the cardiovascular system. Cool water temperatures and direct contact with the water seem to help dissipate body heat more efficiently, further decreasing the strain on the heart.

Fitness experts recommend that this difference in maximal heart rate (13 bpm) be subtracted before determining cardiovascular training intensities. For example, the estimated maximal swimming heart rate for a 20-year old would be 187 bpm (220 – 20 – 13).

To produce better training benefits, gliding periods such as those in the breast stoke and side stroke should be minimized. Achieving proper training intensities with these strokes is difficult. The forward crawl is recommended for better aerobic results.

Overweight individuals need to swim fast enough to achieve an adequate training intensity. Excessive body fat makes the body more buoyant, and often the tendency is to just float along. This may be good for lowering stress and relaxing, but it does not increase caloric expenditure to aid with weight loss. Walking or jogging in waist- or armpit-deep water are better choices for overweight individuals who cannot walk or jog on land for a long time.

Most of the work with swimming is done by the upper body musculature. Although the heart's ability to pump a greater amount of oxygenated blood improves significantly with any type of aerobic activity, the major increase in the ability of cells to utilize oxygen with swimming occurs in the upper body and not the lower extremities. Therefore, fitness improvements with swimming are best attained by comparing changes in distances swum using the swim test.

Water Aerobics

Besides developing fitness, water aerobics provides an opportunity for socialization and fun in a comfortable and refreshing setting. Water aerobics incorporates a combination of rhythmic arm and leg actions performed in a vertical position while submerged in waist- to armpit-deep water. The vigorous limb movements against the water's resistance during water aerobics provide the training stimuli for cardiorespiratory development.

The popularity of water aerobics as an exercise modality to develop the cardiorespiratory system has been on the rise in recent years. This increase in popularity can be attributed to several factors:

1. Water buoyancy reduces weight-bearing stress on joints and therefore reduces the risk for injuries.

2. Water aerobics is a more feasible type of exercise for overweight individuals and those with arthritic conditions who may not be able to participate in weight-bearing activities such as walking, jogging, and aerobics.

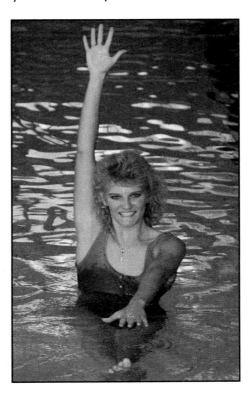

Water aerobics represents fitness, fun, and safety for people of all ages.

3. Heat dissipation in water is beneficial to obese participants who seem to undergo a higher heat strain than individuals of average weight.

4. Water aerobics is available to swimmers and nonswimmers alike.

The exercises used during water aerobics are designed to elevate the heart rate, which contributes to cardiorespiratory development. In addition, the aquatic medium provides increased resistance for strength improvement with virtually no impact. Because of this resistance to movement, strength gains with water aerobics seem to be better than with most land-based aerobic activities.

Another benefit is that weight reduction can be facilitated without the pain and fear of injuries by

> **TERMS**
>
> **Low-impact aerobics (LIA)** Form of aerobics in which at least one foot is in contact with the floor or ground at all times.
>
> **Step aerobics (SA)** Form of aerobics using a combination of stepping and arm movements.
>
> **Moderate-impact aerobics (MIA)** Form of aerobics that requires forceful jumps (plyometrics) of springing off the ground immediately after landing from a previous jump.

many who initiate exercise programs. Water aerobics provides a relatively safe environment for participating in injury-free exercise. The cushioned environment of the water allows patients recovering from leg and back injuries, individuals with joint problems, injured athletes, pregnant women, and obese people to benefit from water aerobics. In water these people can exercise to develop and maintain cardiovascular endurance and yet limit or eliminate the potential for further injury.

Similar to swimming, maximal heart rates achieved during water aerobics are lower than during running. The difference between water aerobics and running, however, is only 10 bpm (as compared to 13 for swimming). The smaller difference is thought to be related to the upright position maintained during water aerobics, which may not facilitate blood flow distribution to the same extent as swimming. This difference of 10 bpm in maximal heart rate also should be considered when prescribing exercise intensities for water aerobics.

Cycling

Cycling is an activity that most people learn in their youth. As a non-weight-bearing activity, it is a good exercise modality for people with lower body or lower back injuries. Cycling helps to develop the cardiorespiratory system, as well as muscular strength and endurance in the lower extremities. With the advent of stationary bicycles, this activity can be done year-round.

Raising the heart rate to the proper training intensity is more difficult with cycling than with the activities discussed thus far. As the amount of muscle

Skill is required for safety and enjoyment of road cycling.

mass involved during aerobic exercise decreases, so does the demand placed on the cardiorespiratory system. In cycling the thigh muscles do most of the work, making a high cardiorespiratory training intensity harder to achieve and maintain.

Maintaining a continuous pedaling motion and eliminating coasting periods helps the participant achieve a higher heart rate. Exercising for longer periods also helps to compensate for the lower heart rate intensity during cycling. In comparing cycling to jogging, similar aerobic benefits take roughly three times the distance at twice the speed of jogging. Cycling, however, puts less stress on muscles and joints than jogging does, making the former a better exercise modality for people who cannot otherwise walk or jog.

To increase riding efficiency, the height of the bike seat should be adjusted so the legs are almost completely extended when the heels are placed on the pedals. The body should not sway from side to side as the person rides. The cycling cadence also is important for maximal efficiency. Bike tension or gears should be set at a moderate level to be able to ride at 70 to 90 revolutions per minute.

Skill is important in road cycling. Cyclists must be in control of the bicycle at all times. They have to be able to maneuver the bike in traffic, maintain balance at slow speeds, switch gears, apply the brakes, watch for pedestrians and stoplights, and ride through congested areas. Stationary cycling does not require special skills. Nearly everyone can do it.

Safety is a key issue in road cycling. More than a million bicycle injuries occur each year. Proper equipment and common sense are necessary. A well-designed and maintained bike is easier to maneuver. Toe clips are recommended to keep the feet from sliding and to maintain equal upward and downward force on the pedals.

Bike riders must follow the same rules as motorists. Many accidents happen because cyclists run traffic lights and stop signs. Some further suggestions are:

- Use bike hand signals to let the traffic around you know of your actions.
- Don't ride side by side with another rider.
- Be aware of turning vehicles and cars backing out of alleys and parking lots; always yield to motorists in these situations.
- Watch out for storm drains. By not crossing them at the proper angle, front wheels can get caught and the rider thrown from the bike.

- Wear a good helmet, certified by the Snell Memorial Foundation or the American National Standards Institute. Many serious accidents and even deaths have been prevented by using helmets. Do not allow fashion, aesthetics, comfort, or price to be a factor when selecting and using a helmet for road cycling. Health and life are too precious to give up because of vanity and thriftiness.

- Wear appropriate clothes and shoes. Special clothing for cycling is not required. Clothing should be lightweight and not restrict movement. Shorts should be long enough to keep the skin from rubbing against the seat. For greater comfort, cycling shorts have extra padding sewn into the seat and crotch areas. Experienced cyclists often wear special shoes with a cleat that snaps directly onto the pedal.

The stationary bike is one of the most popular pieces of equipment sold by sporting good stores. Before buying a stationary bike, though, be sure to try the activity a few days. If you enjoy it, you may want to purchase one. Invest with caution. If you opt to buy a lower-priced model, you may be disappointed. Good stationary bikes have comfortable seats, are stable, and provide a smooth and uniform pedaling motion. A sticky bike that is hard to pedal only leads to discouragement and, along with many others, ends up stored in the corner of a basement.

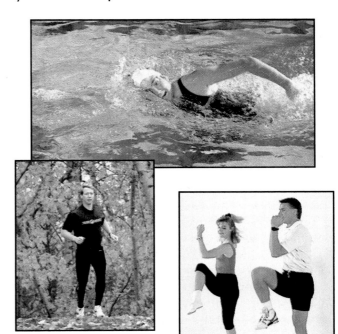

Cross-training enhances fitness, decreases the rate of injuries, and eliminates the monotony of single-activity programs.

Cross-Training

An exercise program that combines two or more activities is referred to as **cross-training**. This type of training is designed to enhance fitness, decrease injuries, and eliminate the monotony of single-activity programs. Cross-training may combine aerobic and nonaerobic activities such as moderate jogging, speed training, and strength training.

Cross-training can produce better workouts than a single activity. For example, jogging develops the lower body and swimming builds the upper body. Rowing contributes to upper body development and cycling builds the legs. Combining activities such as these provides good overall conditioning and at the same time helps to improve or maintain fitness. Cross-training also offers an opportunity to develop skill and have fun with different activities.

Speed training (Chapters 4 and 5) often is coupled with cross-training. Faster performance times in aerobic activities (running, cycling) are generated with speed or interval training. People who want to improve their running times often run shorter intervals at faster speeds than the actual racing pace. For example, a person wanting to run a 6-minute mile may run four 440-yard intervals at a speed of 1 minute and 20 seconds per interval. A 440-yard walk/jog can become a recovery interval between fast runs.

Strength training is used frequently with cross-training. Strength training helps to condition muscles, tendons, and ligaments. In many activities improved strength enhances overall sports performance. For example, research has shown that, although road cyclists who trained with weights showed no improvement in aerobic capacity, the cyclists had a 33% improvement in riding time to exhaustion when exercising at 75% of their maximal capacity.[13]

TERMS   **Cross-training**   Combining two or more activities to achieve a similar training effect.

Rope Skipping

Rope skipping not only contributes to cardiorespiratory fitness, but it also helps to increase reaction time, coordination, agility, dynamic balance, and muscular strength in the lower extremities. At first, rope skipping may seem to be a highly strenuous form of aerobic exercise. Beginners often reach maximal heart rates after only 2 or 3 minutes of jumping. As skill improves, however, the energy demands decrease considerably.

Some people have claimed training benefits equal to a 30-minute jog in as few as 10 minutes of skipping. Although differences in strength and flexibility development are observed among various activities, 10 minutes at a certain heart rate provide similar cardiorespiratory benefits regardless of the nature of the activity. To obtain an adequate aerobic workout, the duration of exercise must be at least 20 minutes.

As with high-impact aerobics, a major concern of rope skipping is the stress placed on the lower extremities. Skipping with one foot at a time decreases the impact somewhat, but it does not eliminate the risk for injuries. Fitness experts recommend that skipping be used sparingly and primarily as a supplement to an aerobic exercise program.

In-Line Skating

Frequently referred to as *blading*, in-line skating has become a highly popular fitness activity in recent years. Suddenly millions of children and adults are trying this activity. In the early 1990s stores could not keep up with the demand for in-line skates.

In-line skating has its origin in ice skating. Because warm-weather ice skating was not feasible, blades were replaced by wheels for summertime participation. Four-wheel roller skates were invented in the mid 1700s, but the activity did not really catch on until the late 1800s. The first in-line skate with five wheels in a row attached to the bottom of a shoe was developed in 1823. The in-line concept took hold in the United States in 1980, when hockey skates were adapted for this road-skating.

In-line skating is an excellent activity to develop cardiorespiratory fitness and lower body strength. The intensity of the activity is regulated by how hard you blade. The key to effective cardiorespiratory training is to maintain a constant and rhythmic pattern, using arms and legs and minimizing the gliding phase of blading. As a weight-bearing activity, in-line bladers also develop superior leg strength.

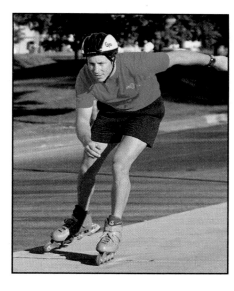

In-line skating is a popular fitness activity in the 1990s.

Instruction is necessary to achieve a minimum level of proficiency in this sport. Bladers commonly encounter hazards. Potholes, cracks, rocks, gravel, sticks, oil, street curbs, and driveways all pose challenges. Unskilled bladers are more prone to falls and injuries.

Good equipment will make the activity safer and more enjoyable. Blades range in price from $40 to $500. Recreational participants need not purchase the more costly competitive skates. An adequate blade should provide strong ankle support. Soft and flexible boots do not provide enough support. Small wheels offer more stability, and larger wheels enable greater speed. Blades should be purchased from stores that understand the sport and can provide sound advice according to skill level and needs.

Protective equipment is a *must* for in-line skating. Similar to road cycling, a good helmet that meets the safety standards set by the Snell Memorial Foundation or the American Standards Institute is important for protection in case of a fall. Wrist guards and knee and elbow pads also are recommended. The kneecap and the elbows are easily injured in any fall. Nighttime bladers should wear light-colored clothing and reflective tape.

Rowing

Rowing is a low-impact activity that provides a complete body workout. It mobilizes most major muscle groups including the arms, legs, hips, abdominals, trunk, and shoulders. Rowing not only is a good form of aerobic exercise but, because of the nature of the activity (constant pushing and pulling against resistance), it also promotes total strength development. To accommodate different fitness levels, workloads can be regulated on most rowing machines.

Rowing is not among the most popular forms of aerobic exercise. Similar to stationary bicycles, a person should try the activity a few weeks before purchasing a unit.

Stair Climbing

If sustained for at least 20 minutes, stair climbing is an extremely efficient form of aerobic exercise. Precisely because of the high intensity of stair climbing, many people in our society stay away from stairs and instead ride elevators. Many people dislike living in two-story homes because they have to climb the stairs frequently.

Not too many places have enough flights of stairs to climb continuously for 20 minutes. Stair-climbing machines offer an alternative. Stair climbing has become so popular that fitness enthusiasts often wait in line at health clubs to use the machines.

In terms of injuries, stair climbing seems to be relatively safe. Because the feet never leave the climbing surface, it is considered a low-impact activity. Joints and ligaments are not strained during climbing. The intensity of exercise is controlled easily because most stair climbers can be programmed to regulate the workload.

Racquet Sports

In racquet sports such as tennis, racquetball, squash, and badminton, the aerobic benefits are dictated by the individual's skill, intensity of the game, and how long the game is played. Skill is crucial to participate effectively in these sports and also to sustain continuous play. Frequent pauses during play do not allow people to maintain the heart rate in the appropriate target zone to stimulate cardiorespiratory development.

Many people who participate in racquet sports do so for enjoyment, social fulfillment, and relaxation. For developing cardiorespiratory fitness, these people supplement the sport with other forms of aerobic exercise such as jogging, cycling, or swimming.

If a racquet sport is the main form of aerobic exercise, participants need to try to run hard, fast, and as constantly as possible during play. They should not have to spend much time retrieving balls (bird or shuttlecock in badminton). Similar to low-impact aerobics, all movements should be accentuated by

Racquet sports require rhythmic and continuous activity to provide aerobic benefits.

reaching out and bending more than usual, for better cardiorespiratory development.

● Rating the Fitness Benefits of Aerobic Activities

The fitness contributions of different aerobic activities to the health-related components of fitness vary. Although an accurate assessment of the contributions to each fitness component is difficult to establish, a summary of likely benefits of several activities is provided in Table 3.1. Instead of a single rating or number, ranges are given for some of the categories. The benefits derived are based on the person's effort while participating in the activity.

The nature of the activity often dictates the potential aerobic development. For example, jogging is much more strenuous than walking. The effort during exercise also has an impact on the amount of physiological development. The training benefits of just going through the motions of a low-impact aerobics routine, as compared to accentuating all motions, are of a different magnitude.

Table 3.1 indicates a starting fitness level for each aerobic activity. Attempting to participate in high-intensity activities without proper conditioning often leads to injuries and discouragement. Beginners should start with low-intensity activities that carry a minimum risk for injuries.

In some cases, such as high-impact aerobics and rope skipping, the risk for injuries remains high even if the participants have adequate conditioning. These

Table 3.1 *Ratings for Selected Aerobic Activities*

Activity	Recommended Starting Fitness Level[1]	Injury Risk[2]	Potential Cardiovascular Endurance Development (VO$_{2max}$)[3, 5]	Upper Body Strength Development[3]	Lower Body Strength Development[3]	Upper Body Flexibility Development[3]	Lower Body Flexibility Development[3]	Weight Control[3]	MET Level[4, 5, 6]	Caloric Expenditure (cal/hour)[5,6]
Walking	B	L	1–2	1	2	1	1	3	4–6	300–450
Walking/Water/Chest-Deep	I	L	2–4	2	3	1	1	3	6–10	450–750
Hiking	B	L	2–4	1	3	1	1	3	6–10	450–750
Jogging	I	M	3–5	1	3	1	1	5	6–15	450–1125
Jogging/Deep Water	A	L	3–5	2	2	1	1	5	8–15	600–1125
High-Impact Aerobics	A	H	3–4	2	4	3	2	4	6–12	450–900
Low-Impact Aerobics	B	L	2–4	2	3	3	2	3	5–10	375–750
Step Aerobics	I	M	2–4	2	3–4	3	2	3–4	5–12	375–900
Moderate-Impact Aerobics	I	M	2–4	2	3	3	2	3	6–12	450–900
Swimming (front crawl)	B	L	3–5	4	2	3	1	3	6–12	450–900
Water Aerobics	B	L	2–4	3	3	3	2	3	6–12	450–900
Stationary Cycling	B	L	2–4	1	4	1	1	3	6–10	450–750
Road Cycling	I	M	2–5	1	4	1	1	3	6–12	450–900
Cross-Training	I	M	3–5	2–3	3–4	2–3	1–2	3–5	6–15	450–1125
Rope Skipping	I	H	3–5	2	4	1	2	3–5	8–15	600–1125
Cross-Country Skiing	B	M	4–5	4	4	2	2	4–5	10–16	750–1200
Aero-belt Exercise	B	M	4–5	4	4	3	2	4–5	10–16	750–1200
In-Line Skating	I	M	2–4	2	4	2	2	3	6–10	450–750
Rowing	B	L	3–5	4	2	3	1	4	8–14	600–1050
Stair Climbing	B	L	3–5	1	4	1	1	4–5	8–15	600–1125
Racquet Sports	I	M	2–4	3	3	3	2	3	6–10	450–750

[1] B = Beginner, I = Intermediate, A = Advanced

[2] L = Low, M = Moderate, H = High

[3] 1 = Low, 2 = Fair, 3 = Average, 4 = Good, 5 = excellent

[4] One MET represents the rate of energy expenditure at rest (3.5 ml/kg/min). Each additional MET is a multiple of the resting value. For example, 5 METs represents an energy expenditure equivalent to five times the resting value or about 17.5 ml/kg/min.

[5] Varies according to the person's effort (exercise intensity) during exercise.

[6] Varies according to body weight.

activities should be supplemental only and are not recommended as the sole mode of exercise. Most exercise-related injuries occur as a result of high-impact activities and not a high exercise intensity.

Physicians who work with cardiac patients frequently use **METs** as an alternative method of prescribing exercise intensity. One MET represents the rate of energy expenditure at rest or the equivalent of an oxygen uptake of 3.5 ml/kg/min. The MET range for the various activities is included in Table 3.1. A 10-MET activity requires a tenfold increase in the resting energy requirement, or approximately 35 ml/kg/min. MET levels for a given activity vary according to the effort expended. The harder a person exercises, the higher is the MET level.

The effectiveness of various aerobic activities in weight management also is provided in Table 3.1. As a general rule, the greater the muscle mass involved in exercise, the better are the results. Rhythmic and continuous activities that involve large amounts of muscle mass are most effective in burning calories.

Higher intensity activities increase caloric expenditure as well. Exercising longer, however, compensates for lower intensities. If carried out long enough (45 to 60 minutes five to six times per week), even walking can be an excellent exercise mode for weight loss. Additional information on a comprehensive weight management program is given in Chapter 8.

● Specific Exercise Considerations

In addition to many of the exercise-related issues discussed to this point, many other concerns require clarification or are somewhat controversial. Let's examine some of these issues.

1. *Does aerobic exercise make a person immune to heart and blood vessel disease?* Although aerobically fit individuals as a whole have a lower incidence of cardiovascular disease, a regular aerobic exercise program by itself does not offer an absolute guarantee against cardiovascular disease. Overall risk factor management is the best way to minimize the risk for cardiovascular disease. Many factors, including a genetic predisposition, can increase the person's risk. Experts believe, however, that a regular aerobic exercise program not only will delay the onset of cardiovascular problems but also will improve the chances of surviving a heart attack.

Even moderate increases in aerobic fitness lower the incidences of premature cardiovascular deaths significantly. Data from the Aerobics Research Institute in Dallas, Texas (see Chapter 1, Figure 1.6) indicate that the decrease in cardiovascular mortality is greatest between the unfit (group 1) and the moderately fit (2 and 3) groups. A further decrease in cardiovascular mortality is observed between the moderately fit and the highly fit groups (4 and 5), but the difference is not as much as that between the unfit and moderately fit groups.

2. *How much aerobic exercise is required to decrease the risk for cardiovascular disease?* Although research has not yet indicated the exact amount of aerobic exercise required to lower the risk for cardiovascular disease, some general recommendations have been set forth. In their study, Dr. Ralph Paffenbarger and co-researchers showed that 2,000 calories expended per week as a result of physical activity yielded the lowest risk for cardiovascular disease among a group of almost 17,000 Harvard alumni.[14] Two thousand calories per week represents about 300 calories per daily exercise session.

3. *Do people get a "physical high" during aerobic exercise?* During vigorous exercise, **endorphines** are released from the pituitary gland in the brain. They can create feelings of euphoria and natural well-being.

Higher levels of endorphines often are seen as a result of aerobic endurance activities and may remain elevated for as long as 30 to 60 minutes following exercise. Many experts believe these higher levels explain the physical high some people get during and after prolonged exercise.

Endorphine levels also have been shown to be elevated during pregnancy and delivery. Endorphines act as pain killers. The higher levels could explain why a woman has more tolerance

---

TERMS • • • • •

MET Represents the rate of resting energy expenditure at rest; one MET is the equivalent of an oxygen uptake of 3.5 ml/kg/min.

Endorphines Morphine-like substances released from the pituitary gland in the brain. They are thought to induce feelings of euphoria and natural well-being. Higher levels of endorphines are released during prolonged aerobic exercise.

for the pain and discomfort of natural childbirth and her pleasant feelings shortly after the baby's birth. Several reports have indicated that well-conditioned women have shorter and easier labor. These women possibly attain higher endorphine levels during delivery, making childbirth less traumatic than it is for untrained women.

4. *Is exercise safe during pregnancy?* Women should not forsake exercise during pregnancy. If anything, they should exercise to strengthen the body and prepare for delivery. Moderate exercise during pregnancy helps to prevent excessive weight gain and speed up recovery following birth.

   Pregnant women in American Indian tribes continue to do all of their difficult work chores up to the very day of delivery, and a few hours after the baby's birth they resume their normal activities. Several women athletes have competed in sports during the early stages of pregnancy. Nevertheless, the woman and her personal physician should make the final decision regarding her exercise program.

   Stretching exercises are to be performed gently because hormonal changes during pregnancy increase the laxity of muscles and connective tissue. These changes facilitate delivery, but they also make women more susceptible to injuries during exercise.

   Among the American College of Obstetricians and Gynecologists recommendations for exercise during pregnancy with no additional risk factors are:[15]

   - Continue to exercise at a mild-to-moderate pace throughout the pregnancy, but decrease exercise intensity by about 25% from the pre-pregnancy program.
   - Exercise regularly a minimum of three times a week instead of doing occasional bouts of exercise.
   - Pay attention to the body's signals of discomfort and distress. Stop exercise when tired. Never exercise to exhaustion. Stop if unusual symptoms arise. These include pain of any kind, cramping, nausea, bleeding or leaking amniotic fluid, faintness, dizziness, palpitations, numbness in any part of the body, or decreased fetal activity.
   - After the first trimester, avoid exercises that require you to lie on your back. This position

can block blood flow to the uterus and the baby.
   - Do non-weight-bearing activities such as cycling, swimming, or water aerobics, which minimize the risk of injury and may allow you to continue exercise throughout the pregnancy.
   - Avoid activities that could lead to a loss of balance or cause even mild trauma to the abdomen.
   - Get proper nourishment. Pregnancy requires approximately 300 extra calories per day.
   - During the first 3 months in particular, avoid exercise in the heat. Wear clothing that allows for proper heat dissipation, and drink plenty of water.

5. *Does exercise help relieve* **dysmenorrhea**? Exercise has not been shown to either cure or aggravate painful menstruation, but it has been shown to relieve menstrual cramps because it improves circulation to the uterus. Less severe menstrual cramps also could be related to higher increased levels of endorphines produced during prolonged physical activity, which may counteract pain. Particularly, stretching exercises of the muscles in the pelvic region seem to reduce and prevent painful menstruation that is not the result of disease.[16]

6. *Does participation in exercise hinder menstruation?* In some instances, highly trained athletes may develop **amenorrhea** during training and competition. This condition is seen most often in extremely lean women who also engage in sports that require strenuous physical effort over a sustained time, but it is by no means irreversible. At present, we do not know whether the condition is caused by physical or emotional stress related to high-intensity training, excessively low body fat, or other factors.

   Although, on the average, women have a lower physical capacity during menstruation, medical surveys at the Olympic games have shown that women have broken Olympic and world records at all stages of the menstrual cycle. Menstruation should not keep a woman from participating in athletics, and it will not necessarily have a negative impact on performance.

7. *Does exercise offset the detrimental effects of cigarette smoking?* Physical exercise often motivates toward smoking cessation but does not

offset any ill effects of smoking. If anything, smoking greatly decreases the ability of the blood to transport oxygen to working muscles.

Oxygen is carried in the circulatory system by hemoglobin, the iron-containing pigment of the red blood cells. Carbon monoxide, a by-product of cigarette smoke, has 210 to 250 times greater affinity for hemoglobin over oxygen. Consequently, carbon monoxide combines much faster with hemoglobin, decreasing the oxygen-carrying capacity of the blood.

Chronic smoking also increases airway resistance, requiring the respiratory muscles to work much harder and consume more oxygen just to ventilate a given amount of air. If a person quits smoking, exercise does help increase the functional capacity of the pulmonary system.

A regular exercise program does seem to be a powerful incentive to quit smoking. A random survey of 1,250 runners conducted at the 6.2-mile Peachtree Road Race in Atlanta provided impressive results. The results indicated that 81% and 75% of the men and women who smoked cigarettes when they started running had quit before the race date.

8. *What type of clothing should I wear when I exercise?* The type of clothing you wear during exercise is important. In general, clothing should fit comfortably and allow free movement of the various body parts. Select clothing according to air temperature, humidity, and exercise intensity. Avoid nylon and rubberized materials and tight clothes that interfere with the cooling mechanism of the human body or obstruct normal blood flow. Fabrics made from polypropylene, Capilene, Thermax, and synthetics are best. These types of fabrics draw moisture away from the skin, enhancing evaporation and cooling of the body. Exercise intensity is also important because the harder you exercise, the more heat the body produces.

When exercising in the heat, avoid the hottest time of the day, between 11:00 a.m. and 5:00 p.m. Surfaces such as asphalt, concrete, and artificial turf absorb heat, which then radiates to the body. Therefore, these surfaces are not recommended. (Also see question 11).

Only a minimal amount of clothing is necessary during exercise in the heat, to allow for maximal evaporation. Clothing should be

Activity-specific shoes are recommended to prevent lower-extremity injuries.

lightweight, light-colored, loose-fitting, airy, and absorbent. Examples of commercially available products that can be used during exercise in the heat include Asci's Perma Plus, Cool-max, and Nike's Dri-F.I.T. Double-layer acrylic socks are more absorbent than cotton and help to prevent blistering and chafing of the feet. A straw-type hat can be worn to protect the eyes and head from the sun. Clothing for exercise in the cold is discussed later in this chapter.

A good pair of shoes is vital to prevent injuries to lower limbs. Shoes manufactured specifically for your choice of activity are a must. When selecting proper footwear, you should consider body type, tendency toward pronation (rotating foot outward) or supination (rotating foot inward), and exercise surfaces. Shoes should have good stability, motion control, and comfortable fit. Purchase shoes in the middle of the day when feet have expanded and might be one-half size larger. For increased breatheability, choose shoes with nylon or mesh uppers. Generally, salespeople at reputable athletic shoe stores are knowledgeable and can help you select a good shoe that fits your needs. After 300 to 500 miles or 6 months, examine your shoes and obtain a new pair if they are worn out. Old shoes frequently are responsible for lower-limb injuries.

9. *How long should a person wait after a meal before exercising strenuously?* The length of

 TERMS

Dysmenorrhea Painful menstruation.
Amenorrhea Cessation of menstruation.

time to wait before exercising after a meal depends on the amount of food eaten. On the average, after a regular meal, you should wait about 2 hours before participating in strenuous physical activity. A walk or some other light physical activity is fine following a meal, though. If anything, it helps burn extra calories and may help the body metabolize fats more efficiently.

10. *What time of the day is best for exercise?* You can do intense exercise almost any time of the day, with the exception of about 2 hours following a heavy meal, or the noon and early afternoon hours on hot and humid days. Moderate exercise seems to be beneficial shortly after a meal, because exercise enhances the **thermo-genic response**. A walk after a meal burns more calories than a walk several hours after a meal.

    Many people enjoy exercising early in the morning because it gives them a boost to start the day. People who exercise in the morning also seem to stick with it more than others. Some prefer the lunch hour for weight-control reasons. By exercising at noon, they do not eat as big a lunch, which helps keep daily caloric intake down. Highly stressed people seem to like the evening hours because of the relaxing effects of exercise.

11. *Why is exercising in hot and humid conditions unsafe?* When a person exercises, only 30% to 40% of the energy the body produces is used for mechanical work or movement. The rest of the energy (60% to 70%) is converted into heat. If this heat cannot be dissipated properly because the weather either is too hot or the relative humidity is too high, body temperature increases and, in extreme cases, can result in death.

    The specific heat of body tissue (the heat required to raise the temperature of the body by 1°C) is .38 calories per pound of body weight per 1°C (.38 cal/lb/°C). This indicates that if no body heat is dissipated, a 150-pound person needs to burn only 57 calories (150 × .38) to increase total body temperature by 1°C. If this person were to conduct an exercise session requiring 300 calories (about 3 miles running) without any heat dissipation, the inner body temperature would increase by 5.3°C, which is the equivalent of going from 98.6°F to 108.1°F.

    This example illustrates clearly the need for caution when exercising in hot or humid weather. If the relative humidity is too high, body heat cannot be lost through evaporation because the atmosphere already is saturated with water vapor. In one instance, a football casualty occurred at a temperature of only 64°F but at a relative humidity of 100%. People must be cautious when air temperature is above 90°F and the relative humidity is above 60%.

The American College of Sports Medicine recommends that individuals should not engage in strenuous physical activity when the readings of a wet-bulb globe thermometer exceed 82.4°F. With this type of thermometer, the wet bulb is cooled by evaporation, and on dry days it shows a lower temperature than the regular (dry) thermometer. On humid days the cooling effect is less because of less evaporation; hence, the difference between the wet and dry readings is not as great.

The American Running and Fitness Association offers the following descriptions and first-aid measures for three signs of trouble when exercising in the heat:

- **Heat cramps.** Symptoms include spasms and muscle twitching in the legs, arms, and abdomen. To relieve heat cramps, stop exercising, get out of the heat, massage the painful area, slowly stretch, and drink plenty of fluids.

- **Heat exhaustion.** Symptoms include fainting, dizziness, profuse sweating, cold, clammy skin, weakness, headache, and a rapid, weak pulse. If you experience any of these symptoms, stop

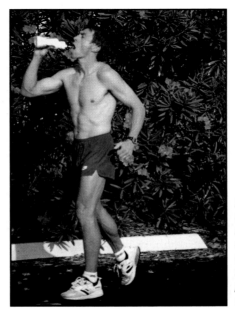

Fluid and carbohydrate replacement are essential during exercise in the heat and of prolonged duration.

and find a cool place to rest. Drink plenty of cool fluids. Loosen or remove clothing, and rub your body with a cool, wet towel. Stay out of the heat for the rest of the day, and possibly for the next 2 or 3 days.

- **Heat stroke.** Symptoms include serious disorientation, warm, dry skin, no sweating, rapid, full pulse, vomiting, diarrhea, unconsciousness, and high body temperature. As the temperature climbs, unexplained anxiety sets in. When the body temperature reaches 104°F to 105°F, the individual may get goosebumps, feel a cold sensation in the trunk of the body, nauseous, throbbing in the temples, and numbness in the extremities. After this stage, most people become incoherent. When body temperature reaches 105°F to 106°F, disorientation, loss of fine-motor control, and muscular weakness set in. If the temperature exceeds 106°F, serious neurologic injury and death may be imminent.

  Heat stroke requires immediate emergency medical attention. Someone should request help (call 911) and get the person out of the sun. While you're waiting for the person to be taken to the hospital's emergency room, spray the person with cool water and rub the body with cool towels. Fan the person and give him or her plenty of cold liquids.

12. *What should a person do to replace fluids lost during prolonged aerobic exercise?* The main objective of fluid replacement during prolonged aerobic exercise is to maintain the blood volume so circulation and sweating can continue at normal levels. Adequate water replacement is the most important factor in preventing heat disorders. Drinking about 6 to 8 ounces of cool water every 15 to 20 minutes during exercise seems to be ideal to prevent **dehydration.** Cold fluids seem to be absorbed more rapidly from the stomach.

    Other relevant points are the following.

- Commercial fluid-replacement solutions (such as Exceed and Gatorade) contain about 6% to 8% glucose, which seems to be optimal for fluid absorption and performance. Sugar does not become available to the muscles until about 30 minutes after drinking a glucose solution.
- Drinks high in fructose or with a glucose concentration above 8% will slow down water absorption when exercising in the heat.

- Most soft drinks (cola, non-cola) contain between 10% and 12% glucose, an amount that is too high for proper rehydration during exercise in the heat.
- Commercially prepared sports drinks are recommended when exercise will be strenuous and carried out for more than an hour. For exercise lasting less than an hour, water is just as effective in replacing fluid loss. The sports drinks you select should be based on your personal preference. Try different drinks at 6% to 8% glucose concentration to see which drink you tolerate best and suits your tastes as well.

13. *What precautions must a person take when exercising in the cold?* When exercising in the cold, the two factors to consider are **frostbite** and **hypothermia.** In contrast to hot and humid conditions, exercising in the cold usually does not threaten one's health because clothing for heat conservation can be selected, and exercise itself increases the production of body heat.

    Most people actually overdress for exercise in the cold. Because exercise increases body temperature, a moderate workout on a cold day makes a person feel that the temperature is 20°–30° warmer than it actually is. Overdressing for exercise can make the clothes damp from excessive perspiration. The risk for hypothermia increases when a person is wet or not moving around sufficiently to increase body heat. Initial warning signs of hypothermia include shivering, loss of coordination, and difficulty speaking. With a continued drop in body temperature, shivering stops, the muscles weaken and stiffen, and the person has feelings of elation or intoxication and eventually loses consciousness. To

TERMS

Thermogenic response The amount of energy required to digest food.

Heat cramps Muscle spasms caused by heat-induced changes in electrolyte balance in muscle cells.

Heat exhaustion Heat-related fatigue.

Heat stroke Heat-related emergency.

Dehydration Loss of body water below normal volume.

Frostbite Damage to the tissues as a result of prolonged exposure to extreme cold.

Hypothermia A breakdown in the body's ability to generate heat with a drop in temperature below 95°F.

prevent hypothermia, use common sense, dress properly, and be aware of environmental conditions.

The popular belief that exercising in cold temperatures (32°F and lower) freezes the lungs is false because the air is warmed properly in the air passages before it reaches the lungs. Cold is not what poses a threat. Rather, wind velocity is what affects the chill factor greatly.

For example, exercising at a temperature of 25°F with adequate clothing is not too cold, but if the wind is blowing at 25 miles per hour, the chill factor lowers the actual temperature to −5°F. This effect is even worse if a person is wet and exhausted. When the weather is windy, exercise (jog, cycle) against the wind on the way out and with the wind when you return.

Even though the lungs are under no risk when exercising in the cold, the face, head, hands, and feet should be protected, as they are subject to frostbite. Watch for signs of frostbite: numbness and discoloration. In cold temperatures, about 30% of the body's heat is lost through the head's surface area if it is unprotected. A wool or synthetic cap, hood, or hat will help to hold in body heat. Mittens are better than gloves because they keep the fingers together, so the surface area from which to lose heat is less. Inner linings of synthetic material to wick (draw) moisture away from the skin are recommended.

Wearing several layers of lightweight clothing is preferable to wearing one single, thick layer because warm air is trapped between layers of clothes, enabling greater heat conservation. As body temperature increases, you can remove layers as necessary. For lengthy or long-distance workouts (cross-country skiing or long runs), take a small backpack to carry the clothing that is removed. You also can carry extra warm and dry clothes in case you stop exercising away from shelter. If you remain outdoors following exercise, added clothing and continuous body movement are essential.

The first layer of clothes should wick moisture away from the skin. Polypropylene, Capilene, and Thermax are recommended materials. Next, a layer of wool, dacron, or polyester fleece insulates well even when wet. Lycra tights or sweatpants help protect the legs. The outer layer should be waterproof, wind-resistant, and breatheable. A synthetic material such as Gortex is best so moisture still can escape from the body. A ski mask or face mask helps protect the face. In extremely cold conditions, exposed skin, such as the nose, cheeks, or around the eyes, can be insulated with petroleum jelly.

● Managing Exercise-Related Injuries

To enjoy and maintain physical fitness, preventing injury during a conditioning program is essential. Exercise-related injuries, nonetheless, are common in individuals who participate in exercise programs. Surveys indicate that more than half of all new participants suffer injuries during the first 6 months of the conditioning program.

The four most common causes of injuries are: (a) high-impact activities, (b) rapid conditioning programs — doing too much too quick, (c) improper shoes or training surfaces, and (d) anatomical predisposition (body propensity). High-impact activities and a significant increase in quantity, intensity, and duration of activities are by far the most common causes of injuries. The body requires time to adapt to more intense activities. Most of these injuries can be prevented through a more gradual and correct conditioning (low-impact) program.

Proper shoes for specific activities are essential. Shoes should be replaced when they show a lot of wear and tear. Softer training surfaces, such as grass and dirt, produce less trauma than asphalt and concrete.

Few people have perfect body alignment, so injuries may occur eventually. These types of injuries often are associated with overtraining. In case of injury, proper treatment can avert a lengthy recovery process. A summary of common exercise-related injuries and how to manage them follows.

Acute Sports Injuries

The best treatment always has been prevention itself. If an activity causes unusual discomfort or chronic irritation, you need to treat the cause by decreasing the intensity, switching activities, substituting equipment, or upgrading clothing, such as proper-fitting shoes.

In cases of acute injury, the standard treatment is rest, cold application, compression or splinting (or both), and elevation of the affected body part. This commonly is referred to as RICE: R = rest, I = ice application, C = compression, and E = elevation. Cold should be applied three to five times a day for 15 to 20 minutes at a time during the first 24 to 36 hours, by submerging the injured area in cold water, using an icebag, or applying ice massage to the affected part. An elastic bandage or wrap can be used for compression. Elevating the body part decreases blood flow to it.

The purpose of these treatment modalities is to minimize swelling in the area, which hastens recovery time. After the first 36 to 48 hours, heat can be used if the injury shows no further swelling or inflammation. If you have doubts regarding the nature or seriousness of the injury (such as suspected fracture), you should seek a medical evaluation.

Obvious deformities (such as in fractures, dislocations, or partial dislocations) call for splinting, cold application with an icebag, and medical attention. Never try to reset any of these conditions by yourself, as muscles, ligaments, and nerves could be damaged further. Treatment of these injuries always should be in the hands of specialized medical personnel. A quick reference guide for the signs or symptoms and treatment of exercise-related problems is provided in Table 3.2.

Muscle Soreness and Stiffness

Individuals who begin an exercise program or participate after a long layoff from exercise often develop muscle soreness and stiffness. The acute soreness that sets in the first few hours after exercise

Table 3.2 *Reference Guide for Exercise-Related Problems*

Injury	Signs/Symptoms	Treatment*
Bruise (contusion)	Pain, swelling, discoloration	Cold application, compression, rest
Dislocations Fractures	Pain, swelling, deformity	Splinting, cold application, seek medical attention
Heat cramps	Cramps, spasms, and muscle twitching in the legs, arms, and abdomen	Stop activity, get out of the heat, stretch, massage the painful area, drink plenty of fluids
Heat exhaustion	Fainting, profuse sweating, cold/clammy skin, weak/rapid pulse, weakness, headache	Stop activity, rest in a cool place, loosen clothing, rub body with cool/wet towel, drink plenty of fluids, stay out of heat for 2–3 days
Heat stroke	Hot/dry skin, no sweating, serious disorientation, rapid/full pulse, vomiting, diarrhea, unconsciousness, high body temperature	**Seek immediate medical attention**, request help and get out of the sun, bathe in cold water/spray with cold water/rub body with cold towels, drink plenty of cold fluids
Joint sprains	Pain, tenderness, swelling, loss of use, discoloration	Cold application, compression, elevation, rest, heat after 36 to 48 hours (if no further swelling)
Muscle cramps	Pain, spasm	Stretch muscle(s), use mild exercises for involved area
Muscle soreness and stiffness	Tenderness, pain	Mild stretching, low-intensity exercise, warm bath
Muscle strains	Pain, tenderness, swelling, loss of use	Cold application, compression, elevation, rest, heat after 36 to 48 hours (if no further swelling)
Shin splints	Pain, tenderness	Cold application prior to and following any physical activity, rest, heat (if no activity is carried out)
Side stitch	Pain on the side of the abdomen below the rib cage	Decrease level of physical activity or stop altogether, gradually increase level of fitness
Tendinitis	Pain, tenderness, loss of use	Rest, cold application, heat after 48 hours

* Cold should be applied three to four times a day for 15 minutes. Heat can be applied three times a day for 15 to 20 minutes.

is thought to be related to a lack of blood (oxygen) flow and general fatigue of the exercised muscles.

Delayed muscle soreness that appears several hours after exercise (usually about 12 hours later) and lasts 2 to 4 days may be related to actual tiny tears in muscle tissue, muscle spasms that increase fluid retention (stimulating the pain nerve endings), and overstretching or tearing of connective tissue in and around muscles and joints.

Mild stretching before and adequately stretching after exercise helps to prevent soreness and stiffness. Gradually progressing into an exercise program is important, too. A person should not attempt to do too much too quickly. To relieve pain, mild stretching, low-intensity exercise to stimulate blood flow, and a warm bath might help.

Exercise Intolerance

When starting an exercise program, participants should stay within the safe limits. The best method to determine whether you are exercising too strenuously — **exercise intolerance** — is to check your heart rate and make sure it does not exceed the limits of your target zone. Exercising above this target zone may not be safe for unconditioned or high-risk individuals. You do not need to exercise beyond your target zone to gain the desired cardiorespiratory benefits.

Several physical signs will tell you when you are exceeding your functional limitations. Signs of intolerance include rapid or irregular heart rate, difficult breathing, nausea, vomiting, lightheadedness, headache, dizziness, pale skin, flushness, extreme weakness, lack of energy, shakiness, sore muscles, cramps, and tightness in the chest. Learn to listen to your body. If you notice any of these symptoms, seek medical attention before continuing your exercise program.

Recovery heart rate is another indicator of overexertion. To a certain extent, recovery heart rate is related to fitness level. The higher your cardiovascular fitness level, the faster your heart rate will decrease following exercise. As a rule of thumb, heart rate should be below 120 beats per minute 5 minutes into recovery. If your heart rate is above 120, you most likely have overexerted yourself or possibly could have some other cardiac abnormality. If you lower the intensity or duration of exercise, or both, and you still have a fast heart rate 5 minutes into recovery, you should consult your physician.

Side Stitch

Side stitch happens primarily in the early stages of exercise participation. The exact cause is unknown. Some experts suggest that it could relate to a lack of blood flow to the respiratory muscles during strenuous physical exertion. Side stitch occurs primarily in unconditioned beginners and in trained individuals when they exercise at higher intensities than usual. As one's physical condition improves, this condition tends to disappear unless training is intensified. Some people, however, encounter side stitch during downhill running. If side stitch is a problem for you, slow down, and if it persists, stop altogether. Lying down on your back and gently bringing both knees to the chest and holding that position for 30 to 60 seconds also helps.

Some people get side stitch if they eat or drink juice shortly before exercise. Drinking only water an hour to two prior to exercise sometimes prevents side stitch. Other individuals have problems with commercially available carbohydrate solutions during high-intensity exercise. Unless carbohydrate replacement is crucial to complete an event (marathon, triathlon), drink cool water for fluid replacement, or try a different carbohydrate solution.

Shin Splints

The **shin splint**, one of the most common injuries to the lower limbs, usually results from one or more of the following: (a) lack of proper and gradual conditioning, (b) doing physical activities on hard surfaces (wooden floors, hard tracks, cement, and asphalt), (c) fallen arches in the feet, (d) chronic overuse, (e) muscle fatigue, (f) faulty posture, (g) improper shoes, and (h) participating in weight-bearing activities when excessively overweight.

To manage shin splints:

1. Remove or reduce the cause (exercise on softer surfaces, wear better shoes or arch supports, or completely stop exercise until the shin splints heal).
2. Do stretching exercises before and after physical activity.
3. Use ice massage for 10 to 20 minutes before and after physical exercise.
4. Apply active heat (whirlpool and hot baths) for 15 minutes, two to three times a day.

5. Use supportive taping during physical activity (the proper taping technique can be learned readily from a qualified athletic trainer).

Muscle Cramps

Muscle cramps are caused by the body's depletion of essential electrolytes or a breakdown in the coordination between opposing muscle groups. If you have a muscle cramp, you should attempt first to stretch the muscles involved. For example, in the case of the calf muscle, pull your toes up toward the knees. After stretching the muscles, rub them down gently, and, finally, do some mild exercises requiring the use of those muscles.

In pregnant and lactating women, muscle cramps often are related to a lack of calcium. If women get cramps during these times, calcium supplements usually relieve the problem. Tight clothing also can cause cramps, by decreasing blood flow to active muscle tissue.

● Leisure-Time Physical Activity

Although individuals have notable differences, the average person in developed countries has about 3.5 hours of "free" or leisure time daily. Unfortunately, in our current automated society, most of this time is spent in sedentary living. People would be better off doing some physical activities, based on personal interests. Motivational factors include health, aesthetics, weight control, competition and challenge, fun, social interaction, mental arousal, relaxation, and stress management.

Frequently, **leisure-time physical activity** does not include exercise performed during a regular exercise program. It consists of activities such as walking, hiking, gardening, yard work, occupational work and chores, and moderate sports such as tennis, table tennis, badminton, golf, or croquet.

Every small increase in daily physical activity contributes to better health and wellness. Small increases in physical activity have a large impact in decreasing early risk for disease and premature death. Therefore, a new, concerted effort must be made to spend leisure-time in activities that will promote the expenditure of energy, provide a break from daily tasks, and contribute to health-related fitness.

● Getting Started and Adhering to a Lifetime Exercise Program

Having learned the basic principles of cardiorespiratory exercise prescription, you can fill out your own prescription. This exercise prescription calls for a gradual increase in intensity, duration, and frequency.

If you have not been exercising regularly, you might begin by attempting to train five or six times a week for 30 minutes at a time. You may find this discouraging, however, and may drop out before getting too far because you probably will develop some muscle soreness and stiffness and possibly incur minor injuries.

Muscle soreness and stiffness and the risk for injuries can be lessened or eliminated by increasing the intensity, duration, and frequency of exercise progressively as outlined in Figure 3.9. Or, if using the computer software available with this book, you can obtain a printout of your personalized cardiorespiratory exercise prescription (see Figure 3.7). You also can create and regularly update a computer file to keep a record of your activity program (see Figure 3.8). This file is based on the EXLOG computer program.

Once you have determined your exercise prescription, the difficult part begins: starting and sticking to a lifetime exercise program. Although you may be motivated after reading the benefits to be gained from physical activity, lifelong dedication and perseverance are necessary to reap and maintain good fitness.

The first few weeks are probably the most difficult, but where there's a will, there's a way. Once you begin to see positive changes, it won't be as hard. Soon you will develop a habit for exercise that

TERMS

Exercise intolerance Inability to function during exercise, leading to symptoms such as very rapid or irregular heart rate, labored breathing, nausea, vomiting, light-headedness, headaches, dizziness, pale skin, flushness, excessive weakness, lack of energy, shakiness, sore muscles, cramps, and tightness in the chest.

Side stitch A sharp pain in the side of the abdomen.

Shin splints Injury to the lower leg characterized by pain and irritation in the shin region or front of the leg.

Leisure-time physical activity Any activity undertaken during an individual's discretionary time that helps to increase energy or caloric expenditure.

PERSONALIZED CARDIORESPIRATORY EXERCISE PRESCRIPTION
Fitness and Wellness Series - Ver 3.96

Jane K. Johnston   Age: 18   Date: 04-11-1996
Maximal heart rate: 202 bpm   Resting heart rate: 74 bpm
Present cardiorespiratory fitness level: Fair

The following is your personal program for cardiorespiratory fitness development and maintenance. If you have been
exercising regularly and you are in the average or good
category, you may start at week five. If you are in the
excellent category, you can start at week nine.

Week	Time (min.)	Frequency (per week)	Training Intensity (beats per minute)	Pulse (10 sec. count)
1	15	3	About 138	23 beats
2	15	4	About 138	23 beats
3	20	4	About 138	23 beats
4	20	5	About 138	23 beats
5	20	4	138 to 164	23 to 27
6	20	5	138 to 164	23 to 27
7	30	4	138 to 164	23 to 27
8	30	5	138 to 164	23 to 27
9	30	4	164 to 183	27 to 31
10	30	5	164 to 183	27 to 31
11	30--40	5	164 to 183	27 to 31
12	30--40	5-6	164 to 183	27 to 31

You may participate in any combination of activities which
are aerobic and continuous in nature, such as walking, jogging, swimming, cross country skiing, rope skipping, cycling, aerobic dancing, racquetball, stair climbing, stationary running or cycling, etc. As long as the heart rate
reaches the desired rate, and it stays at that level for
the period of time indicated, the cardiorespiratory system
will improve.

Following the twelve week program, in order to maintain
your fitness level, you should exercise between 164 and 183
bpm for about 30 minutes, a minimum of three times per week
on nonconsecutive days.

When you exercise, allow about 5 minutes for a gradual
warm-up period and another 5 for gradual cool-down. Also,
when you check your exercise heart rate, only count your
pulse for 10 seconds (start counting with 0) and then refer
to the above 10 sec. pulse count. You may also multiply by
6 to obtain your rate in beats per minute.

Good cardiorespiratory fitness will greatly contribute toward the enhancement and maintenance of good health. It is
especially important in the prevention of cardiovascular
disease. We encourage you to be persistent in your exercise
program and to participate regularly.

Figure 3.7 • *Sample computerized exercise prescription.*

FITNESS & WELLNESS SERIES
by Werner W.K. Hoeger and Sharon A. Hoeger
Morton Publishing Company - Englewood, Colorado
Ver 3.96

MONTHLY EXERCISE LOG

Jim R. Johnson

Month of October 1996

Date	Body Weight	Type of Exercise	Exercise Heart Rate	Duration of Exercise	Distance (miles)	Calories Burned
1	179.5	Walking (4.5 mph)	120	30 min.	2.0	242
		Running (11 min/mile)	156	34 min.	3.0	427
3	179.0	Running (11 min/mile)	156	33 min.	3.0	413
5	179.0	Tennis/Moderate	126	60 min.		483
		Running (11 min/mile)	162	38 min.	3.5	476
7	178.5	Running (8.5 min/mile)	180	12 min.	1.5	193
9	178.0	Water Aerobics/Vigorous	156	45 min.		561
11	177.5	Running (8.5 min/mile)	174	28 min.	3.0	447
12	177.0	Racquetball	144	60 min.		690
		Swimming (25 yds/min)	138	25 min.	0.5	177
14	176.0	Running (8.5 min/mile)	174	29 min.	3.0	459
16	176.0	Aero-belt Step-Aerobics	144	45 min.		832
		Calisthenics	102	15 min.		87
18	175.5	Running (8.5 min/mile)	174	26 min.	3.0	411
19	175.0	Soccer	136	60 min.		620
		Golf	102	90 min.		473
21	175.0	Running (7 min/mile)	172	18 min.	2.5	321
23	174.5	Step-Aerobics	144	60 min.		733
24	175.0	Bowling	102	90 min.		473
25	174.5	Basketball/Moderate	150	60 min.		482
		Dance/Moderate	102	120 min.		628
26	174.0	Running (7 min/mile)	168	30 min.	4.0	532
		Skiing/Downhill	114	60 min.		626
28	174.0	Running (7 min/mile)	168	30 min.	4.0	532
		Strength Training	138	60 min.		522
30	173.5	Stationary Cycling/Vig.	156	60 min.		729

MONTHLY SUMMARY

Average body weight:	176.2 lbs.
Average exercise heart rate:	145 bpm
Total number of days exercised:	18 days
Average exercise time/day:	68 min.
Total number of calories burned:	12,570
Average number of calories per day exercised:	698
Total number of miles jogged:	30.5
Total number of miles swum:	0.5
Total number of miles walked:	2.0

Figure 3.8 • *Sample monthly exercise record using the EXLOG (Exercise Log) computer program.*

will be deeply satisfying and will bring about a sense of self-accomplishment. The following suggestions have been used successfully to help change behavior and adhere to a lifetime exercise program.

Tips to Start and Adhere to an Exercise Program

1. *Select aerobic activities you enjoy.* If you pick an activity you don't enjoy, you will be less likely to keep exercising. Don't be afraid to try out a new activity, even if that means learning new skills.

2. *Combine different activities.* You can train by doing two or three different activities the same week. This cross-training may deter the monotony of repeating the same activity every day. Try lifetime sports. Many endurance sports such as racquetball, basketball, soccer, badminton, roller skating, cross-country skiing, and body surfing (paddling the board) provide a nice break from regular workouts.

3. *Set aside a regular time for exercise.* If you don't plan ahead, it is a lot easier to skip. Holding your exercise hour "sacred" helps you adhere to the program.

4. *Use the proper clothing and equipment for exercise.* A poor pair of shoes, for example, can make you more prone to injury, discouraging you from the beginning.

5. *Find a friend or group of friends to exercise with.* Social interaction will make exercise more fulfilling. Besides, it's harder to skip if someone else is waiting for you.

6. *Set goals, and share them with others.* Quitting is tougher when someone else knows what you are trying to accomplish. When you reach a targeted goal, reward yourself with a new pair of shoes or a jogging suit.

7. *Don't become a chronic exerciser.* Learn to listen to your body. Overexercising can lead to chronic fatigue and injuries. Exercise should be enjoyable, and in the process you should *stop and smell the roses.*

8. *Exercise in different places and facilities.* This will add variety to your workouts.

9. *Keep a regular record of your activities.* Keeping a record allows you to monitor your progress and compare it against previous months and years (see Figures 3.8 and 3.10).

10. *Conduct periodic assessments.* Improving to a higher fitness category is a reward in itself.

11. *If a health problem arises, see a physician.* When in doubt, it's better to be safe than sorry.

● A Lifetime Commitment to Fitness

The benefits of fitness can be maintained only through a regular lifetime program. Exercise is not like putting money in the bank. It does not help much to exercise 4 or 5 hours on Saturday and not do anything else the rest of the week. If anything, exercising only once a week is unsafe for unconditioned adults.

Even the greatest athletes on earth, if they were to stop exercising, would be, after just a few years, at a risk for disease similar to someone who never has done any physical activity. Staying with a physical fitness program long enough brings about positive physiological and psychological changes, and once you are there, you will not want to have it any other way.

The time involved in losing the benefits of exercise varies among the different components of physical fitness and also depends on the person's condition before the interruption. In regard to cardiorespiratory endurance, it has been estimated that 4 weeks of aerobic training are completely reversed in 2 consecutive weeks of physical inactivity. On the other hand, if you have been exercising regularly for months or years, 2 weeks of inactivity will not hurt you as much as it will someone who has exercised only a few weeks.

As a rule of thumb, after 48 to 72 hours of aerobic inactivity, the cardiorespiratory system starts to lose some of its capacity. Flexibility can be maintained with two or three stretching sessions per week. Strength is easily retained with just one maximal training session per week.

To maintain fitness, you should keep up a regular exercise program, even during vacations. If you have to interrupt your program for reasons beyond your control, you should not attempt to resume training at the same level you left off but, rather, build up gradually again.

Notes

1. W. M. Bortz II, "Disuse and Aging," *Journal of the American Medical Association*, 248 (1982), 1203–1208.
2. American College of Sports Medicine, *Guidelines for Exercise Testing and Prescription* (Baltimore: Williams & Wilkins, 1995).
3. American College of Sports Medicine, "The Recommended Quantity and Quality of Exercise for Developing and Maintaining Cardiorespiratory and Muscular Fitness in Healthy Adults," *Medicine and Science in Sports and Exercise*, 22 (1990), 265–274.
4. W. W. K. Hoeger, M. L. Chupurdia, W. J. Nurge, and D. E. Van Zee, "Physiologic Responses to Step Aerobics and Aero-Belt Step Aerobics," *Medicine and Science in Sports and Exercise*, 26 (1994), S43, 246.
5. D. R. Hopkins, W. W. K. Hoeger, D. E. Van Zee, and W. J. Nurge, "Physiologic Responses to Aero-belt Walking," *Medicine and Science in Sports and Exercise*, 26 (1994), 243:245.

6. W. J. Nurge, D. E. Van Zee, and W. W. K. Hoeger. "Physiologic Responses to Aero-belt Walking and Jogging," *Medicine and Science in Sports and Exercise*, 26 (1994), 243:247.
7. R. F. DeBusk, U. Stenestrand, M. Sheehan, and W. L. Haskell. "Training Effects of Long Versus Short Bouts of Exercise in Healthy Subjects," *American Journal of Cardiology*, 65 (1990), 1010-1013.
8. U. S. Centers for Disease Control and Prevention and American College of Sports Medicine, "Summary Statement: Workshop on Physical Activity and Public Health," *Sports Medicine Bulletin*, 28 (1993), 7.
9. U. S. Department of Agriculture and U. S. Department of Health and Human Services, "Nutrition and Your Health: Dietary Guidelines for Americans," *Home and Garden Bulletin No. 232*, December 1995.
10. U. S. Department of Health and Human Services, *Physical Activity and Health: A Report of the Surgeon General*, Atlanta, GA: U. S. Department of Health and Human Services, Centers for Disease Control and Prevention, National Center for Chronic Disease Prevention and Health Promotion, 1996.

11. W. L. Haskell, "Scanning Sports," *Physician and Sportsmedicine*, 21:11 (1993), 34.
12. U. S. Department of Health and Human Services.
13. E. J. Marcinick, J. Potts, G. Schlabach, S. Will, P. Dawson, and B. F. Hurley, "Effects of Strength Training on Lactate Threshold and Endurance Performance," *Medicine and Science in Sports and Exercise*, 23 (1993), 739–743.
14. R. S. Paffenbarger, Jr., R. T. Hyde, A. L. Wing, and C. H. Steinmetz, "A Natural History of Athleticism and Cardio-vascular Health," *Journal of the American Medical Association*, 252 (1984), 491–495.
15. American College of Obstetricians and Gynecologists, *Guidelines for Exercise During Pregnancy*, 1994.
16. University of California at Berkeley, *The Wellness Guide to Lifelong Fitness* (New York: Random House, 1993), p. 198.

Suggested Readings

Arnheim, D. D., and W. Prentice. *Modern Principles of Athletic Training*. St. Louis: Mosby Year Book, 1993.

Borg, G. "Perceived Exertion: A Note on History and Methods." *Medicine and Science in Sports and Exercise*, 5 (1993), 90–93.

Coleman, E. *Eating for Endurance*. Palo Alto, CA: Bull Publishing, 1992.

Cooper, K. H. *The Aerobics Program for Total Well-Being*. New York: Mount Evans and Co., 1982.

Fox, E. L., R. W. Bowers, and M. L. Fossand. *The Physiological Basis for Exercise and Sport*. Philadelphia: Saunders College Publishing, 1993.

Heyward, V. H. *Advanced Fitness Assessment & Exercise Prescription*. Champaign, IL: Human Kinetic, 1991.

Karvonen, M. J., E. Kentala, and O. Mustala. "The Effects of Training on the Heart Rate, a Longitudinal Study." *Annales Medicinae Experimetalis et Biologiae Fenniae*, 35 (1957), 307-315.

McArdle, W. D., F. I. Katch, and V. L. Katch. *Essentials of Exercise Physiology*. Philadelphia: Lea & Febiger, 1994.

Metcalf, J. A. "Exercising During Pregnancy." *Certified News*, 5:2 (1995), 10–11.

Pfeiffer, R. P, and B. C. Mangus. *Concepts of Athletic Training*. Boston: Jones and Bartlett Publishers, 1995.

Teitz, C. C. "Overuse Injuries," in *Scientific Foundations of Sports Medicine* (C. C. Teitz Editor) (pp. 299–328). Philadelphia: B. C. Decker, 1989.

Wilmore, J. H., and D. L. Costill. *Physiology of Sport and Exercise*. Champaign, IL: Human Kinetics, 1994.

Name:_____Date: _____

Intensity of Exercise

1. Estimate your own maximal heart rate (MHR)

    MHR = 220 minus age (220 − age)

    MHR = 220 − _____ = _____ bpm

2. Resting Heart Rate (RHR) = _____ bpm

3. Heart Rate Reserve (HRR) = MHR − RHR

    HRR = _____ − _____ = _____ beats

4. Training Intensities (TI) = HRR × TI + RHR

    50 Percent TI = _____ × .50 + _____ = _____ bpm

    70 percent TI = _____ × .70 + _____ = _____ bpm

    85 Percent TI = _____ × .85 + _____ = _____ bpm

5. Cardiorespiratory Training Zone. The optimum cardiorespiratory training zone is found between the 70% and 85% training intensities. Individuals who have been physically inactive or are in the poor or fair cardiorespiratory fitness categories, however, should use a 50% training intensity during the first few weeks of the exercise program.

    Cardiorespiratory Training Zone: _____ (70% TI) to _____ (85% TI)

    Rate of Perceived Exertion (see Figure 3.1): _____ to _____

Mode of Exercise

Select any activity or combination of activities that you enjoy doing. The activity has to be continuous in nature and must get your heart rate up to the cardiorespiratory training zone and keep it there for as long as you exercise. Indicate your preferred mode(s) of exercise:

1. _____   2. _____   3. _____

4. _____   5. _____   6. _____

Cardiorespiratory Exercise Program

The following is your weekly program for developing cardiorespiratory endurance. If you are in the average, good, or excellent fitness category, you may start at week 5. After completing this 12-week program, for you to maintain your fitness level, you should exercise in the 70% to 85% training zone for about 20 to 30 minutes, a minimum of three times per week, on nonconsecutive days. You also should recompute your target zone periodically because you will experience a significant reduction in resting heart rate with aerobic training (approximately 10 to 20 beats in about 8 to 12 weeks).

Week	Duration (min)	Frequency	Training Intensity	10-Sec. Pulse Count*
1	15	3	Approximately 50%	
2	15	4	Approximately 50%	
3	20	4	Approximately 50%	_____ beats
4	20	5	Approximately 50%	
5	20	4	About 70%	
6	20	5	About 70%	
7	30	4	About 70%	_____ beats
8	30	5	About 70%	
9	30	4	Between 70% and 85%	
10	30	5	Between 70% and 85%	
11	30–40	5	Between 70% and 85%	_____ to _____ beats
12	30–40	5	Between 70% and 85%	

*Fill out your own 10-second pulse count under this column.

Figure 3.9 ● *Cardiorespiratory exercise prescription form.*

Month _____

Date	Body Weight	Exercise Heart Rate	Type of Exercise	Distance In Miles	Time Hrs/Min	RPE*
1						
2						
3						
4						
5						
6						
7						
8						
9						
10						
11						
12						
13						
14						
15						
16						
17						
18						
19						
20						
21						
22						
23						
24						
25						
26						
27						
28						
29						
30						
31						
			Total			

*Rate of perceived exertion.

Month _____

Date	Body Weight	Exercise Heart Rate	Type of Exercise	Distance In Miles	Time Hrs/Min	RPE*
1						
2						
3						
4						
5						
6						
7						
8						
9						
10						
11						
12						
13						
14						
15						
16						
17						
18						
19						
20						
21						
22						
23						
24						
25						
26						
27						
28						
29						
30						
31						
			Total			

*Rate of perceived exertion.

Figure 3.10 • *Cardiorespiratory exercise record form.*

Month _____

Date	Body Weight	Exercise Heart Rate	Type of Exercise	Distance In Miles	Time Hrs/Min	RPE*
1						
2						
3						
4						
5						
6						
7						
8						
9						
10						
11						
12						
13						
14						
15						
16						
17						
18						
19						
20						
21						
22						
23						
24						
25						
26						
27						
28						
29						
30						
31						
Total						

*Rate of perceived exertion.

Month _____

Date	Body Weight	Exercise Heart Rate	Type of Exercise	Distance In Miles	Time Hrs/Min	RPE*
1						
2						
3						
4						
5						
6						
7						
8						
9						
10						
11						
12						
13						
14						
15						
16						
17						
18						
19						
20						
21						
22						
23						
24						
25						
26						
27						
28						
29						
30						
31						
Total						

*Rate of perceived exertion.

Figure 3.10 ● *Cardiorespiratory exercise record form.*

Muscular Strength Assessment and Prescription

*A*lthough evidence of the benefits of strength training in enhancing health and well-being is well-documented, many people still have the impression that strength is necessary only for highly trained athletes and other individuals who hold jobs that require heavy muscular work. To the contrary, strength is a basic component of fitness and wellness and is crucial for optimal performance in daily activities such as sitting, walking, running, lifting and carrying objects, doing housework, and enjoying recreational activities. Strength also is of great value in improving posture, personal appearance, and self-image, in developing sports skills, and in meeting certain emergencies in life in which strength is necessary to cope effectively. From a health standpoint, strength helps to maintain muscle tissue and a higher resting metabolism, lessens the risk for injury, helps to

Objectives

- Understand the importance of adequate strength levels in maintaining good health and well-being.
- Clarify misconceptions about women who engage in strength-training programs.
- Define *muscular strength* and *muscular endurance*.
- Be able to assess muscular strength and endurance through two different strength testing protocols.
- Learn to interpret strength testing results according to health fitness and physical fitness standards.
- Identify the factors that affect strength.
- Name the different types of muscle fibers.
- Understand the overload principle for strength development.
- Recognize the principles that govern muscular strength and muscular endurance development (mode, resistance, sets, and frequency).
- Become acquainted with two distinct strength-training programs.

87

prevent and eliminate chronic low-back pain, and is a key factor in childbearing.

Muscular strength also seems to be the most important health-related component of physical fitness in the older-adult population. While proper cardiorespiratory endurance helps maintain a healthy heart, good strength levels will do more toward independent living than any other fitness component. More than anything else, older adults want to enjoy good health and function independently. Many of them are, however, confined to nursing homes because they lack sufficient strength to move about. They cannot walk very far and many need to be helped in and out of beds, chairs, and tubs.

A strength-training program can have a tremendous impact in enhancing quality of life. Research has shown leg strength improvements as high as 200% in previously inactive adults over age 90.[1] As strength improves, so does the ability to move about, the capacity for independent living, and enjoyment of life during the "golden years."

Relationship Between Strength and Metabolism

Perhaps one of the most significant benefits of maintaining a good strength level is its relationship to human **metabolism**. A primary outcome of a strength-training program is an increase in muscle mass or size (lean body mass), known as muscle **hypertrophy**.

Muscle tissue uses energy even at rest. In contrast, fatty tissue uses very little energy and may be considered metabolically inert from the point of view of caloric use. As muscle size increases, so does the **resting metabolism**, the amount of energy (calories) an individual requires during resting conditions to sustain proper cell function. Even small increases in muscle mass may affect resting metabolism.

Estimates indicate that each additional pound of muscle tissue increases resting metabolism by 35 calories per day.[2] All other factors being equal, if two individuals both weigh 150 pounds but have different amounts of muscle mass, let's say 5 pounds, the one with more muscle mass will have a higher resting metabolic rate, allowing this person to ingest more calories to maintain the muscle tissue.

Loss of lean tissue also is thought to be the main reason for the decrease in metabolism as people grow older. Contrary to some beliefs, metabolism does not have to slow down significantly with aging.

It is not so much that metabolism slows down. It's that we slow down.

Lean body mass decreases with sedentary living, which, in turn, slows down the resting metabolic rate. If people continue eating at the same rate, body fat increases. The average decrease in resting metabolism from age 26 to age 60 is about 360 calories per day.[3] Hence, participating in a strength training program is important in preventing and reducing excess body fat.

Gender Differences

One of the most common misconceptions about physical fitness is related to women and strength training. Because of the increase in muscle mass commonly seen in men, some women think a strength training program will be counterproductive because they, too, will develop large musculature. Even though the quality of muscle in men and women is the same, endocrinological differences do not allow women to achieve the same amount of muscle hypertrophy (size) as men. Men also have more muscle fibers, and because of the male sex-specific hormones, each individual fiber has more potential for hypertrophy.

The idea that strength training allows women to develop muscle hypertrophy to the same extent as men do is as false as the notion that playing basketball will turn women into giants. *Masculinity and femininity are established by genetic inheritance*, not by the amount of physical activity. Variations in the extent of masculinity and femininity are determined by individual differences in hormonal secretions of androgen, testosterone, estrogen, and progesterone. Women with a bigger-than-average build often are inclined to participate in sports because of their natural physical advantage. As a result, many women have associated participation in sports and strength training with large muscle size.

As the number of females who participate in sports has increased steadily during the last few years, the myth that strength training in women leads to large increases in muscle size has been abated somewhat. For example, per pound of body weight, female gymnasts are considered to be among the strongest athletes in the world. These athletes engage regularly in serious strength-training programs. Yet, female gymnasts have some of the most well-toned and graceful figures of all women.

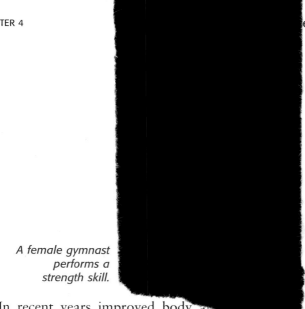

A female gymnast performs a strength skill.

In recent years improved body ap̶̶̶̶̶ become the rule rather than the exception for women who participate in strength-training programs. Some of the most attractive female movie stars also train with weights to further improve their personal image. In his book *Weight Training for Life*, James Hesson points out that many beauty pageant participants engage in some sort of strength training program as they prepare for the pageant. A survey at a recent state beauty pageant revealed that 86% of the participants (38 of 44 contestants) exercised with weights![4]

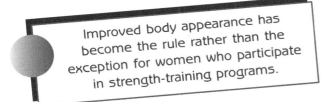

Improved body appearance has become the rule rather than the exception for women who participate in strength-training programs.

At the same time, you may ask, "If weight training does not masculinize women, why do so many women body builders develop such heavy musculature?" In the sport of body building, the athletes follow intense training routines consisting of two or more hours of constant weight lifting with short rest intervals between sets. Many times body building training routines call for back-to-back exercises using the same muscle groups. The objective of this type of training is to "pump" extra blood into the muscles, which makes the muscles appear much bigger than they are in a resting condition. Based on the intensity and the length of the training session, the muscles can remain filled with blood, appearing measurably larger for several hours after completing the training session. Therefore, in real life, these women are not as muscular as they seem when they are "pumped up" for a contest.

In the sport of body building, a big point of controversy is the use of **anabolic steroids** and human growth hormones, even among women participants. Anabolic steroids are synthetic versions of the male sex hormone testosterone, which promotes muscle development and hypertrophy. These hormones, however, produce detrimental and undesirable side effects (e.g., hypertension, fluid retention, decreased breast size, deepening of the voice, facial whiskers, and body hair growth), which some women deem tolerable. Anabolic steroid use in general, except for medical reasons and when carefully monitored by a physician, can lead to serious health consequences.

Anabolic steroid use among female body builders is widespread. According to several sports medicine physicians and female body builders, about 80% of female body builders have used steroids. Furthermore, according to several female track-and-field coaches, as many as 95% of female athletes around the world in this sport had used anabolic steroids to remain competitive at the international level.

Women who take steroids undoubtedly will build heavy musculature, and, if the steroids are taken long enough, will produce masculinizing effects. As a result, the International Federation of Body Building instituted a mandatory steroid-testing program for females participating in the Miss Olympia contest. When drugs are not used to promote development, improved body image is the rule rather than the exception among females who participate in body building, strength training, or sports in general.

● Body Composition Changes

Another benefit of strength training, accentuated even more when combined with aerobic exercise, is a decrease in adipose or fatty tissue around muscle fibers

TERMS

Metabolism All energy and material transformations that occur within living cells necessary to sustain life.

Hypertrophy An increase in the size of the cell (for example, muscle hypertrophy).

Resting metabolism The amount of energy (expressed in milliliters of oxygen per minute or total calories per day) an individual requires during resting conditions to sustain proper body function.

Anabolic steroids Synthetic versions of the male sex hormone testosterone, which promotes muscle development and hypertrophy.

SELECTED DETRIMENTAL EFFECTS OF ANABOLIC STEROID USE

- Liver tumors
- Hepatitis
- Hypertension
- Reduction of high density lipoprotein (HDL)
- Elevation of low density lipoprotein (LDL)
- Hyperinsulinism
- Impaired pituitary function
- Impaired thyroid function
- Mood swings
- Aggressive behavior
- Increased irritability
- Acne
- Fluid retention
- Decreased libido
- HIV infection (via injectable steroids)
- Prostate problems (men)
- Testicular atrophy (men)
- Reduced sperm count (men)
- Clitoral enlargement (women)
- Decreased breast size (women)
- Increased body and facial hair (nonreversible in women)
- Deepening of the voice (nonreversible in women)

regularly to monitor
ther than simply mea-
ight (see Chapter 6).

scular
urance

nd endurance are inter-
owing ways.

ined as the ability to
inst resistance.

e ability of a muscle to
epeatedly over time.

endurance (also referred to as localized muscular endurance) depends to a large extent on muscular strength. Weak muscles cannot repeat an action several times or sustain it for a long time. Keeping these principles in mind, strength tests and training programs have been designed to measure and develop absolute muscular strength or muscular endurance, or a combination of the two.

Muscular strength usually is determined by the maximal amount of resistance (**one repetition maximum, or 1 RM**) *an individual is able to lift in a single effort.* This assessment yields a good measure of absolute strength, but it does require a considerable amount of time, as the 1 RM is determined through trial and error. For example, strength of the chest muscles frequently is measured through the bench press exercise. If an individual has not trained with weights, he may try 100 pounds and lift this resistance quite easily. After adding 50 pounds, he fails to lift the resistance. The resistance then is decreased by 10 or 20 pounds. Finally, after several trials the 1 RM is established.

A true 1 RM might be difficult to obtain the first time an individual is tested because fatigue becomes

themselves. The decrease in fatty tissue often is greater than the amount of muscle hypertrophy (see Figure 4.1). Therefore, losing inches but not body weight is common.

Because muscle tissue is more dense than fatty tissue, and despite the fact that inches are lost during a combined strength training and aerobic program, people, especially women, often become discouraged because they cannot see the results readily on the scale. They can offset this discouragement by

Figure 4.1 • *Changes in body composition from a combined aerobic and strength-training program.*

a factor. By the time the 1 RM is established, the person already has made several maximal or near-maximal attempts.

Muscular endurance typically is established by the number of repetitions an individual can perform against a submaximal resistance or by the length of time a given contraction can be sustained. For example: How many push-ups can an individual do? Or how many times can he or she lift 50 pounds? Or how long can a person hold the chin above a bar while holding on to it?

In strength testing, several body sites should be tested. Because different body parts have different strength levels, no single strength test provides a good assessment of overall body strength. As a minimum, a strength profile should include the upper body, the lower body, and the abdominal muscles.

If time is a factor and only one test item can be done, the Hand Grip Test commonly is used to assess strength. Even this test, though, provides only a weak correlation with overall body strength. (A description of this test is provided in Figure 4.8 on page 98.)

As with cardiorespiratory endurance, you will have the opportunity to assess your own level of muscular strength or endurance, or both. Four tests are provided in this chapter. Your test selection should be based on the time and facilities available. Because individuals who have not been lifting regularly have a small increased risk for injury when attempting a maximal contraction, these individuals probably should avoid an absolute strength test (1 RM test).

After you have selected your test, go directly to the procedure that explains the respective test. For safety reasons, always take a friend or group of friends with you whenever you train with weights or conduct any type of strength assessment. Also, these are four different tests, so to make valid comparisons the same test should be used for pre- and post-assessments. The following are your options:

Muscular Strength and Endurance Test

On this test you will lift a submaximal resistance as many times as possible on six different strength-training exercises. The resistance for each lift is determined according to selected percentages of body weight (see Figure 4.2). If you are not familiar with the different lifts, illustrations are provided at the end of this chapter.

Strength/endurance ratings are determined according to the maximum number of repetitions you are able to do on each exercise. A 16-station, fixed-resistance, Universal Gym apparatus is necessary to administer all but the abdominal crunch exercise on this test (see Mode of Training, later in this chapter, for an explanation of fixed-resistance equipment).

For individuals who do only a few repetitions, the test will primarily measure absolute strength. For those who are able to do a lot of repetitions, the test will be an indicator of muscular endurance. A percentile rank for each exercise is given based on the number of repetitions performed (see Table 4.1), and an overall muscular strength/endurance rating can be determined by totalling the number of points obtained on each exercise. A form to record your data for this test is provided on Figure 4.3 on page 95.

If no fixed resistance Universal Gym equipment is available, you still can perform the test using different equipment. In that case, though, the percentile rankings and strength fitness categories may not be accurate because a certain resistance (for example, 50 pounds) is seldom the same on two different weight machines. The industry has no standard calibration procedure for strength equipment. Consequently, if you lift a certain weight on one machine, you may or may not be able to lift the same amount on a different piece of equipment.

Even though the percentile ranks may not be valid when using different equipment, test results still can be used to evaluate changes in fitness. For example, you may be able to do 7 repetitions on the equipment available to you (whereas you might have done 10 on Universal Gym fixed resistance), but if you can perform 14 repetitions after 12 weeks of training, that's a measure of improvement. When performing this test on different equipment, you should disregard the percentile ranks and use the test results to assess *changes* in fitness only.

TERMS

Muscular strength The ability of a muscle to exert maximum force against resistance (for example, 1 repetition maximum or 1 RM).

Muscular endurance The ability of a muscle to exert submaximal force repeatedly over time.

One repetition maximum (1 RM) The maximum amount of resistance an individual is able to lift in a single effort.

MUSCULAR STRENGTH AND ENDURANCE TEST

A 16-station, fixed resistance, Universal Gym apparatus is required to perform this test, along with a partner.

1. Familiarize yourself with the six lifts used for this test: lat pull-down, leg extension, bench press, bent-leg curl-up or abdominal crunch,* leg curl, and arm curl. Graphic illustrations for each lift are given at the end of this chapter. For the leg curl exercise, the knees should be flexed to 90°. A description and illustration of the bent-leg curl-up and the abdominal crunch exercises is provided in Figure 4.4. For the lateral pull-down exercise, use a sitting position and have your partner hold you down by the waist or shoulders. On the leg extension lift, maintain the trunk in an upright position.

2. Determine your body weight in pounds.

3. Determine the amount of resistance to be used on each lift. To obtain this number, multiply your body weight by the percent given below for each lift.

Lift	Percent of Body Weight	
	Men	Women
Lat Pull-Down	.70	.45
Leg Extension	.65	.50
Bench Press	.75	.45
Bent-Leg Curl-Up or Abdominal Crunch*	NA**	NA**
Leg Curl	.32	.25
Arm Curl	.35	.18

*The abdominal crunch exercise should be used only by individuals who suffer or are susceptible to low-back pain.
**NA = not applicable — see Figure 4.4

4. Perform the maximum continuous number of repetitions possible and record this information in Figure 4.3 on page 95.

5. Based on the number of repetitions performed, look up the percentile rank for each lift in the far left column of Table 4.1.

6. The individual strength fitness category for each lift is determined according to the following classification:

Percentile Rank	Fitness Category	Points
≥90	Excellent	5
70–80	Good	4
50–60	Average	3
30–40	Fair	2
≤20	Poor	1

7. Look up the number of points assigned for each fitness category under item 6 above. Total the number of points and determine your overall strength fitness category according to the following ratings:

Total Points	Strength Category
≥25	Excellent
19–24	Good
13–18	Average
7–12	Fair
≤6	Poor

Figure 4.2 • *Procedure for the Muscular Strength and Endurance Test.*

Table 4.1 *Muscular Strength and Endurance Scoring Table*

Percentile Rank	MEN							WOMEN						
	Lat Pull-Down	Leg Extension	Bench Press	Bent-Leg Curl-Up	Abdominal Crunch	Leg Curl	Arm Curl	Lat Pull-Down	Leg Extension	Bench Press	Bent-Leg Curl-Up	Abdominal Crunch	Leg Curl	Arm Curl
99	30	25	26	100	100	24	25	30	25	27	100	100	20	25
95	25	20	21	81	100	20	21	25	20	21	100	100	17	21
90	19	19	19	65	100	19	19	21	18	20	97	69	12	20
80	16	15	16	51	66	15	15	16	13	16	77	49	10	16
70	13	14	13	44	45	13	12	13	11	13	57	37	9	14
60	11	13	11	31	38	11	10	11	10	11	45	34	7	12
50	10	12	10	28	33	10	9	10	9	10	37	31	6	10
40	9	10	7	25	29	8	8	9	8	5	28	27	5	8
30	7	9	5	22	26	6	7	7	7	3	22	24	4	7
20	6	7	3	17	22	4	5	6	5	1	17	21	3	6
10	4	5	1	10	18	3	3	3	3	0	9	15	1	3
5	3	3	0	3	16	1	2	2	1	0	4	0	0	2

■ High physical fitness standard   ■ Health fitness standard

Muscular Endurance Test

Three exercises were selected to assess the endurance of the upper body, lower body, and mid-body muscle groups (see Figure 4.4). The advantage of this test is that it does not require strength training equipment.

For this test you will need a stopwatch, a metronome, a bench or gymnasium bleacher 16¼" high, a cardboard strip 3½" wide by 30" long, and a partner. As with the Muscular Strength and Endurance Test, a percentile rank is given for each exercise according to the number of repetitions performed (see Table 4.2). An overall endurance rating can be obtained by totalling the number of points obtained on each exercise. The data recording form for this test is given in Figure 4.5 on page 95.

MUSCULAR ENDURANCE TEST

Three exercises are conducted on this test: bench-jumps, modified dips (men) or modified push-ups (women), and bent-leg curl-ups or abdominal crunches. All exercises should be conducted with the aid of a partner. The correct procedure for performing each exercise is as follows:

Bench-jump. Using a bench or gymnasium bleacher 16¼" high, attempt to jump up and down the bench as many times as possible in 1 minute. If you cannot jump the full minute, you may step up and down. A repetition is counted each time both feet return to the floor.

Bench jump.

Modified dip. Men only: Using a bench or gymnasium bleacher, place the hands on the bench with the fingers pointing forward. Have a partner hold your feet in front of you. Bend the hips at approximately 90° (you also may use three sturdy chairs, put your hands on two chairs placed by the sides of your body, and place your feet on the third chair in front of you). Lower your body by flexing the elbows until you reach a 90° angle at this joint, then return to the starting position (see Exercise 6 at the end of this chapter). Perform the repetitions to a two-step cadence (down-up) regulated with a metronome set at 56 beats per minute. Perform as many continuous repetitions as possible. Do not count any more repetitions if you fail to follow the metronome cadence.

Modified dip.

Modified push-up. Women: Lie down on the floor (face down), bend the knees (feet up in the air), and place the hands on the floor by the shoulders with the fingers pointing forward. The lower body will be supported at the knees (as opposed to the feet) throughout the test (*see*

Exercise 3). The chest must touch the floor on each repetition. As with the modified-dip exercise, perform the repetitions (above) to a two-step cadence (up-down) regulated with a metronome set at 56 beats per minute. Perform as many continuous repetitions as possible. Do not count any more repetitions if you fail to follow the metronome cadence.

Bent-leg curl-up. Lie down on the floor (face up) and bend both legs at the knees at approximately 100°. The feet should be on the floor, and you must hold them in place yourself throughout the test. Cross the arms in front of the chest, each hand on the opposite shoulder. Now raise the head off the floor, placing the chin against the chest. This is the starting and finishing position for each curl-up (see Exercise 4a). **The back of the head may not come in contact with the floor, the hands cannot be removed from the shoulders, nor may the feet or hips be raised off the floor at any time during the test. The test is terminated if any of these four conditions occur.** When you curl up, the upper body must come to an upright position before going back down (see Exercise 4c). The repetitions are performed to a two-step cadence (up-down) regulated with the metronome set at 40 beats per minute. For this exercise, you should allow a brief practice period of 5 to 10 seconds to familiarize yourself with the cadence (the *up* movement is initiated with the first beat, then you must wait for the next beat to initiate the *down* movement; one repetition is accomplished every two beats of the metronome). Count as many repetitions as you are able to perform following the proper cadence. The test is also terminated if you fail to maintain the appropriate cadence or if you accomplish 100 repetitions. Have your partner check the angle at the knees throughout the test to make sure to maintain the 100° angle as close as possible.

Abdominal crunch. This test is recommended only for individuals who are unable to perform the bent-leg curl-up test because susceptibility to low-back injury. Exercise form must be carefully monitored during the test. Several authors and researchers[5,6,7,8] have indicated

(Continued)

Figure 4.4 ● *Procedure for the Muscular Endurance Test.*

that proper form during this test is extremely difficult to control. Subjects often slide their bodies, bend their elbows, or shrug their shoulders during the test. Such actions facilitate the performance of the test and misrepresent the actual test results. Biomechanical factors also limit the ability to perform this test.[9] Further, lack of spinal flexibility keeps some individuals from being able to move the full 3½" range of motion.[10,11] Others are unable to keep their heels on the floor during the test. The validity of this test as an effective measure of abdominal strength or abdominal endurance has also been questioned in recent research.[12,13]

Tape a 3½ x 30" strip of cardboard onto the floor. Lie down on the floor in a supine position (face up) with the knees bent at approximately 100° and the legs slightly apart. The feet should be on the floor and you must hold them in place yourself throughout the test. Straighten out your arms and place them on the floor alongside the trunk with the palms down and the fingers fully extended. The fingertips of both hands should barely touch the closest edge of the cardboard (see Figure 4.4a). Bring the head off the floor until the chin is 1" to 2" away from your chest. Keep the head in this position during the entire test (do not move the head by flexing or extending the neck). You are now ready to begin the test.

Abdominal crunch test.

Perform the repetitions to a two-step cadence (up-down) regulated with a metronome set at 60 beats per minute. As you curl up, slide the fingers over the cardboard until the fingertips reach the far end (3½") of the board (see Figure 4.4b), then return to the starting position.

Allow a brief practice period of 5 to 10 seconds to familiarize yourself with the cadence. Initiate the up movement with the first beat and the down movement with the next beat. Accomplish one repetition every two beats of the metronome. Count as many repetitions as you are able to perform following the proper cadence. You may not count a repetition if the fingertips fail to reach the distant end of the cardboard.

Terminate the test if: (a) you fail to maintain the appropriate cadence, (b) bend the elbows, (c) shrug the shoulders, (d) slide the body, (e) the heels come off the floor, (f) the chin is not kept close to the chest, (g) you accomplish 100 repetitions, or (h) you no longer can perform the test. Have your partner check the angle at the knees throughout the test to make sure that the 100° angle is maintained as close as possible.

For this test you may also use a Crunch-Ster Curl-Up Tester, available from Novel Products.* An illustration of the test performed with this equipment is provided in Figures 4.4c and 4.4d.

Abdominal crunch test performed with a Crunch-ster curl-up tester.

You may record your test results in Figure 4.5, page 95. According to the results, look up your percentile rank for each exercise in the far left column of Table 4.2 and determine your muscular endurance fitness category according to the following classification:

Percentile Rank	Fitness Category	Points
≥90	Excellent	5
70–80	Good	4
50–60	Average	3
30–40	Fair	2
≤20	Poor	1

Look up the number of points assigned for each fitness category above. Total the number of points and determine your overall strength endurance fitness category according to the following ratings:

Total Points	Strength Endurance Category
≥13	Excellent
10–12	Good
7–9	Average
4–6	Fair
≤3	Poor

*Novel Products, Inc. Figure Finder Collection. P.O. Box 408, Rockton, IL 61072-0408. 1-800-323-5143, FAX 815-624-4866.

Figure 4.4 ● *Procedure for Muscular Endurance Test (Continued).*

Name:_____ Sex: _____ Date: _____

Body Weight:_____

Lift	% Body Weight		Resistance	Repetitions	Fitness Category	Points
	Men	Women				
Lat Pull-Down	.70	.45	☐	☐	☐	☐
Leg Extension	.65	.50	☐	☐	☐	☐
Bench Press	.75	.45	☐	☐	☐	☐
Bent-Leg Curl-Up or Abdominal Crunch	NA*	NA*	☐	☐	☐	☐
Leg Curl	.32	.25	☐	☐	☐	☐
Arm Curl	.35	.18	☐	☐	☐	☐

Total Points: ☐

Overall Strength Category: ☐

*NA = Not Applicable. See Figure 4.4.

Figure 4.3 ● *Data form for Muscular Strength and Endurance test results.*

Name:_____ Sex: _____ Date: _____

	Exercise	Metronome Cadence	Repetitions	Fitness Category	Points
Men	Bench-Jumps	NA*	☐	☐	☐
	Modified-Dips	56	☐	☐	☐
	Bent-Leg Curl-Up or Abdominal Crunches	60	☐	☐	☐
Women	Bench-Jumps	NA*	☐	☐	☐
	Modified Push-Ups	56	☐	☐	☐
	Bent-Leg Curl-Up or Abdominal Crunches	60	☐	☐	☐

*NA = No cadence required. Perform as many jumps as possible in one minute

Total Points: ☐

Overall Strength Endurance Category: ☐

Figure 4.5 ● *Data form for Muscular Endurance test results.*

Table 4.2   *Muscular Endurance Scoring Table*

Percentile Rank	MEN				WOMEN			
	Bench Jumps	Modified Dips	Bent-Leg Curl-Ups	Abdominal Crunches	Bench Jumps	Modified Push-ups	Bent-Leg Curl-Ups	Abdominal Crunches
99	66	54	100	100	58	95	100	100
95	63	50	81	100	54	70	100	100
90	62	38	65	100	52	50	97	69
80	58	32	51	66	48	41	77	49
70	57	30	44	45	44	38	57	37
60	56	27	31	38	42	33	45	34
50	54	26	28	33	39	30	37	31
40	51	23	25	29	38	28	28	27
30	48	20	22	26	36	25	22	24
20	47	17	17	22	32	21	17	21
10	40	11	10	18	28	18	9	15
5	34	7	3	16	26	15	4	0

▨ High physical fitness standard   ▨ Health fitness standard

Strength-to-Body Weight Ratio Test

This is an absolute strength test that will require you to determine your 1 RM on six different lifts (see Figure 4.6). Each 1 RM is expressed as a percentage of your body weight (1 RM divided by body weight), and points are awarded based on the ratio obtained for each lift (see Table 4.3). The final strength score is obtained by totaling the points received for each lift (see Figure 4.7 on page 101).

Because the 1 RM is determined through trial and error, individual assessments require about 20 to 30 minutes or longer. As with the Muscular Strength and Endurance Test (the first test), a 16-station, fixed-resistance, Universal Gym apparatus is necessary.

STRENGTH-TO-BODY WEIGHT RATIO TEST

1. Familiarize yourself with the six lifts used for this test: bench press, arm curl, lat pull-down, leg press, leg extension, and leg curl (an illustration of each lift is given at the end of this chapter).

2. Determine your body weight in pounds.

3. Determine your one repetition maximum (1 RM) for each lift. This is done through trial and error. Estimate the amount of resistance (weight) that you think you will be able to lift. If the load is too light, increase the resistance by 5 to 10 pounds; if it is too heavy, decrease by the same amount. Allow 2 to 3 minutes between trials. Continue the process until you have determined the maximal amount of resistance you can lift in one single effort. Record this information under the 1 RM column in Figure 4.7, page 101.

4. Express each 1 RM as a percentage of your body weight. To obtain this number, divide the 1 RM for each lift by your weight. Enter this number under the ratio column in Figure 4.7, page 101. For example, the strength-to-body weight ratio for a 150-pound male who bench-presses 180 pounds is 1.20 (180 ÷ 150).

5. Using Table 4.3, look up on the far right column the number of points scored for the ratio obtained on each lift. In the previous example, a ratio of 1.2 on the bench press for a male would score seven points. Record this information in the appropriate points column in Figure 4.7, page 101.

6. Total the number of points obtained on each lift, and determine your overall strength fitness category according to the following ratings:

Total Points	Strength Category
≥49	Excellent
37–48	Good
25–36	Average
13–24	Fair
≤12	Poor

Figure 4.6 ● *Procedure for the Strength-to-Body Weight Ratio test.*

Table 4.3 Strength-to-Body Weight Ratio Test Scoring Table

MEN						
Bench Press	Arm Curl	Lat. Pull-Down	Leg Press	Leg Extension*	Leg Curl	Points
1.50	0.70	1.20	3.00	1.30	0.70	10
1.40	0.65	1.15	2.80	1.35	0.65	9
1.30	0.60	1.10	2.60	1.20	0.60	8
1.20	0.55	1.05	2.40	1.10	0.55	7
1.10	0.50	1.00	2.20	1.00	0.50	6
1.00	0.45	0.95	2.00	0.90	0.45	5
0.90	0.40	0.90	1.80	0.80	0.40	4
0.80	0.35	0.85	1.60	0.70	0.35	3
0.70	0.30	0.80	1.40	0.60	0.30	2
0.60	0.25	0.75	1.20	0.50	0.25	1
WOMEN						
0.90	0.50	0.85	2.70	1.05	0.60	10
0.85	0.45	0.80	2.50	1.00	0.55	9
0.80	0.42	0.75	2.30	0.95	0.52	8
0.70	0.38	0.73	2.10	0.90	0.50	7
0.65	0.35	0.70	2.00	0.85	0.45	6
0.60	0.32	0.65	1.80	0.80	0.40	5
0.55	0.28	0.63	1.60	0.75	0.35	4
0.50	0.25	0.60	1.40	0.70	0.30	3
0.45	0.21	0.55	1.20	0.65	0.25	2
0.35	0.18	0.50	1.00	0.60	0.20	1

▨ High physical fitness standard
▨ Health fitness standard

*leg extension ratios adapted with permission by author.

From *Advanced Fitness and Exercise Prescription* (p. 108) by Vivian H. Heyward, 1991, Champaign, IL: Human Kinetics. Copyright © 1991 by Vivian H. Heyward. Reprinted by permission.

Hand Grip Test

As indicated earlier, when time is a factor, the Hand Grip Test can be used to provide a rough estimate of strength. Unlike the previous three tests, this is an isometric* (static contraction) test. If the proper grip is used, no finger or body movement is visible during the test. The test procedure is given in Figure 4.8 and you can record your test results in Figure 4.9 on page 101.

Changes in strength may be more difficult to evaluate with this test. Most strength-training programs are dynamic in nature (body segments are

---

*A muscle contraction producing little or no movement. Also see Mode of Training later in this chapter.

The hand grip test provides a rough estimate of strength.

HAND GRIP STRENGTH TEST

1. Adjust the width of the dynamometer* so the middle bones (middle phalanges) of your fingers rest on the distant end of the dynamometer grip (see Figure 4.8a).

FIGURE 4.8a Proper grip size for the hand grip test.

2. Use your dominant hand for this test. Place your elbow at a 90° angle and about 2" away from the body.

3. Grip as hard as you can for a few seconds. Do not move any other body part as you perform the test (do not flex or extend the elbow, do not move the elbow away or toward the body, and do not lean forward or backward during the test).

4. Record the dynamometer reading in pounds (if reading is in kilograms, multiply by 2.2046).

5. Three trials are allowed for this test. Use the highest reading for your final test score. Record your test results in Figure 4.9, page 101, and look up your percentile rank in Table 4.4.

6. Based on your percentile rank, obtain the hand grip strength fitness category according to the following guidelines:

Percentile Rank	Fitness Category
≥90	Excellent
70–80	Good
50–60	Average
30–40	Fair
≤20	Poor

* A Lafayette model 78010 dynamometer is recommended for this test. Lafayette Instruments Co., Sagamore and North 9th Street, Lafayette, IN 47903.

Figure 4.8 ● Procedure for the Hand Grip Strength Test.

Table 4.4 *Grip Strength Scoring Table*

Percentile Rank	Men	Women
99	153	101
95	145	94
90	141	91
80	139	86
70	132	80
60	124	78
50	122	74
40	114	71
30	110	66
20	100	64
10	91	60
5	76	58

▢ High physical fitness standard
▢ Health fitness standard

moved through a range of motion), and this test provides an isometric assessment. Further, grip strength exercises seldom are used in strength training, and increases in strength are specific to the body parts exercised. This test also can be used to supplement the other three strength tests in this chapter.

Recording Your Strength Fitness Category

After you have established your own strength fitness category, record this information on Figure 4.10 on page 101 and on your fitness and wellness profile in Appendix A. If you wish to conduct periodic strength assessments, extra blanks are included in Figure 4.10 for you to monitor your improvements.

● Strength Training Prescription

Muscle cells increase and decrease their capacity to exert force according to the demands placed upon the muscular system. If muscle cells are overloaded beyond their normal use, such as in strength training programs, the cells increase in size (hypertrophy) and strength. If the demands placed on the muscle cells decrease, such as in sedentary living or required rest because of illness or injury, the cells **atrophy** and lose strength. A good level of muscular strength is

important to develop and maintain fitness, health, and total well-being.

● Factors That Affect Strength

Several physiological factors are related to muscle contraction and subsequent strength gains: neural stimulation, type of muscle fiber, the overload principle, and specificity of training. Basic knowledge of these concepts is important in understanding the principles involved in strength training.

Neural Stimulation

Within the neuromuscular system single **motor neurons** (nerves traveling from the central nervous system to the muscle) branch and attach to multiple muscle fibers. The combination of the motor neuron and the fibers it innervates is called a *motor unit*. The number of fibers a motor neuron can innervate varies from just a few in muscles that require precise control (eye muscles, for example) to as many as 1,000 or more in large muscles that do not perform refined or precise movements.

Muscular strength seems to be the most important health-related component of physical fitness in the older-adult population.

Stimulation of a motor neuron causes the muscle fibers to contract maximally or not at all. Variations in the number of fibers innervated and the frequency of their stimulation determine the strength of the muscle contraction. As the number of fibers innervated and frequency of stimulation increases, so does the strength of the muscular contraction.

Types of Fiber

Two basic types of muscle fibers determine muscle response: (a) slow-twitch or red fibers, and (b) fast-twitch or white fibers. **Slow-twitch fibers** have a

TERMS

Atrophy Decrease in the size of a cell.
Motor neurons Nerves traveling from the central nervous system to the muscle.
Slow-twitch fibers Muscle fibers with greater aerobic potential and slow speed of contraction.

greater capacity for aerobic work. **Fast-twitch fibers** have a greater capacity for anaerobic work and produce more overall force. The latter are important for quick and powerful movements commonly used in strength training activities.

The proportion of slow- and fast-twitch fibers is determined genetically, and consequently varies from one person to another. Nevertheless, training increases the functional capacity of both types of fiber, and more specifically, strength training increases their ability to exert force.

During muscular contraction slow-twitch fibers always are recruited first. As the force and speed of muscle contraction increase, the relative importance of the fast-twitch fibers also increases. To activate the fast-twitch fibers, an activity must be intense and powerful.

Overload Principle

Strength gains are achieved in two ways:

1. Through increased ability of individual muscle fibers to generate a stronger contraction.

2. By recruiting a greater proportion of the total available fibers for each contraction.

These two factors combine in the **overload principle**. This principle states that for strength to improve, the demands placed on the muscle must be increased systematically and progressively over time, and the resistance must be of a magnitude significant enough to cause physiologic adaptation. In simpler terms, just like all other organs and systems of the human body, to increase in physical capacity, muscles have to be taxed beyond their accustomed loads. Because of this principle, strength training also is called *progressive resistance training*.

Specificity of Training

The principle of **specificity of training** states that, for a muscle to increase in strength or endurance, the training program must be specific to obtain the desired effects. In like manner, to increase static (isometric) versus dynamic strength, an individual must use static against dynamic training to achieve the desired results.

● Principles Involved in Strength Training

Because muscular strength and endurance are important in developing and maintaining overall fitness

and well-being, the principles necessary to develop a strength-training program have to be followed, as in the prescription of cardiorespiratory exercise. These principles are: mode, resistance, sets, and frequency of training.

Mode of Training

Two basic types of training methods are used to improve strength: **isometric** (static) and **dynamic**. *Isometric training* refers to a muscle contraction that produces little or no movement, such as pushing or pulling against an immovable object. *Dynamic training* refers to a muscle contraction with movement, such as extending the knees with resistance (weight) on the ankles (leg extension exercise).

Isometric training does not require much equipment. It was popular several years ago, but its popularity has waned. Because strength gains with isometric training are specific to the angle of muscle contraction, this type of training is beneficial in a sport such as gymnastics, which requires regular static contractions during routines.

Dynamic training programs can be conducted without weights or with **free weights** (barbells and dumbbells), fixed-resistance machines, variable-resistance machines, and **isokinetic** equipment. When

TERMS
•••••

Fast-twitch fibers Muscle fibers with greater anaerobic potential and fast speed of contraction.

Overload principle Training concept stating that the demands placed on a system (cardiorespiratory, muscular) must be increased systematically and progressively over a period of time to cause physiologic adaptation (development or improvement).

Specificity of training A principle stating that training must be done with the specific muscle the person is attempting to improve.

Isometric strength training Strength training method referring to a muscle contraction that produces little or no movement, such as pushing or pulling against an immovable object.

Dynamic strength training Strength training method referring to a muscle contraction with movement.

Free weights Barbells and dumbbells.

Isokinetic strength training Strength-training method in which the speed of the muscle contraction is kept constant because the equipment (machine) provides an accommodating resistance to match the user's force (maximal) through the range of motion.

Name:_____ Sex: _____ Date: _____

Body Weight:_____ lbs.

Lift	1 RM	Ratio	Points
Bench Press			
Leg Press			
Arm Curl			
Lat Pull-Down			
Leg Extension			
Leg Curl			

Total Points: [   ]

Overall Strength Category [   ]

Figure 4.7 ● *Data form for Strength-to-Body Weight Ratio test results.*

Name:_____ Sex: _____ Date: _____

Grip Strength Score: [   ]   % Rank: [   ]   Strength Category: [   ]

Figure 4.9 ● *Data form for Hand Grip Strength test results.*

Name:_____ Age: _____ Sex:_____

Date	Test Used	Score	Fitness Classification

Figure 4.10 ● *Muscular strength report.*

In isometric training, muscle contraction produces little or no movement.

Strength-training can be done using free weights.

performing dynamic exercises without weights (for example, pull-ups, push-ups), with free weights, or with **fixed-resistance** machines, a constant resistance is moved through a joint's full **range of motion**. The greatest resistance that can be lifted equals the maximum weight that can be moved at the weakest angle of the joint. This is because of changes in muscle length and angle of pull as the joint moves through its range of motion.

As strength training became more popular, new strength-training machines were developed. This technology brought about isokinetic and **variable-resistance** training programs, which require special machines equipped with mechanical devices that provide differing amounts of resistance, with the intent of overloading the muscle group maximally through the entire range of motion. A distinction of isokinetic training is that the speed of the muscle

In dynamic training, the muscle contracts with movement.

contraction is kept constant because the machine provides resistance to match the user's force through the range of motion. The mode of training an individual selects depends mainly on the type of equipment available and the specific objective the training program is attempting to accomplish.

Dynamic training is the most popular mode for strength training. The primary advantage is that strength is gained through the full range of motion. Most daily activities are dynamic in nature. We are constantly lifting, pushing, and pulling objects, and strength is needed through a complete range of motion. Another advantage is that improvements are measured easily by the amount lifted.

The benefits of isokinetic and variable-resistance training are similar to the other dynamic training methods. Theoretically, strength gains should be better because maximum resistance is applied at all angles. Research, however, has not shown this type of training to be more effective than other modes of dynamic training. A possible advantage, though, is that specific speeds used in various sport skills can be duplicated more closely with isokinetic strength training, which may enhance performance (specificity of training). A disadvantage is that the equipment is not readily available to many people.

TERMS

Fixed resistance Type of exercise in which a constant resistance is moved through a joint's full range of motion.

Range of motion Movement around a given joint.

Variable resistance Training using special machines equipped with mechanical devices that provide differing amounts of resistance through the range of motion.

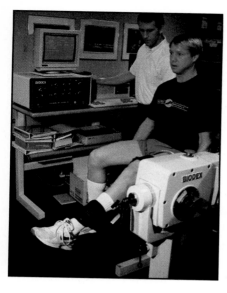

In isokinetic training, the speed of muscle contraction is constant.

Resistance

Resistance in strength training is the equivalent of intensity in cardiorespiratory exercise prescription. The amount of resistance, or weight lifted, depends on whether the individual is trying to develop muscular strength or muscular endurance.

To stimulate strength development, a resistance of approximately 80% of the maximum capacity (1 RM) is recommended.[14] For example, a person who can press 150 pounds should work with at least 120 pounds (150 × .80). Less than 80% will help increase muscular endurance rather than strength.

Because of the time factor involved in constantly determining the 1 RM on each lift to ensure that the person is indeed working above 80%, a rule of thumb widely accepted by many authors and coaches is that individuals should perform between 3 and 12 repetitions maximum (3 to 12 RM) for adequate strength gains. For example, if a person is training with a resistance of 120 pounds and cannot lift it more than 12 times, the training stimulus is adequate for strength development.

Once the person can lift the resistance more than 12 times, the resistance should be increased by 5 to 10 pounds and the person again should build up to 12 repetitions. If training is conducted with more than 12 repetitions, primarily muscular endurance will be developed.

Strength research indicates that the closer a person trains to the 1 RM, the greater are the strength gains. A disadvantage of working constantly at or near the 1 RM is that it increases the risk for injury.

Highly trained athletes seeking maximum strength development often use 1 to 6 repetitions maximum. Working around 10 repetitions maximum seems to produce the best results in terms of muscular hypertrophy.

Body builders tend to work with moderate resistance levels (60% to 85% of the 1 RM) and perform 8 to 20 repetitions to near fatigue. A foremost objective of body building is to increase muscle size. Moderate resistance promotes blood flow to the muscles, "pumping up the muscles" (also known as "the pump") and making them look much larger than they are in a relaxed state.

From a health-fitness point of view, 8 to 12 repetitions maximum are ideal for adequate development. We live in a dynamic world in which muscular strength and endurance are both required to lead an enjoyable life. Therefore, working near a 10 repetition threshold seems best to improve overall performance.

Sets

In strength training a **set** is the number of repetitions performed for a given exercise. For example, a person lifting 120 pounds eight times has performed one set of eight repetitions (1 × 8 × 120).

When working with 8 to 12 repetitions maximum, three sets per exercise are recommended. Because of the characteristics of muscle fiber, the number of sets that can be done is limited. As the number of sets increases, so does the amount of muscle fatigue and subsequent recovery time. Therefore, strength gains may be lessened by performing too many sets.

A recommended program for beginners in their first year of training is three heavy sets, up to the maximum number of repetitions, preceded by one or two light warm-up sets using about 50% of the 1 RM (no warm-up sets are necessary for subsequent exercises that use the same muscle group). Because of the lower resistances used in body building, four to eight sets can be done for each exercise.

To avoid muscle soreness and stiffness, new participants ought to build up gradually to the three sets of maximal repetitions. This can be done by performing only one set of each exercise with a lighter resistance on the first day, two sets of each exercise on the second day — one light and the second with the regular resistance — and three sets on the third day — one light and two heavy. After that, a person should be able to do all three heavy sets.

The time necessary to recover between sets depends mainly on the resistance used during each set. In strength training, the energy to lift heavy weights is derived primarily from the ATP-CP or phosphagen system (see Chapter 7 discussion on energy production). Ten seconds of maximal exercise pretty much depletes the CP stores in the exercised muscle(s). These stores are replenished in about 3 minutes of recovery.

Based on this principle, a rest period of about 3 minutes between sets is necessary for people who are trying to maximize their strength gains. Individuals training for health-fitness purposes might allow 2 minutes of rest between sets. Body builders should rest no more than a minute to maximize the "pumping" effect.

The exercise program will be more time-effective by alternating two or three exercises that require different muscle groups, called **circuit training**. In this way, an individual will not have to wait 2 to 3 minutes before proceeding to a new set on a different exercise. For example, bench press, leg extensions, and abdominal crunches may be combined so the person can go almost directly from one set to the next.

> One strength-training session per week is sufficient to maintain strength.

Frequency of Training

Strength training should be done either through a total body workout three times a week, or more frequently if using a split body routine (upper body one day, lower body the next). After a maximum strength workout, the muscles should be rested for about 2 to 3 days to allow adequate recovery. If not completely recovered in 2 to 3 days, the person most likely is overtraining and therefore not reaping the full benefits of the program. In that case, the person should do fewer sets or exercises than in the previous workout. A summary of strength training guidelines for health-fitness purposes is provided in Figure 4.11.

To achieve significant strength gains, a minimum of 8 weeks of consecutive training is necessary. After achieving an ideal strength level, one training session per week will be sufficient to maintain the new strength level.

Mode:	8 to 10 isotonic strength-training exercises involving the body's major muscle groups.
Resistance:	Enough resistance to perform 8 to 12 repetitions to near fatigue.
Sets:	A minimum of one set.
Frequency:	At least two times per week.

Source: "The Recommended Quantity and Quality of Exercise for Developing and Maintaining Cardiorespiratory and Muscular Fitness in Healthy Adults by the American College of Sports Medicine," *Medicine Science in Sports and Exercise*, 22 (1990), 265–274.

Figure 4.11 • *Strength training guidelines.*

Frequency of strength training for body builders varies from person to person. Because they use moderate resistances, daily or even two-a-day workouts are common. The frequency depends on the amount of resistance, number of sets performed per session, and the person's ability to recover from the previous exercise bout (see Table 4.5). The latter often is dictated by level of conditioning.

Table 4.5 — *Guidelines for Various Strength Training Programs*

Strength Training Program	Resistance	Sets	Rest Between Sets*	Frequency (workouts per week)**
Health fitness	8–12 reps max	3	2 min	2–3
Maximal strength	1–6 reps max	3–6	3 min	2–3
Muscular endurance	10–30 reps	3–6	2 min	3–6
Body building	8–20 reps near max	3–8	0–1 min	4–12

* Recovery between sets can be decreased by alternating exercises that use different muscle groups.

** Weekly training sessions can be increased by using a split body routine.

TERMS

Resistance Amount of weight that is lifted.

Set Number of repetitions performed for a given exercise.

Circuit training Alternating exercises by performing them in sequence of three to six or more.

● Plyometrics

Strength, speed, and explosiveness are all crucial for success in athletics. All three of these factors are enhanced with a progressive resistance training program, but greater increases in speed and explosiveness are thought possible with plyometric training.

Plyometric exercise is defined best as explosive jump training, incorporating speed and strength training to enhance explosiveness. The objective is to generate the greatest amount of force in the shortest time. A sound strength base is necessary before attempting plyometric exercises.

Plyometric training is popular in sports that require powerful movements, such as basketball, volleyball, sprinting, jumping, and tumbling. A typical plyometric exercise involves jumping off and back onto a box, attempting to rebound as quickly as possible on each jump. Box heights are increased progressively from about 12" to 22".

The bounding action attempts to take advantage of the stretch-recoil and stretch reflex characteristics of muscle. The rapid stretch applied to the muscle during ground contact is thought to augment muscle contraction, leading to more explosiveness. Plyometrics can be used, too, for strengthening upper body muscles. An example is push-ups with a forceful extension of the arms to drive the hands (and body) completely off the floor during each repetition.

A drawback of plyometric training is the higher risk for injuries compared to conventional modes of progressive resistance training. The potential for injury escalates as the box height increases.

Plyometric training requires powerful movements.

● Strength Training Exercises

The two strength training programs introduced next provide a complete body workout. The major muscles of the human body referred to in the exercises are pointed out in Figure 4.12.

Only a minimum of equipment is required for the first program, Strength Training Exercises Without Weights (Exercises 1 through 12). This program can be conducted within the walls of your own home. Your body weight is used as the primary resistance for most exercises. A few exercises call for a friend's help or some basic implements from around your house, to provide greater resistance.

Strength Training Exercises with Weights (Exercises 13 through 32), require machines such as those shown in the accompanying photographs. These exercises can be conducted on either fixed-resistance or variable-resistance equipment. Many of these exercises also can be performed with free weights. The first 12 exercises (13 to 24) are recommended to get a complete workout. You can do these exercises as circuit training. If time is a factor, as a minimum, perform the first eight (13 through 20) exercises. Exercises 25 to 32 are supplemental or can be used to replace some of the basic 12 (Exercise 25 or 26 for 13, 27 for 14, 28 for 17, 29 for 18, 30 for 21, 31 or 32 for 23).

● Setting Up Your Own Strength-Training Program

Depending on the facilities available, you can choose one of the training programs outlined in this chapter. Once you begin your strength-training program, you may use the form provided in Figure 4.13 to keep a record of your training sessions.

The resistance and the number of repetitions you use with your program should be based on whether you want to increase muscular strength or muscular endurance. Do up to 12 repetitions maximum for strength gains, and more than 12 for muscular endurance. For most people, three training sessions per week on nonconsecutive days is an ideal arrangement for proper development.

Because both strength and endurance are required in daily activities, three sets of about 12 repetitions maximum for each exercise are recommended. In doing this, you will obtain good strength gains and yet be close to the endurance threshold. If you are training for reasons other than health fitness, a summary of the guidelines is provided in Table 4.5.

Perhaps the only exercise that calls for more than 12 repetitions is the abdominal group of exercises. The abdominal muscles are considered primarily anti-gravity or postural muscles. Hence, a little more endurance may be required. When doing abdominal work, most people perform about 20 repetitions.

If time is a concern in completing a strength training exercise program, the American College of Sports Medicine[15] recommends as a minimum: (a) one set of 8 to 12 repetitions performed to near fatigue, and (b) 8 to 10 exercises involving the major muscle groups of the body, conducted twice a week. The recommendation is based on research showing that this training generates 70% to 80% of the improvements reported in other programs using three sets of about 10 RM.

TERMS **Plyometric exercise** Explosive jump training, incorporating speed and strength training to enhance explosiveness.

Notes

1. W. J. Evans, "Exercise, Nutrition and Aging," *Journal of Nutrition*, 122 (1992), 796–801.
2. W. W. Campbell, M. C. Crim, V. R. Young, and W. J. Evans, "Increased Energy Requirements and Changes in Body Composition with Resistance Training in Older Adults," *American Journal of Clinical Nutrition*, 60 (1994), 167–175.
3. P. E. Allsen, *Strength Training* (Dubuque, IA: Kendall/Hunt Publishing Company, 1996).
4. J. L. Hesson, *Weight Training for Life* (Englewood, CO: Morton Publishing, 1995).
5. R. A. Faulkner, E. J. Sprigings, A. McQuarrie, and R. D. Bell, "A Partial Curl-Up Protocol for Adults Based on Analysis of Two Procedures," *Canadian Journal of Sports Science*, 14 (1989), 135–141.
6. P. A. Macfarlane, "Out with the Sit-Up, in with the Curl-Up!" *JOPERD*, 64 (1993), 62–66.
7. D. Knudson and D. Johnston, "Validity and Reliability of a Bench Trunk-Curl-Up test of Abdominal Endurance," *Journal of Strength and Conditioning Research*, 9 (1995), 165–169.
8. R. Kjorstad. "Validity of Two Field Tests of Abdominal Strength and Muscular Endurance," Unpublished Master's Thesis, Boise State University, 1997.
9. T. McNeill, D. Warwick, G. Anderson, and A. Schultz, "Trunk Strengths in Attempted Flexion, Extension, and Lateral Bending in Healthy Subjects and Patients with Low-Back Pain Disorders," *Spine*, 5 (1980), 529–536.
10. L. D. Robertson and H. Magnusdottir, "Evaluation of Criteria Associated with Abdominal Fitness Testing," *Research Quarterly for Exercise and Sport*, 58 (1987), 355–359.
11. Macfarlane.
12. Kjorstad.
13. G. L. Hall, R. K. Hetzler, D. Perrin, and A. Weltman, "Relationship of Timed Sit-Up Tests to Isokinetic Abdominal Strength," *Research Quarterly for Exercise and Sport*, 63 (1992), 80–84.
14. W. W. K. Hoeger, D. R. Hopkins, S. L. Barette, and D. F. Hale, "Relationship Between Repetitions and Selected Percentages of One Repetition Maximum: A Comparison Between Untrained and Trained Males and Females," *Journal of Applied Sport Science Research*, 4:2 (1990), 47-51.
15. "The Recommended Quantity and Quality of Exercise for Developing and Maintaining Cardiorespiratory and Muscular Fitness in Healthy Adults," *Medicine and Science in Sports and Exercise*, 22 (1990), 265–274.

Suggested Readings

Allsen, P. E. *Strength Training*. Dubuque IA: Kendall/Hunt Publishing, 1996.

Fox, E. L., R. W. Bowers, and M. L. Fossand. *The Physiological Basis for Exercise and Sport*. Philadelphia: Saunders College Publishing, 1993.

Getchell, B. *Physical Fitness: A Way of Life*. New York: Macmillan, 1992.

Hesson, J. L. *Weight Training for Life*. Englewood, CO: Morton Publishing, 1991.

Heyward, V. H. *Advanced Fitness Assessment & Exercise Prescription*. Champaign, IL: Human Kinetics, 1991.

Hoeger, W. W. K., and S. A. Hoeger. *Principles and Labs for Fitness and Wellness: A Personalized Program*. Englewood, CO: Morton Publishing, 1997.

McArdle, W. D., F. I. Katch, and V. L. Katch. *Exercise Physiology: Energy, Nutrition and Human Performance*. Philadelphia: Lea and Febiger, 1995.

O'Shea, J. P. *Scientific Principles and Methods of Strength Fitness*. Reading, MA: Addison-Wesley, 1976.

Silvester, L. J. *Weight Training for Strength and Fitness*. Boston: Jones and Bartlett Publishers, 1992.

Temporalis
(closes jaw)

Masseter
(flexes jaw)
(closes)

Sterno-cleido-mastoid
(rotates head)

Intercostals
(breathing)

Pectoralis minor
(abducts ribs)

Biceps brachii
(flexes elbow)

Serratus
(adducts shoulder)

Rectus abdominus

Deep flexors
(flexes fingers)

Internal oblique
(flattens abdomen)

Tendons from
forearm flexors
to fingers

Sartorius
(rotates thigh)

Rectus femoris
(extends knee)

Gastrocnemius
(points toe, flexes knee)

Soleus
(points toe)

Tendons of toes

Frontalis
(raises eyebrow)

Orbicularis oculi
(closes eye)

Orbicularis oris
(purses lips)

Throat muscles
(aids swallowing)

Pectoralis major
(adducts arm)

Deltoid
(abducts arm)

Brachialis
(flexes arm)

External oblique
(flattens abdomen)

Superficial flexors
(flexes fingers)

Vastus lateralis
(extends knee)

Vastus medialis
(extends knee)

Tibialis anterior
(raises feet)

Splenius capitus

Sternomastoid

Trapezius

Deltoid

Triceps

Latissimus dorsi

Serratus posterior
inferior

Extensors
of forearm

Gluteus
maximus

Tendons
from forearm,
extensors
to fingers

Biceps femoris

Semitendonosus

Gastrocnemius

Tendon of Achilles

THE MUSCULAR SYSTEM

From *Basic Physiology and Anatomy* by E. Chaffee and F. Lytle (Philadelphia: Lippincott Co., 1980). Reproduced by permission.

Figure 4.12 ● *Major muscles of the human body.*

Name _____

Date									
Exercise	St/Reps/Res*	St/Reps/Res*	St/Reps/Res*	St/Reps/Res*	St/Reps/Res*	St/Reps/Res*	St/Reps/Res*	St/Reps/Res*	St/Reps/Res*

*St/Reps/Res = Sets, Repetitions, and Resistance (e.g., 1/6/125 = 1 set of 6 repetitions with 125 pounds)

Figure 4.13 • *Strength training record form.*

Name _____

Date									
Exercise	St/Reps/Res*	St/Reps/Res*	St/Reps/Res*	St/Reps/Res*	St/Reps/Res*	St/Reps/Res*	St/Reps/Res*	St/Reps/Res*	St/Reps/Res*

*St/Reps/Res = Sets, Repetitions, and Resistance (e.g., 1/6/125 = 1 set of 6 repetitions with 125 pounds)

Figure 4.13 ● Strength training record form.

Strength-Training Exercise without Weights

Step-Up

Action   Step up and down using a box or chair approximately 12 to 15 inches high (a). Conduct one set using the same leg each time you go up, and then conduct a second set using the other leg. You also could alternate legs on each step-up cycle. You may increase the resistance by holding an object in your arms (b). Hold the object close to the body to avoid increased strain in the lower back.

Muscles Developed   Gluteal muscles, quadriceps, gastrocnemius, and soleus

High-Jumper

Action   Start with the knees bent at approximately 150° (a) and jump as high as you can, raising both arms simultaneously (b).

Muscles Developed   Gluteal muscles, quadriceps, gastrocnemius, and soleus

Push-Up

Action   Maintaining your body as straight as possible (a), flex the elbows, lowering the body until you almost touch the floor (b), then raise yourself back up to the starting position. If you are unable to perform the push-up as indicated, decrease the resistance by supporting the lower body with the knees rather than the feet (c) or using an incline plane and supporting your hands at a higher point than the floor (d). If you wish to increase the resistance, have someone else add resistance to your shoulders as you are coming back up (e).

Muscles Developed   Triceps, deltoid, pectoralis major, erector spinae, and abdominals

4 Abdominal Crunch and Bent-Leg Curl-Up

Action Start with your head and shoulders off the floor, arms crossed on your chest, and knees slightly bent (a). The greater the flexion of the knee, the more difficult the curl-up. Now curl up to about 30° (**abdominal crunch** — illustration b) or curl up all the way (**bent-leg curl-up** — illustration c), then return to the starting position without letting the head or shoulders touch the floor or allowing the hips to come off the floor. If you allow the hips to raise off the floor and the head and shoulders to touch the floor, you most likely will "swing up" on the next crunch or curl-up, which minimizes the work of the abdominal muscles. If you cannot curl up with the arms on the chest, place the hands by the side of the hips or even help yourself up by holding on to your thighs (illustrations d and e). Do not perform the curl-up exercise with your legs completely extended, as this will strain the lower back. For additional resistance during the abdominal crunch, have a partner add slight resistance to your shoulders as you "crunch up."

Muscles Developed Abdominal muscles and hip flexors

NOTE: The bent-leg curl-up exercise should be used only by individuals of at least average fitness without a history of lower back problems. New participants and those with a history of lower back problems should use the abdominal crunch exercise in its place.

5 Leg Curl

Action Lie on the floor face down. Cross the right ankle over the left heel (a). Apply resistance with your right foot while you bring the left foot up to 90° at the knee joint (b). Apply enough resistance so the left foot can only be brought up slowly. Repeat the exercise, crossing the left ankle over the right heel.

Muscles Developed Hamstrings (and quadriceps)

6 Modified Dip

Action Place your hands and feet on opposite chairs with knees slightly bent (make sure that the chairs are well stabilized). Dip down at least to a 90° angle at the elbow joint, then return to the initial position. To increase the resistance, have someone else hold you down by the shoulders on the way up (see illustration c). You may also perform this exercise using a gymnasium bleacher or box and with the help of a partner, as illustrated in photo d.

Muscles Developed Triceps, deltoid, and pectoralis major

7   Pull-Up

Action   Suspend yourself from a bar with a pronated (thumbs in) grip (a). Pull your body up until your chin is above the bar (b), then lower the body slowly to the starting position. If you are unable to perform the pull-up as described, either have a partner hold your feet to push off and facilitate the movement upward (illustrations c and d) or use a lower bar and support your feet on the floor (e).

Muscles Developed   Biceps, brachioradialis, brachialis, trapezius, and latissimus dorsi

8   Arm Curl

Action   Using a palms-up grip, start with the arm completely extended, and with the aid of a sandbag or bucket filled (as needed) with sand or rocks (a), curl up as far as possible, then return to the initial position (b). Repeat the exercise with the other arm.

Muscles Developed   Biceps, brachioradialis, and brachialis

9   Heel Raise

Action   From a standing position with feet flat on the floor (a), raise and lower your body weight by moving at the ankle joint only (b). For added resistance, have someone else hold your shoulders down as you perform the exercise.

Muscles Developed   Gastrocnemius and soleus

10 Leg Abduction and Adduction

Action   Both participants sit on the floor. The person on the left places the feet on the inside of the other person's feet. Simultaneously, the person on the left presses the legs laterally (to the outside — abduction), while the person on the right presses the legs medially (adduction). Hold the contraction for 5 to 10 seconds. Repeat the exercise at all three angles, and then reverse the pressing sequence. The person on the left places the feet on the outside and presses inward, while the person on the right presses outward.

Muscles Developed   Hip abductors (rectus femoris, sartori, gluteus medius and minimus), and adductors (pectineus, gracilis, adductor magnus, adductor longus, and adductor brevis)

11 Reverse Crunch

Action   Lie on your back with arms crossed on your chest and knees and hips flexed at 90° (a). Now attempt to raise the pelvis off the floor by lifting vertically from the knees and lower legs (b). This is a challenging exercise that may be difficult for beginners to perform.

Muscles Developed   Abdominals

12 Pelvic Tilt

Action   Lie flat on the floor with the knees bent at about a 90° angle (a). Tilt the pelvis by tightening the abdominal muscles, flattening your back against the floor, and raising the lower gluteal area ever so slightly off the floor (b). Hold the final position for several seconds. The exercise can also be performed against a wall (c).

Areas Stretched   Low-back muscles and ligaments

Areas Strengthened   Abdominal and gluteal muscles

Strength-Training Exercises with Weights

Bench Press

Action Lie down on the bench with the head by the weight stack, the bench press bar above the chest, and the knees bent so the feet rest on the far end of the bench (a). Grasp the bar handles and press upward until the arms are completely extended (b), then return to the original position. Do not arch the back during this exercise.

Muscles Developed Pectoralis major, triceps, and deltoid

Leg Press

Action From a sitting position with the knees flexed at about 90° and both feet on the footrest (a), extend the legs fully (b), then return slowly to the starting position.

Muscles Developed Quadriceps and gluteal muscles

Abdominal Crunch

Action Sit in an upright position. Grasp the handles over your shoulders and crunch forward. Return slowly to the original position.

Muscles Developed Abdominals

Rowing Torso

Action Sit in the machine with your arms in front of you, elbows bent and resting against the padded bars (a). Press back as far as possible, drawing the shoulder blades together (b). Return to the original position.

Muscles Developed Posterior deltoid, rhomboids, and trapezius

17. Arm Curl

Action Using a supinated or palms-up grip, start with the arms almost completely extended (a). Curl up as far as possible (b), then return to the starting position.

Muscles Developed Biceps, brachioradialis, and brachialis

18. Leg Curl

Action Lie with the face down on the bench, legs straight, and place the back of the feet under the padded bar (a). Curl up to at least 90° (b), and return to the original position.

Muscles Developed Hamstrings

19. Seated Back

Action Sit in the machine with your trunk flexed and the upper back against the shoulder pad. Place the feet under the padded bar and hold on with your hands to the bars on the sides (a). Start the exercise by pressing backward, simultaneously extending the trunk and hip joints (b). Slowly return to the original position.

Muscles Developed Erector spinae and gluteus maximus

20. Heel Raise

Action Start with your feet either flat on the floor or the front of the feet on an elevated block (a), then raise and lower yourself by moving at the ankle joint only (b). If additional resistance is needed, you can use a squat strength-training machine.

Muscles Developed Quadriceps

21. Lat Pull-Down

Action Starting from a sitting position, hold the exercise bar with a wide grip (a). Pull the bar down until it touches the base of the neck (b), then return to the starting position. (If heavy resistance is used, stabilization of the body may be required either by using equipment as shown or by having someone else hold you down by the waist or shoulders.

Muscles Developed Latissimus dorsi, pectoralis major, and biceps

22. Rotary Torso

Action Sit upright into the machine and place the elbows behind the padded bars (a). Rotate the torso as far as possible to one side (b) and then return slowly to the starting position. Repeat the exercise to the opposite side.

Muscles Developed Internal and external obliques (abdominal muscles).

23. Triceps Extension

Action Sit in an upright position, arms up, elbows bent, and place the little finger side of the hands and wrists against the pads, palms of the hands facing each other (a). Fully extend one arm at a time (b), and then return to the original position. Repeat with the other arm.

Muscles Developed Triceps

Leg Extension

Action   Sit in an upright position with the feet under the padded bar and grasp the handles at the sides (a). Extend the legs until they are completely straight (b), then return to the starting position.

Muscles Developed   Quadriceps

Shoulder Press

Action   Sit in an upright position and grasp the bar wider than shoulder width (a). Press the bar all the way up until the arms are fully extended (b), then return to the initial position.

Muscles Developed   Triceps, deltoid, and pectoralis major

Chest Press

Action   Start with the arms up to the side, hands resting against the handle bars, and elbows bent at 90° (a). Press the movement arms forward as far as possible, leading with the elbows (b). Slowly return to the starting position.

Muscles Developed   Pectoralis major and deltoid

27 Squat

Action Sit in an upright position with the feet under the padded bar and grasp the handles at the sides (a). Extend the legs until they are completely straight (b), then return to the starting position.

Muscles Developed Quadriceps

28 Upright Rowing

Action Start with the arms extended and grip the handles with the palms down (a). Pull all the way up to the chin (b), then return to the starting position.

Muscles Developed Biceps, brachioradialis, brachialis, deltoid, and trapezius

29 Seated Leg Curl

Action Sit in the unit and place the strap over the upper thighs. With legs extended, place the back of the feet over the padded rollers (a). Flex the knees until you reach a 90° to 100° angle (b). Slowly return to the starting position.

Muscles Developed Hamstrings

30 Bent-Arm Pullover

Action Sit back into the chair and grasp the bar behind your head (a). Pull the bar over your head all the way down to your abdomen (b), and slowly return to the original position.

Muscles Developed Latissimus dorsi, pectoral muscles, deltoid, and serratus anterior

31 Triceps Extension

Action Using a palms-down grip, grasp the bar slightly closer than shoulder width, and start with the elbows almost completely bent (a). Extend the arms fully (b), then return to starting position.

Muscles Developed Triceps

32 Dip

Action Start with the elbows flexed (a), then extend the arms fully and return slowly to the initial position.

Muscles Developed Triceps, deltoid, and pectoralis major

Muscular Flexibility Assessment and Prescription

5

*F*lexibility is defined as the ability of a joint to move freely through its full range of motion. Health-care professionals and practitioners generally have underestimated and overlooked the contribution of good muscular **flexibility** to overall fitness and preventive health care. In daily life we often have to make rapid or strenuous movements we are not accustomed to making, which may cause injury. Sports medicine specialists believe that many muscular/skeletal problems and injuries are related to a lack of flexibility.

Approximately 80% of all low back problems in the United States stems from improper alignment of the vertebral column and pelvic girdle, a direct result of inflexible and weak muscles. This backache syndrome costs American industry billions of dollars each year in lost productivity, health services, and workers compensation.[1]

Objectives

- Understand the importance of muscular flexibility to adequate fitness and preventive health care.
- Identify the factors that affect muscular flexibility.
- Become familiar with a battery of muscular flexibility tests to assess overall body flexibility (Modified Sit-and-Reach Test, Total Body Rotation Test, Shoulder Rotation Test).
- Learn to interpret flexibility test results according to health fitness and physical fitness standards.
- Define ballistic stretching, slow-sustained stretching, and proprioceptive neuromuscular facilitation stretching.
- Understand the factors that contribute to the development of muscular flexibility.
- Be introduced to a program for the prevention and rehabilitation of low back pain.

Photo by Doug Olmstead. Courtesy of United Spirit Association, Sunnyvale, CA.

Improving and maintaining good range of motion in the joints is important to enhance the quality of life. Participating in a regular flexibility program will help a person maintain good joint mobility, increase resistance to muscle injury and soreness, prevent low-back and other spinal column problems, improve and maintain good postural alignment, promote proper and graceful body movement, improve personal appearance and self-image, and help to develop and maintain motor skills throughout life. In addition, flexibility exercises have been prescribed successfully to treat dysmenorrhea[2] (painful menstruation) and general neuromuscular tension (stress).

Further, **stretching** exercises, in conjunction with calisthenics, are helpful in warm-up routines to prepare the human body for more vigorous aerobic or strength-training exercises, as well as cool-down routines following exercise to help the person return to a normal resting state. Fatigued muscles tend to contract to a shorter than average resting length, and stretching exercises help fatigued muscles reestablish their normal resting length.

Similar to muscular strength, good range of motion is critical in older life. Because of a lack of flexibility, some older adults are unable to perform simple daily tasks such as bending forward or turning. Many older adults do not turn their head or rotate their trunk to look over their shoulder but, rather, step around 90° to 180° to see behind them.

Physical activity and exercise also can be hampered severely by lack of good range of motion.

Lack of physical conditioning frequently leads to chronic back pain.

Because of the pain involved with activity, older people who have tight hip flexors (muscles) cannot jog or walk very far. A vicious circle then ensues, because the condition usually worsens with further inactivity. A simple stretching program can alleviate or prevent this problem and help people return to an exercise program.

● Factors Affecting Flexibility

Total range of motion around a joint is highly specific and varies from one joint to another (hip, trunk, shoulder), as well as from one individual to the next. Muscular flexibility relates primarily to genetic factors and to physical activity. Beyond that, factors such as joint structure, ligaments, tendons, muscles, skin, tissue injury, adipose tissue (fat), body temperature, age, and sex influence range of motion about a joint. Because of the specificity of flexibility, indicating what constitutes an ideal level of flexibility is difficult. Nevertheless, flexibility is important to health and independent living.

Plastic elongation is permanent lengthening of soft tissue.
Elastic elongation is the temporary lengthening of soft tissue.

The range of motion about a given joint depends mostly on the structure of that joint. Greater range of motion, however, can be attained through plastic and elastic elongation. **Plastic elongation** is the permanent lengthening of soft tissue. Even though joint capsules, ligaments, and tendons are basically non-elastic, they can undergo plastic elongation. This permanent lengthening, accompanied by increases in range of motion, is best attained through slow-sustained stretching exercises.

Elastic elongation is the temporary lengthening of soft tissue. Muscle tissue has elastic properties and responds to stretching exercises by undergoing elastic or temporary lengthening. Elastic elongation increases the extensibility of the muscles.

Changes in muscle temperature can increase or decrease flexibility by as much as 20%. Properly warmed-up individuals have better flexibility than non-warmed-up people. Cool temperatures have the opposite effect, impeding joint range of motion. Because of the effects of temperature on muscular flexibility, many people prefer to do their stretching exercises after the aerobic phase of their workout. Aerobic activities raise body temperature, facilitating plastic elongation.

Another factor that influences flexibility is the amount of adipose (fat) tissue in and around joints and muscle tissue. A lot of adipose tissue not only increases resistance to movement but the added bulk also hampers joint mobility because of the contact between body surfaces.

On the average, women have more flexibility than men do, and they seem to retain this advantage throughout life. Aging does decrease the extensibility of soft tissue, though, resulting in less flexibility in both sexes.

The two most significant contributors to lower flexibility levels are sedentary living and lack of exercise. With less physical activity muscles lose their elasticity, and tendons and ligaments tighten and shorten. Inactivity also tends to be accompanied by an increase in adipose tissue, which further decreases joint range of motion. Finally, injury to muscle tissue and tight skin from excessive scar tissue have negative effects on joint range of motion.

● Assessment of Flexibility

Most of the flexibility tests developed over the years are specific to certain sports and are not practical for the general population. Their application in health and fitness programs is limited. For example, the Front-to-Rear Splits Test and the Bridge-Up Test have applications in sports such as gymnastics and several track-and-field events, but they do not represent actions most people encounter in daily life.

Because of the lack of practical flexibility tests, most health/fitness centers have relied strictly on the Sit-and-Reach Test as an indicator of overall flexibility.

This test measures flexibility of the hamstring muscles (back of the thigh) and, to a lesser extent, the lower back muscles.

Flexibility is joint-specific, and a lot of flexibility in one joint does not necessarily indicate the same is true in other joints. Therefore, two additional tests — indicators of everyday movements such as reaching, bending, and turning — are included to determine your flexibility profile. These tests are the Total Body Rotation Test and the Shoulder Rotation Test.

The Sit-and-Reach Test has been modified from the traditional test. Unlike the traditional Sit-and-Reach Test, arm and leg lengths are taken into consideration to determine the score (see Figure 5.1). In the original Sit-and-Reach Test, the 15" mark of the yardstick used to measure flexibility always is set at the edge of the box where the feet are placed. This does not take into consideration an individual with long arms and/or short legs or one with short arms and/or long legs.[3,4,5] All other factors being equal, an individual with longer arms or shorter legs, or both, receives a better rating because of the structural advantage.

The procedures and norms for the battery of flexibility tests are described in Figures 5.1 through 5.3 and Tables 5.1 through 5.3. For the flexibility profile, instead of a choice of tests, you should take all three tests.

> **TERMS**
>
> **Flexibility** The ability of a joint to move freely through its full range of motion.
>
> **Stretching** Moving the joints beyond the accustomed range of motion.
>
> **Plastic elongation** Permanent lengthening of soft tissue.
>
> **Elastic elongation** Temporary lengthening of soft tissue.

Front-to-Rear Splits (a) and Bridge-Up (b) tests.

MODIFIED SIT-AND-REACH TEST

To perform this test, you will need the Acuflex I* Sit-and-Reach Flexibility Tester, or you may simply place a yardstick on top of a box approximately 12" or 30 cm high.

1. Warm up properly before the first trial.

2. Remove your shoes for the test. Sit on the floor with the hips, back, and head against a wall; the legs fully extended; and the bottom of the feet against the Acuflex I or sit-and-reach box.

3. Place the hands one on top of the other, and reach forward as far as possible without letting the head and back come off the wall (the shoulders may be rounded as much as possible, but neither the head nor back should come off the wall at this time). The technician then can slide the reach indicator on the Acuflex I (or yardstick) along the top of the box until the end of the indicator touches the participant's fingers. The indicator then must be held firmly in place throughout the rest of the test.

4. Now your head and back can come off the wall. Gradually reach forward three times, the third time stretching forward as far as possible on the indicator (or yardstick) and holding the final position for at least 2 seconds. Be sure that during the test you keep the backs of the knees flat against the floor.

Determining the starting position for the Modified Sit-and-Reach Test.

5. Record the final number of inches reached to the nearest one-half inch or centimeter.

You are allowed two trials, and an average of the two scores is used as the final test score. The respective percentile ranks and fitness categories for this test are given in Tables 5.1 and 5.4.

*The Acuflex I Flexibility Tester for the Modified Sit-and-Reach Test can be obtained from Figure Finder Collection, Novel Products, P. O. Box 408, Rockton, IL 61072-0480. Phone: 800-323-5143, FAX 815-624-4866.

Figure 5.1 ● *Procedure for the Modified Sit-and-Reach Test.*

Table 5.1 *Percentile Ranks for the Modified Sit-and-Reach Test*

	MEN									WOMEN							
Percentile Rank	**Age Category**								**Percentile Rank**	**Age Category**							
	≤18		19–35		36–49		≥50			≤18		19–35		36–49		≥50	
	in.	cm	in.	cm	in.	cm	in.	cm		in.	cm	in.	cm	in.	cm	in.	cm
99	20.8	52.8	20.1	51.1	18.9	48.0	16.2	41.1	99	22.6	57.4	21.0	53.3	19.8	50.3	17.2	43.7
95	19.6	49.8	18.9	48.0	18.2	46.2	15.8	40.1	95	19.5	49.5	19.3	49.0	19.2	48.8	15.7	39.9
90	18.2	46.2	17.2	43.7	16.1	40.9	15.0	38.1	90	18.7	47.5	17.9	45.5	17.4	44.2	15.0	38.1
80	17.8	45.2	17.0	43.2	14.6	37.1	13.3	33.8	80	17.8	45.2	16.7	42.4	16.2	41.1	14.2	36.1
70	16.0	40.6	15.8	40.1	13.9	35.3	12.3	31.2	70	16.5	41.9	16.2	41.1	15.2	38.6	13.6	34.5
60	15.2	38.6	15.0	38.1	13.4	34.0	11.5	29.2	60	16.0	40.6	15.8	40.1	14.5	36.8	12.3	31.2
50	14.5	36.8	14.4	36.6	12.6	32.0	10.2	25.9	50	15.2	38.6	14.8	37.6	13.5	34.3	11.1	28.2
40	14.0	35.6	13.5	34.3	11.6	29.5	9.7	24.6	40	14.5	36.8	14.5	36.8	12.8	32.5	10.1	25.7
30	13.4	34.0	13.0	33.0	10.8	27.4	9.3	23.6	30	13.7	34.8	13.7	34.8	12.2	31.0	9.2	23.4
20	11.8	30.0	11.6	29.5	9.9	25.1	8.8	22.4	20	12.6	32.0	12.6	32.0	11.0	27.9	8.3	21.1
10	9.5	24.1	9.2	23.4	8.3	21.1	7.8	19.8	10	11.4	29.0	10.1	25.7	9.7	24.6	7.5	19.0
05	8.4	21.3	7.9	20.1	7.0	17.8	7.2	18.3	05	9.4	23.9	8.1	20.6	8.5	21.6	3.7	9.4
01	7.2	18.3	7.0	17.8	5.1	13.0	4.0	10.2	01	6.5	16.5	2.6	6.6	2.0	5.1	1.5	3.8

  High physical fitness standard   Health fitness standard

TOTAL BODY ROTATION TEST

An Acuflex II* Total Body Rotation Flexibility Tester or a measuring scale with a sliding panel is needed to administer this test. The Acuflex II or scale is placed on the wall at shoulder height and should be adjustable to accommodate individual differences in height. If you need to build your own scale, use two measuring tapes and glue them above and below the sliding panel centered at the 15" (38 cm) mark. Each tape should be at least 30" (76 cm) long. If no sliding panel is available, simply tape the measuring tapes onto a wall. A line also must be drawn on the floor and centered with the 15" (38 cm) mark.

1. Warm up properly before beginning this test.

2. Stand sideways, an arm's length away from the wall, with the feet straight ahead, slightly separated, and the toes right up to the corresponding line drawn on the floor. Hold out the arm opposite to the wall horizontally from the body, making a fist with the hand. The Acuflex II, measuring scale, or tapes should be shoulder height at this time.

3. Rotate the trunk, the extended arm going backward (always maintaining a horizontal plane) and making contact with the panel, gradually sliding it forward as far as possible. If no panel is available, slide the fist alongside the tapes as far as possible. Hold the final position at least 2 seconds. Position the hand with the little finger side forward during the entire sliding movement. **Proper hand position is crucial. Many people attempt to open the hand, or push with extended fingers, or slide the panel with the knuckles — none of which is acceptable.** During the test the knees can be slightly bent, but **the feet cannot be moved, always pointing straight forward.** The body must be kept as straight (vertical) as possible.

4. Conduct the test on either the right or the left side of the body. Perform two trials on the selected side. Record the farthest point reached, measured to the nearest half inch or centimeter and held for at least 2 seconds. Use the average of the two trials as the final test score. Referring to Tables 5.2 and 5.4, determine the percentile rank and flexibility fitness classification for this test.

Acuflex II measuring device for the Total Body Rotation Test.

Homemade measuring device for the Total Body Rotation Test.

* The Acuflex II Flexibility Tester for the Total Body Rotation Test can be obtained from Figure Finder Collection, Novel Products, P.O. Box 408, Rockton, IL 61072-0408. Phone: 800-323-5143, FAX 815-624-4866.

Measuring tapes for the Total Body Rotation Test.

Total Body Rotation Test.

Proper hand position for the Total Body Rotation Test.

Figure 5.2 ● *Procedure for Total Body Rotation Test.*

Table 5.2 *Percentile Ranks for the Total Body Rotation Test*

Percentile Rank	Left Rotation								Right Rotation							
	≤18		19–35		36–49		≥50		≤18		19–35		36–49		≥50	
	in.	cm	in.	cm	in.	cm	in.	cm	in.	cm	in.	cm	in.	cm	in.	cm
MEN																
99	29.1	73.9	28.0	71.1	26.6	67.6	21.0	53.3	28.2	71.6	27.8	70.6	25.2	64.0	22.2	56.4
95	26.6	67.6	24.8	63.0	24.5	62.2	20.0	50.8	25.5	64.8	25.6	65.0	23.8	60.5	20.7	52.6
90	25.0	63.5	23.6	59.9	23.0	58.4	17.7	45.0	24.3	61.7	24.1	61.2	22.5	57.1	19.3	49.0
80	22.0	55.9	22.0	55.9	21.2	53.8	15.5	39.4	22.7	57.7	22.3	56.6	21.0	53.3	16.3	41.4
70	20.9	53.1	20.3	51.6	20.4	51.8	14.7	37.3	21.3	54.1	20.7	52.6	18.7	47.5	15.7	39.9
60	19.9	50.5	19.3	49.0	18.7	47.5	13.9	35.3	19.8	50.3	19.0	48.3	17.3	43.9	14.7	37.3
50	18.6	47.2	18.0	45.7	16.7	42.4	12.7	32.3	19.0	48.3	17.2	43.7	16.3	41.4	12.3	31.2
40	17.0	43.2	16.8	42.7	15.3	38.9	11.7	29.7	17.3	43.9	16.3	41.4	14.7	37.3	11.5	29.2
30	14.9	37.8	15.0	38.1	14.8	37.6	10.3	26.2	15.1	38.4	15.0	38.1	13.3	33.8	10.7	27.2
20	13.8	35.1	13.3	33.8	13.7	34.8	9.5	24.1	12.9	32.8	13.3	33.8	11.2	28.4	8.7	22.1
10	10.8	27.4	10.5	26.7	10.8	27.4	4.3	10.9	10.8	27.4	11.3	28.7	8.0	20.3	2.7	6.9
05	8.5	21.6	8.9	22.6	8.8	22.4	0.3	0.8	8.1	20.6	8.3	21.1	5.5	14.0	0.3	0.8
01	3.4	8.6	1.7	4.3	5.1	13.0	0.0	0.0	6.6	16.8	2.9	7.4	2.0	5.1	0.0	0.0
WOMEN																
99	29.3	74.4	28.6	72.6	27.1	68.8	23.0	58.4	29.6	75.2	29.4	74.7	27.1	68.8	21.7	55.1
95	26.8	68.1	24.8	63.0	25.3	64.3	21.4	54.4	27.6	70.1	25.3	64.3	25.9	65.8	19.7	50.0
90	25.5	64.8	23.0	58.4	23.4	59.4	20.5	52.1	25.8	65.5	23.0	58.4	21.3	54.1	19.0	48.3
80	23.8	60.5	21.5	54.6	20.2	51.3	19.1	48.5	23.7	60.2	20.8	52.8	19.6	49.8	17.9	45.5
70	21.8	55.4	20.5	52.1	18.6	47.2	17.3	43.9	22.0	55.9	19.3	49.0	17.3	43.9	16.8	42.7
60	20.5	52.1	19.3	49.0	17.7	45.0	16.0	40.6	20.8	52.8	18.0	45.7	16.5	41.9	15.6	39.6
50	19.5	49.5	18.0	45.7	16.4	41.7	14.8	37.6	19.5	49.5	17.3	43.9	14.6	37.1	14.0	35.6
40	18.5	47.0	17.2	43.7	14.8	37.6	13.7	34.8	18.3	46.5	16.0	40.6	13.1	33.3	12.8	32.5
30	17.1	43.4	15.7	39.9	13.6	34.5	10.0	25.4	16.3	41.4	15.2	38.6	11.7	29.7	8.5	21.6
20	16.0	40.6	15.2	38.6	11.6	29.5	6.3	16.0	14.5	36.8	14.0	35.6	9.8	24.9	3.9	9.9
10	12.8	32.5	13.6	34.5	8.5	21.6	3.0	7.6	12.4	31.5	11.1	28.2	6.1	15.5	2.2	5.6
05	11.1	28.2	7.3	18.5	6.8	17.3	0.7	1.8	10.2	25.9	8.8	22.4	4.0	10.2	1.1	2.8
01	8.9	22.6	5.3	13.5	4.3	10.9	0.0	0.0	8.9	22.6	3.2	8.1	2.8	7.1	0.0	0.0

▨ High physical fitness standard   ▨ Health fitness standard

SHOULDER ROTATION TEST

This test can be done using the Acuflex III* Flexibility Tester, which consists of a shoulder caliper and a measuring device for shoulder rotation. If unavailable, you can construct your own device quite easily. The caliper can be built with three regular yardsticks. Nail and glue two of the yardsticks at one end at a 90° angle, and use the third one as the sliding end of the caliper. Construct the rotation device by placing a 60" (150 cm) measuring tape on an aluminum or wood stick, starting at about 6" (15 cm) from the end of the stick.

1. Warm up before the test.

2. Using the shoulder caliper, measure the biacromial width to the nearest fourth inch or half centimeter (use the top scale on the Acuflex III). Measure biacromial width between the lateral edges of the acromion processes of the shoulders.

Measuring biacromial width.

Starting position for the Shoulder Rotation Test (note the reverse grip used for this test).

3. Place the Acuflex III or homemade device behind the back and **use a reverse grip (thumbs out)** to hold on to the device. Place the right hand next to the zero point of the scale or tape (lower scale on the Acuflex III) and hold it firmly in place throughout the test. Place the left hand on the other end of the measuring device, as wide as needed.

4. Standing straight up and extending both arms to full length, with elbows locked, slowly bring the measuring device over the head until it reaches forehead level. For subsequent trials, depending on the resistance encountered when rotating the shoulders, move the left grip in ½" to 1" (1 to 2 cm) at a time, and repeat the task until you no longer can rotate the shoulders without undue strain or start bending the elbows to do so. Always keep the right-hand grip against the zero point of the scale. Measure the last successful trial to the nearest half inch or centimeter. Take this measurement right at the inner edge of the left hand on the side of the little finger.

6. Determine the final score for this test by subtracting the biacromial width from the best score (shortest distance) between both hands on the rotation test. For example, if the best score is 35" and the biacromial width is 15", the final score is 20" (35 − 15 = 20). Using Tables 5.3 and 5.4, determine the percentile rank and flexibility fitness classification for this test.

Shoulder Rotation Test.

* The Acuflex III Flexibility Tester for the Shoulder Rotation Test can be obtained from Figure Finder Collection, Novel Products, Inc., P. O. Box 408, Rockton, IL 61072-0408. Phone: (800) 323-5143, FAX 815-624-4866.

Figure 5.3 ● *Procedure for the Shoulder Rotation Test.*

Table 5.3 — Percentile Ranks for the Shoulder Rotation Test

Percentile Rank	≤18 in.	≤18 cm	19–35 in.	19–35 cm	36–49 in.	36–49 cm	≥50 in.	≥50 cm
MEN								
99	2.2	5.6	−1.0	−2.5	18.1	46.0	21.5	54.6
95	15.2	38.6	10.4	26.4	20.4	51.8	27.0	68.6
90	18.5	47.0	15.5	39.4	20.8	52.8	27.9	70.9
80	20.7	52.6	18.4	46.7	23.3	59.2	28.5	72.4
70	23.0	58.4	20.5	52.1	24.7	62.7	29.4	74.7
60	24.2	61.5	22.9	58.2	26.6	67.6	29.9	75.9
50	25.4	64.5	24.4	62.0	28.0	71.1	30.5	77.5
40	26.3	66.8	25.7	65.3	30.0	76.2	31.0	78.7
30	28.2	71.6	27.3	69.3	31.9	81.0	31.7	80.5
20	30.0	76.2	30.1	76.5	33.3	84.6	33.1	84.1
10	33.5	85.1	31.8	80.8	36.1	91.7	37.2	94.5
05	34.7	88.1	33.5	85.1	37.8	96.0	38.7	98.3
01	40.8	103.6	42.6	108.2	43.0	109.2	44.1	112.0
WOMEN								
99	2.6	6.6	−2.4	−6.1	11.5	29.2	13.1	33.3
95	8.0	20.3	6.2	15.7	15.4	39.1	16.5	41.9
90	10.7	27.2	9.7	24.6	16.8	42.7	20.9	53.1
80	14.5	36.8	14.5	36.8	19.2	48.8	22.5	57.1
70	16.1	40.9	17.2	43.7	21.5	54.6	24.3	61.7
60	19.2	48.8	18.7	47.5	23.1	58.7	25.1	63.8
50	21.0	53.3	20.0	50.8	23.5	59.7	26.2	66.5
40	22.2	56.4	21.4	54.4	24.4	62.0	28.1	71.4
30	23.2	58.9	24.0	61.0	25.9	65.8	29.9	75.9
20	25.0	63.5	25.9	65.8	29.8	75.7	31.5	80.0
10	27.2	69.1	29.1	73.9	31.1	79.0	33.1	84.1
05	28.0	71.1	31.3	79.5	33.4	84.8	34.1	86.6
01	32.5	82.5	37.1	94.2	34.9	88.6	35.4	89.9

▨ High physical fitness standard
▨ Health fitness standard

Modified Sit-and-Reach Test.

Interpreting Flexibility Test Results

After obtaining your scores and fitness ratings for each test, you can determine the fitness category for each flexibility test using the guidelines given in Table 5.4. You should also look up the number of points assigned for each fitness category in this table. The overall flexibility fitness classification is obtained by totaling the number of points from all three tests and using the ratings given in Table 5.5. You can use Figure 5.4 to record your flexibility fitness results. If you test your flexibility more than once, additional space is provided in this figure to record three separate sets of data. You also should record your overall flexibility results in the fitness and wellness profile given in Appendix A.

Principles of Muscular Flexibility Prescription

Even though genetics play a crucial role in body flexibility, range of joint mobility can be increased and maintained through a regular flexibility exercise program. Because range of motion is highly specific to each body part (ankle, trunk, shoulder), a comprehensive stretching program should include all body parts and follow the basic guidelines for flexibility development.

Table 5.4 — Flexibility Fitness Categories According to Percentile Ranks

Percentile Rank	Fitness Category	Points
≥90	Excellent	5
70–80	Good	4
50–60	Average	3
30–40	Fair	2
≤20	Poor	1

Table 5.5 — Overall Flexibility Fitness Category

Total Points	Flexibility Category
≥13	Excellent
10–12	Good
7–9	Average
4–6	Fair
≤3	Poor

Name: _____ Age: _____ Sex: _____

Date: _____

Test	Score	Fitness Category	Points
Modified Sit-and-Reach			
Total Body Rotation ☐ Right ☐ Left			
Shoulder Rotation			

Total Points: _____

Overall Flexibility Category: _____

Date: _____

Test	Score	Fitness Category	Points
Modified Sit-and-Reach			
Total Body Rotation ☐ Right ☐ Left			
Shoulder Rotation			

Total Points: _____

Overall Flexibility Category: _____

Date: _____

Test	Score	Fitness Category	Points
Modified Sit-and-Reach			
Total Body Rotation ☐ Right ☐ Left			
Shoulder Rotation			

Total Points: _____

Overall Flexibility Category: _____

Figure 5.4 ● *Muscular flexibility report.*

The overload and specificity of training principles discussed in conjunction with strength development in Chapter 4 apply as well to the development of muscular flexibility. To increase the total range of motion of a joint, the specific muscles surrounding that joint have to be stretched progressively beyond their accustomed length. The principles of mode, intensity, repetitions, and frequency of exercise also can be applied to flexibility programs.

Mode of Training

Three modes of stretching exercises can increase flexibility:

1. Ballistic stretching.
2. Slow-sustained stretching.
3. Proprioceptive neuromuscular facilitation stretching.

Although research has indicated that all three types of stretching are effective in improving flexibility, each technique has certain advantages.

Ballistic (or dynamic) **stretching** exercises are done with jerky, rapid, and bouncy movements that provide the necessary force to lengthen the muscles. This type of stretching helps to develop flexibility, but the ballistic actions may cause muscle soreness and injury from small tears to the soft tissue.

Precautions must be taken not to overstretch ligaments, because they undergo plastic or permanent elongation. If the stretching force cannot be controlled, as in fast, jerky movements, ligaments easily can be overstretched. This, in turn, leads to excessively loose joints, increasing the risk for injuries, including joint dislocation and **subluxation** (partial dislocation). Slow-ballistic stretching (instead of jerky, rapid, and bouncy movements), however, is quite effective in developing flexibility and can be performed safely by most individuals.

With the **slow-sustained stretching** technique, muscles are lengthened gradually through a joint's complete range of motion, and the final position is held for a few seconds. A slow-sustained stretch causes the muscles to relax and thereby achieve greater length. This type of stretch causes little pain and has a low risk for injury. Slow-sustained stretching exercises are the most frequently used and recommended for flexibility development programs.

Proprioceptive neuromuscular facilitation (PNF) stretching has become more popular in the last few years. This technique, based on a "contract and relax" method, requires the assistance of another person. The procedure is as follows:

1. The person assisting with the exercise provides initial force by pushing slowly in the direction of the desired stretch. This first stretch does not cover the entire range of motion.

2. The person being stretched then applies force in the opposite direction of the stretch, against the assistant, who tries to hold the initial degree of stretch as close as possible. An isometric contraction is being performed at that angle.

3. After 4 or 5 seconds of isometric contraction, the muscle being stretched is relaxed completely. The assistant then increases the degree of stretch slowly to a greater angle.

Proprioceptive neuromuscular facilitation (PNF) stretching technique (a) isometric phase; (b) stretching phase.

TERMS

Ballistic stretching Exercises done with jerky, rapid, bouncy movements, or slow-short and sustained movements.

Subluxation Partial dislocation of a joint.

Slow-sustained stretching Exercises in which the muscles are lengthened gradually through a joint's complete range of motion.

Proprioceptive neuromuscular facilitation (PNF) A stretching technique involving systematic contraction and relaxation of muscles.

4. The isometric contraction is repeated for another 4 or 5 seconds, following which the muscle is relaxed again. The assistant then can increase the degree of stretch slowly one more time. Steps 1 through 4 are repeated two to five times, until the exerciser feels mild discomfort. On the last trial the final stretched position should be held for several seconds.

Theoretically, with the PNF technique, the isometric contraction helps relax the muscle being stretched, which results in greater muscle length. Some fitness leaders believe PNF is more effective than slow-sustained stretching. Another benefit of PNF is an increase in strength of the muscle(s) being stretched. Recent research showed an approximate 17% and 35% increase in absolute strength and muscular endurance, respectively, in the hamstring muscle group through 12 weeks of PNF stretching.[6] The results were consistent in both men and women. These increases are attributed to the isometric contractions performed during PNF. The disadvantages are more pain with PNF, a second person, preferably, has to assist, and more time is necessary to conduct each session.

Intensity of Exercise

The **intensity**, or degree of stretch, when doing flexibility exercises, should be only to a point of mild discomfort. Pain does not have to be part of the stretching routine. Excessive pain is an indication that the load is too high and may lead to injury.

All stretching should be done to slightly below the pain threshold. As participants reach this point, they should try to relax the muscle being stretched as much as possible. After completing the stretch, the body part is brought back gradually to the starting point.

Repetitions

The time required for an exercise session for flexibility development is based on the number of repetitions and the length of time each repetition (final stretched position) is held. The general recommendation is that each exercise be done four or five times, holding the final position each time about 10 to 30 seconds.

As flexibility increases, a person can gradually increase the time each repetition is held, to a maximum of 1 minute. Individuals who are susceptible to flexibility injuries, however, should limit each stretch to 20 seconds.

Frequency of Exercise

Flexibility exercises should be conducted five to six times a week in the early stages of the program. After a minimum of 6 to 8 weeks of almost daily stretching, flexibility levels can be maintained with only two or three sessions per week, doing about three repetitions of 10 to 15 seconds each. Figure 5.5 summarizes the flexibility development guidelines.

● When to Stretch?

Many people do not differentiate a warm-up from stretching. Warming up means starting a workout slowly with walking, slow jogging, or light calisthenics. Stretching implies movement of joints through their range of motion.

Before performing flexibility exercises, the muscles should be warmed up properly. Failing to warm up increases the risk for muscle pulls and tears. Surveys have shown that individuals who stretch before workouts without an adequate warm-up actually have a higher rate of injuries than those who do not stretch at all.

A good time to do flexibility exercises is after aerobic workouts. Higher body temperature in itself helps to increase joint range of motion. Muscles also are fatigued following exercise. A fatigued muscle tends to shorten, which can lead to soreness and spasms. Stretching exercises help fatigued muscles reestablish their normal resting length and prevent unnecessary pain.

● Flexibility Exercises

To improve body flexibility, each major muscle group should be subjected to at least one stretching exercise.

Mode	Static stretching or proprioceptive neuromuscular facilitation (PNF) to include every major joint of the body
Intensity	Stretch to the point of mild discomfort
Repetitions	Repeat each exercise three to five times and hold the final stretched position for 10 to 30 seconds
Frequency	At least 3 days per week

Source: ACSM's Guidelines for Exercise Testing and Prescription. (Baltimore: Williams & Wilkins, 1995).

Figure 5.5 ● *Guidelines for flexibility development.*

A complete set of exercises for developing muscular flexibility is presented at the end of this chapter.

You may not be able to hold a final stretched position with some of these exercises (examples: lateral head tilts and arm circles), but you still should perform the exercise through the joint's full range of motion. Depending on the number and length of repetitions, a complete workout will last between 15 and 30 minutes.

● Preventing and Rehabilitating Low Back Pain

Few people make it through life without having low back pain at some point. An estimated 75 million Americans currently suffer from chronic low back pain each year. About 80% of the time, backache syndrome is preventable and is caused by: (a) physical inactivity, (b) poor postural habits and body mechanics, and (c) excessive body weight.

Lack of physical activity is the most common reason for chronic low back pain. Deterioration or weakening of the abdominal and gluteal muscles, along with tightening of the lower back (erector spine) muscles, brings about an unnatural forward tilt of the pelvis (Figure 5.6). This tilt puts extra pressure on the spinal vertebrae, causing pain in the lower back. Accumulation of fat around the midsection of the body contributes to the forward tilt of the pelvis, which further aggravates the condition.

> Faulty posture and weak and inelastic muscles are the leading causes of chronic low-back problems in the United States.

Low back pain frequently is associated with faulty posture and improper body mechanics (body positions in all of life's daily activities, including sleeping, sitting, standing, walking, driving, working, and exercising). Incorrect posture and poor mechanics, as explained in Figure 5.7, increase strain not only on the lower back but on many other bones, joints, muscles, and ligaments as well.

Low back pain can be reduced greatly by including some specific stretching and strengthening exercises in the regular fitness program. In most cases back pain is present only with movement and physical activity. If the pain is severe and persists even at rest, the first step is to consult a physician, who can rule out any disc damage and most likely will prescribe proper bed rest using several pillows under the knees for leg support (see Figure 5.7). This position helps release muscle spasms by stretching the muscles involved. In addition, a physician may prescribe a muscle relaxant or anti-inflammatory medication (or both) and some type of physical therapy.

Once a person is pain-free in the resting state, he or she needs to start correcting the muscular imbalance by stretching the tight muscles and strengthening the weak ones. Stretching exercises always are performed first.

Several exercises for preventing and rehabilitating the backache syndrome are given at the end of this chapter. These exercises can be done twice or more daily when a person has back pain. Under normal circumstances, doing these exercises three to four times a week is enough to prevent the syndrome.

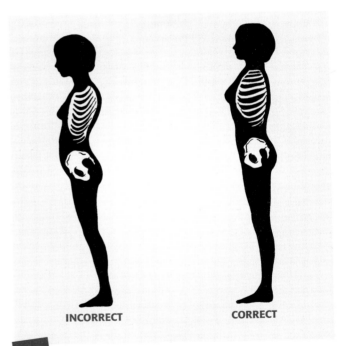

INCORRECT   CORRECT

Figure 5.6 ● *Incorrect and correct pelvic alignment.*

Intensity Degree of stretch when doing flexibility exercises.

Notes

1. S. A. Plowman, "Physical Fitness and Healthy Low Back Function," *President's Council on Physical Fitness and Sports: Physical Activity and Fitness Research Digest*, Series 1 (3):3, 1993.
2. American College of Obstetricians and Gynecologists, *Guidelines for Exercise During Pregnancy*, 1994.
3. W. W. K. Hoeger and D. R. Hopkins, "A Comparison Between the Sit and Reach and the Modified Sit and Reach in the Measurement of Flexibility in Women," *Research Quarterly for Exercise and Sport*, 63:191-195.
4. W. W. K. Hoeger, D. R. Hopkins, S. Button, and T. A. Palmer, "Comparing the Sit and Reach with the Modified Sit and Reach in Measuring Flexibility in Adolescents," *Pediatric Exercise Science*, 2 (1990), 156-162.
5. D. R., Hopkins and W. W. K. Hoeger, "A Comparison of the Sit and Reach and the Modified Sit and Reach in the Measurement of Flexibility for Males," *Journal of Applied Sports Science Research*, 6 (1992), 7-10.
6. J. Kokkonen and S. Lauritzen, "Isotonic Strength and Endurance Gains Through PNF Stretching," *Medicine and Science in Sports and Exercise*, 27 (1995), S22:127.

Suggested Readings

Billing, H., and E. Loewendahl. *Mobilization of the Human Body.* Palo Alto, CA: Stanford University Press, 1949.

Chapman, E. A., H. A. deVries, and R. Swezey. "Joint Stiffness: Effects of Exercise on Young and Old Men." *Journal of Gerontology* 27 (1972), 218-221.

Dickerson, R. V. "The Specificity of Flexibility." *Research Quarterly,* 33 (1962), 222-229.

Fleishman, E. A. *Examiners Manual for Basic Fitness Tests.* Englewood Cliffs, NJ: Prentice-Hall, 1964.

Heyward, V. H. *Advanced Methods for Physical Fitness Assessment and Exercise Prescription.* Champaign, IL: Human Kinetic Publishers, 1991.

Hoeger, W. W. K., S. Button, D. R. Hopkins, and T. A. Palmer. "Relationship Among Four Selected Flexibility Tests for High School-Age Students." *Northwest Journal for Health, Physical Education, Recreation and Dance,* 1:2 (1989), 6-10.

Hoeger, W. W. K., and D. R. Hopkins. "Assessing Muscular Flexibility." *Fitness Management,* 6:2 (1990), 34-36, 42.

Holt, L. E., T. M. Travis, and T. Okita. "Comparative Study of Three Stretching Techniques." *Perceptual and Motor Skills,* 31 (1970), 611-616.

Johnson, B. L., and J. K. Nelson. *Practical Measurements for Evaluation in Physical Education.* Minneapolis: Burgess Publishing, 1979.

Sapega, A. A., T. C. Quedenfeld, R. A. Moyer, and R. A. Butler. "Biophysical Factors in Range-of-Motion Exercise." *Physician and Sportsmedicine,* 9 (1981), 57-65.

Wright, V., and R. J. Johns. "Physical Factors Concerned with Stiffness of Normal and Diseased Joints." *Bulletin of Johns Hopkins Hospital,* 106 (1960), 215-231.

Your back and how to care for it

Whatever the cause of low back pain, part of its treatment is the correction of faulty posture. But good posture is not simply a matter of "standing tall." It refers to correct use of the body at all times. In fact, for the body to function in the best of health it must be so used that no strain is put upon the muscles, joints, bones, and ligaments. To prevent low back pain, avoiding strain must become a way of life, practiced while lying, sitting, standing, walking, working, and exercising. When body position is correct, internal organs have enough room to function normally and blood circulates more freely.

With the help of this guide, you can begin to correct the positions and movements which bring on or aggravate backache. Particular attention should be paid to the positions recommended for resting, since it is possible to strain the muscles of the back and neck even while lying in bed. By learning to live with good posture, under all circumstances, you will gradually develop the proper carriage and stronger muscles needed to protect and support your hard-working back.

HOW TO STAY ON YOUR FEET WITHOUT TIRING YOUR BACK

To prevent strain and pain in everyday activities, it is restful to change from one task to another before fatigue sets in. Housewives can lie down between chores; others should check body position frequently, drawing in the abdomen, flattening the back, bending the knees slightly.

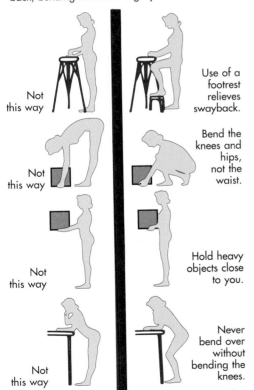

Not this way

Not this way

Not this way

Not this way

Use of a footrest relieves swayback.

Bend the knees and hips, not the waist.

Hold heavy objects close to you.

Never bend over without bending the knees.

CHECK YOUR CARRIAGE HERE

In correct, fully erect posture, a line dropped from the ear will go through the tip of the shoulder, middle of hip, back of kneecap, and front of anklebone.

Incorrect
Lower back is arched or hollow.

Incorrect
Upper back is stooped, lower back is arched, abdomen sags.

Incorrect
Note how, in strained position pelvis tilts forward, chin is out, and ribs are down, crowding internal organs.

Correct
In correct position, chin is in, head up back flattened, pelvis held straight.

To find the correct standing position: Stand one foot away from wall. Now sit against wall, bending knees slightly. Tighten abdominal and buttock muscles. This will tilt the pelvis back and flatten the lower spine. Holding this position, inch up the wall to standing position, by straightening the legs. Now walk around the room, maintaining the same posture. Place back against wall again to see if you have held it.

HOW TO SIT CORRECTLY

A back's best friend is a straight, hard chair. If you can't get the chair you prefer, learn to sit properly on whatever chair you get. <u>To correct sitting position from forward slump:</u> Throw head well back, then bend it forward to pull in the chin. This will straighten the back. Now tighten abdominal muscles to raise the chest. Check position frequently.

Relieve strain by sitting well forward, flatten back by tightening abdominal muscles, and cross knees.

Use of footrest relieves swayback. Aim is to have knees higher than hips.

Correct way to sit while driving, close to pedals. Use seat belt or hard backrest, available commercially.

TV slump leads to "dowager's hump," strains neck and shoulders.

If chair is too high, swayback is increased.

Keep neck and back in as straight a line as possible with the spine. Bend forward from hips.

Driver's seat too far from pedals emphasizes curve in lower back.

Strained reading position. Forward thrusting strains muscles of neck and head.

Figure 5.7 ● *Exercises to alleviate low back pain.*

HOW TO PUT YOUR BACK TO BED

For proper bed posture, a firm mattress is essential. Bed-boards, sold commercially, or devised at home, may be used with soft mattresses. Bedboards, preferably, should be made of 3/4 inch plywood. Faulty sleeping positions intensify sway-back and result not only in backache but in numbness, tingling, and pain in arms and legs.

Incorrect:
Lying flat on back makes swayback worse.

Correct:
Lying on side with knees bent effectively flattens the back. Flat pillow may be used to support neck, especially when shoulders are broad.

Use of high pillow strains neck, arms, shoulders.

Sleeping on back is restful and correct when knees are properly supported.

Sleeping face down exaggerates swayback, strains neck and shoulders.

Raise the foot of the mattress eight inches to discourage sleeping on the abdomen.

Bending one hip and knee does not relieve sway-back.

Proper arrangement of pillows for resting or reading in bed.

A straight-back chair used behind a pillow makes a serviceable backrest.

WHEN DOING NOTHING, DO IT RIGHT

Rest is the first rule for the tired, painful back. The following positions relieve pain by taking all pressure and weight off the back and legs.

Note pillows under knees to relieve strain on spine.

For complete relief and relaxing effect, these positions should be maintained from 5 to 25 minutes.

EXERCISE — WITHOUT GETTING OUT OF BED

Exercises to be performed while lying in bed are aimed not so much at strengthening muscles as at teaching correct positioning. But muscles used correctly become stronger and in time are able to support the body with the least amount of effort.

Do all exercises in this position. Legs should not be straightened.

Bring knee up to chest. Lower slowly but do not straighten leg. Relax. Repeat with each leg 10 times.

Bring both knees slowly up to chest. Tighten muscles of abdomen, press back flat against bed. Hold knees to chest 20 seconds, then lower slowly. Relax. Repeat 5 times. This exercise gently stretches the shortened muscles of the lower back, while strengthening abdominal muscles. Clasp knees, bring them up to chest, at the same time coming to a sitting position. Rock back and forth.

RULES TO LIVE BY - FROM NOW ON

1. Never bend from the waist only; bend the hips and knees.
2. Never lift a heavy object higher than your waist.
3. Always turn and face the object you wish to lift.
4. Avoid carrying unbalanced loads; hold heavy objects close to your body.
5. Never carry anything heavier than you can manage with ease.
6. Never lift or move heavy furniture. Wait for someone to do it who knows the principles of leverage.
7. Avoid sudden movements, sudden "overloading" of muscles. Learn to move deliberately, swinging the legs from the hips.
8. Learn to keep the head in line with the spine, when standing, sitting, lying in bed.
9. Put soft chairs and deep couches on your "don't sit" list. During prolonged sitting, cross your legs to rest your back.
10. Your doctor is the only one who can determine when low back pain is due to faulty posture. He is the best judge of when you may do general exercises for physical fitness. when you do, omit any exercise which arches or overstrains the lower back: backward bends, or forward bends, touching the toes with the knees straight.
11. Wear shoes with moderate heels, all about the same height. Avoid changing from high to low heels.
12. Put a footrail under the desk, and a footrest under the crib.
13. Diaper the baby sitting next to him or her on the bed.
14. Don't stoop and stretch to hand the wash; raise the clothesbasket and lower the washline.
15. Beg or buy a rocking chair. Rocking rests the back by changing the muscle groups used.
16. Train yourself vigorously to use your abdominal muscles to flatten your lower abdomen. In time, this muscle contraction will become habitual, making you the envied possessor of a youthful body-profile!
17. Don't strain to open windows or doors.
18. For good posture, concentrate on strengthening "nature's corset" — the abdominal and buttock muscles. The pelvic roll exercise is especially recommended to correct the postural relation between the pelvis and the spine.

EXERCISE — WITHOUT ATTRACTING ATTENTION

Use these inconspicuous exercises whenever you have a spare moment during the day, both to relax tension and improve the tone of important muscle groups.

1. Rotate shoulders, forward and backward.
2. Turn head slowly side to side.
3. Watch an imaginary plane take off, just below the right shoulder. Stretch neck, follow it slowly as it moves up, around and down, disappearing below the other shoulder. Repeat, starting on left side.
4. Slowly, slowly, touch left ear to left shoulder, right ear to right shoulder. Raise both shoulders to touch ears, drop them as far down as possible.
5. At any pause in the day — waiting for an elevator to arrive, for a specific traffic light to change — pull in abdominal muscles, tighten, hold it for the count of eight without breathing. Relax slowly. Increase the count gradually after the first week, practice breathing normally with the abdomen flat and contracted. Do this sitting, standing, and walking.

Figure 5.7 • *Exercises to alleviate low back pain (continued).*

Flexibility Exercises

1 Lateral Head Tilt

Action Slowly and gently tilt the head laterally. Repeat several times to each side.

Areas Stretched Neck flexors and extensors and ligaments of the cervical spine.

2 Arm Circles

Action Gently circle your arms all the way around. Conduct the exercise in both directions.

Areas Stretched Shoulder muscles and ligaments.

3 Side Stretch

Action Stand straight up, feet separated to shoulder width, and place your hands on your waist. Now move the upper body to one side and hold the final stretch for a few seconds. Repeat on the other side.

Areas Stretched Muscles and ligaments in the pelvic region.

4 Body Rotation

Action Place your arms slightly away from your body, and rotate the trunk as far as possible, holding the final position for several seconds. Conduct the exercise for both the right and left sides of the body. You also can perform this exercise by standing about 2 feet away from the wall (back toward the wall) and then rotating the trunk, placing the hands against the wall.

Areas Stretched Hip, abdominal, chest, back, neck, and shoulder muscles; hip and spinal ligaments.

5 Chest Stretch

Action Kneel down behind a chair and place both hands on the back of the chair. Gradually push your chest downward and hold for a few seconds.

Areas Stretched Chest (pectoral) muscles and shoulder ligaments.

6 Shoulder Hyperextension Stretch

Action Have a partner grasp your arms from behind by the wrists and slowly push them upward. Hold the final position for a few seconds.

Areas Stretched Deltoid and pectoral muscles, and ligaments of the shoulder joint.

7 Shoulder Rotation Stretch

Action With the aid of surgical tubing or an aluminum or wood stick, place the tubing or stick behind your back and grasp the two ends using a reverse (thumbs-out) grip. Slowly bring the tubing or stick over your head, keeping the elbows straight. Repeat several times (bring the hands closer together for additional stretch).

Areas Stretched Deltoid, latissimus dorsi, and pectoral muscles; shoulder ligaments.

9 Heel Cord Stretch

Action Stand against the wall or at the edge of a step, and stretch the heel downward, alternating legs. Hold the stretched position for a few seconds.

Areas Stretched Heel cord (Achilles tendon), gastrocnemius and soleus muscles.

11 Sitting Adductor Stretch

Action Sit on the floor and bring your feet in close to you, allowing the soles of the feet to touch each other. Now place your forearms (or elbows) on the inner part of the thigh and push the legs downward, holding the final stretch for several seconds.

Areas Stretched Hip adductor muscles.

8 Quad Stretch

Action Lie on your side and move one foot back by flexing the knee. Grasp the front of the ankle and pull the ankle toward the gluteal region. Hold for several seconds. Repeat with the other leg.

Areas Stretched Quadriceps muscle, and knee and ankle ligaments.

10 Adductor Stretch

Action Stand with your feet about twice shoulder width and place your hands slightly above the knee. Flex one knee and slowly go down as far as possible, holding the final position for a few seconds. Repeat with the other leg.

Areas Stretched Hip adductor muscles.

12 Sit-and-Reach Stretch

Action Sit on the floor with legs together and gradually reach forward as far as possible. Hold the final position for a few seconds. This exercise also may be performed with the legs separated, reaching to each side as well as to the middle.

Areas Stretched Hamstrings and lower back muscles, and lumbar spine ligaments.

13. Triceps Stretch

Action Place the right hand behind your neck. Grasp the right arm above the elbow with the left hand. Gently pull the elbow backward. Repeat the exercise with the opposite arm.

Areas Stretched Back of upper arm (triceps muscle) and shoulder joint.

NOTE: Exercises 14 through 20 are also flexibility exercises and can be added to your stretching program.

Exercises for the Prevention and Rehabilitation of Low-Back Pain

14. Single-Knee to Chest Stretch

Action Lie down flat on the floor. Bend one leg at approximately 100° and gradually pull the opposite leg toward your chest. Hold the final stretch for a few seconds. Switch legs and repeat the exercise.

Areas Stretched Lower back and hamstring muscles, and lumbar spine ligaments.

15. Double-Knee to Chest Stretch

Action Lie flat on the floor and then curl up slowly into a fetal position. Hold for a few seconds.

Areas Stretched Upper and lower back and hamstring muscles; spinal ligaments.

16. Upper and Lower Back Stretch

Action Sit on the floor and bring your feet in close to you, allowing the soles of the feet to touch each other. Holding on to your feet, bring your head and upper chest gently toward your feet.

Areas Stretched Upper and lower back muscles and ligaments

17. Sit-and-Reach Stretch

(see Exercise 12 on page 132)

18. Gluteal Stretch

Action Sit on the floor, bend your right leg and place your right ankle slightly above the left knee. Grasp the left thigh with both hands and gently pull the leg toward your chest. Repeat the exercise with the opposite leg.

Areas Stretched Buttock area (gluteal muscles).

19 Back Extension Stretch

Action Lie face down on the floor with the elbows by the chest, forearms on the floor, and the hands beneath the chin. Gently raise the trunk by extending the elbows until you reach an approximate 90° angle at the elbow joint. Be sure the forearms remain in contact with the floor at all times. DO NOT extend the back beyond this point. Hyperextension of the lower back may lead to or aggravate an existing back problem. Hold the stretched position for about 10 seconds.

Areas Stretched Abdominal region.

Additional Benefits Restore lower back curvature.

20 Trunk Rotation and Lower Back Stretch

Action Sit on the floor and bend the right leg, placing the right foot on the outside of the left knee. Place the left elbow on the right knee and push against it. At the same time, try to rotate the trunk to the right (clockwise). Hold the final position for a few seconds. Repeat the exercise with the other side.

Areas Stretched Lateral side of the hip and thigh; trunk and lower back.

21 Pelvic Tilt

Action Lie flat on the floor with the knees bent at about a 90° angle (a). Tilt the pelvis by tightening the abdominal muscles, flattening your back against the floor, and raising the lower gluteal area ever so slightly off the floor (b). Hold the final position for several seconds. The exercise can also be performed against a wall (c).

Areas Stretched Low-back muscles and ligaments.

Areas Strengthened Abdominal and gluteal muscles.

22 Cat Stretch

Action Kneel on the floor and place your hands in front of you (on the floor) about shoulder width apart. Relax your trunk and lower back (a). Now arch the spine and pull in your abdomen as far as you can and hold this position for a few seconds (b). Repeat the exercise 4–5 times.

Areas Stretched Low back muscles and ligaments.

Areas Strengthened Abdominal and gluteal muscles.

23 Abdominal Crunch or Bent-Leg Curl-Up
(see Exercise 4 in Chapter 4, page 106)

It is important that you do not stabilize your feet when performing either of these exercises, because doing so decreases the work of the abdominal muscles. Also, remember not to "swing up" but, rather, to curl up as you perform these exercises.

Body Composition Assessment

6

Obesity is a health hazard of epidemic proportions in most developed countries around the world. An estimated 35% of the adult population in industrialized nations is obese. In the United States, 30 million people are obese. Furthermore, according to 1993 estimates, 65% of adults in the United States were at least 10% above recommended body weight. The prevalence continues to increase. When Yankee Stadium in New York was renovated several years ago, total seating capacity had to be reduced to accommodate the wider bodies of the spectators. During the last decade, the average weight of American adults increased by about 15 pounds.

Obesity by itself has been associated with several serious health problems and may account for 15% to 20% of the annual mortality rate (about 300,000 deaths) in the United States. Obesity is a risk factor for diseases of the cardiovascular system, including coronary heart disease, hypertension, congestive heart failure, high levels of blood lipids, atherosclerosis, and thromboembolitic disease.

Objectives

- Define body composition and its relationship to recommended body weight assessment.
- Identify the difference between essential and storage fat.
- Name various techniques used in assessing body composition.
- Be able to assess body composition using the skinfold thickness technique.
- Be able to assess body composition using the girth measurements technique.
- Understand the importance of waist-to-hip ratio and body mass index.
- Be able to determine recommended weight according to recommended percent body fat values.

Other research points toward a possible link between obesity and cancer of the colon, rectum, prostate, gallbladder, breast, uterus, and ovaries. In addition, obesity has been associated with diabetes, osteoarthritis, varicose veins, intermittent claudication, ruptured intervertebral discs, gallstones, gout, respiratory insufficiency, and complications during pregnancy and delivery. Furthermore, it is implicated in psychological maladjustment and a higher accidental death rate.

> During the last decade, the average weight of American adults increased by about 15 pounds.

The same is true for underweight people. Although the social pressure to be thin has retreated slightly in recent years, the pressure to attain model-like thinness is still with us and contributes to the gradual increase in the number of people who develop eating disorders (anorexia nervosa and bulimia, discussed in Chapter 8). Extreme weight loss can lead to medical conditions such as heart damage, gastrointestinal problems, shrinkage of internal organs, immune system abnormalities, disorders of the reproductive system, loss of muscle tissue, damage to the nervous system, and even death.

• What Does "Body Composition" Mean?

To understand body composition, we must recognize first that the human body consists of fat and nonfat components. The fat component usually is called fat mass or **percent body fat**. The nonfat component is termed **lean body mass**.

For many years people relied on height/weight charts to determine recommended body weight. We now know, however, that these tables can be highly inaccurate and they fail to identify critical fat values associated with higher risk for disease. The proper way to determine recommended weight is by finding out what percent of total body weight is fat and what amount is lean tissue — determining body composition.

Once the fat percentage is known, recommended body weight can be calculated from recommended

body fat. **Recommended body weight**, also called *healthy weight*, implies the absence of any medical condition that would improve with weight loss and a fat distribution pattern that is not associated with higher risk for illness.

Although various techniques for determining percent body fat were developed several years ago, many people still are unaware of these procedures and continue to depend on height/weight charts to find out their recommended body weight. The standard height/weight tables, first published in 1912, were based on average weights (including shoes and clothing) for men and women who obtained life insurance policies between 1888 and 1905. The recommended body weight on these tables is obtained according to sex, height, and frame size. Because no scientific guidelines are given to determine frame size, most people choose their frame size based on the column in which the weight comes closest to their own!

To determine whether people are truly overweight or falsely at recommended body weight, **body composition** must be established. Obesity is related to an excess of body fat. If body weight is the only criterion, an individual can easily be overweight, according to height/weight charts, yet not have too much body fat. Football players, body builders, weight lifters, and other athletes with large muscle size are typical examples. Some of these athletes who appear to be 20 or 30 pounds overweight really have little body fat.

> Recommended body weight, also called healthy weight, is defined as the body weight at which there seems to be no harm to human health.

The inaccuracy of height/weight charts was illustrated clearly when a young man who weighed about 225 pounds applied to join a city police force but was turned down without having been granted an interview. The reason? He was "too fat," according to the height/weight charts. When this young man's body composition later was assessed at a preventive medicine clinic, he was shocked to find out that only 5% of his total body weight was in the form of fat — considerably lower than the recommended standard. In the words of the technical director of the clinic, "The only way this fellow could come down to the chart's target weight would have been through surgical removal of a large amount of his muscle tissue."

At the other end of the spectrum, some people who weigh very little and may be viewed as skinny or underweight actually can be classified as obese because of their high body fat content. People who weigh as little as 100 pounds but are more than 35% fat (about one-third of their total body weight) are not uncommon. These cases are found more readily in the sedentary population and among people who are always dieting. Physical inactivity and constant negative caloric balance both lead to a loss in lean body mass (see Chapter 8). From these examples, body weight alone clearly does not always tell the true story.

● Essential and Storage Fat

Total fat in the human body is classified into two types: essential fat and storage fat. **Essential fat** is needed for normal physiological functions, and without it human health deteriorates. This type of fat is found in tissues such as muscles, nerve cells, bone marrow, intestines, heart, liver, and lungs. This essential fat constitutes about 3% of the total weight in men and 12% in women. The percentage is higher in women because it includes sex-specific fat, such as that found in the breast tissue, the uterus, and other sex-related fat deposits.

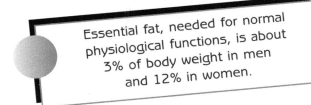

Essential fat, needed for normal physiological functions, is about 3% of body weight in men and 12% in women.

Storage fat is the fat stored in adipose tissue, mostly beneath the skin (subcutaneous fat) and around major organs in the body. This fat serves three basic functions:

1. As an insulator to retain body heat.
2. As energy substrate for metabolism.
3. As padding against physical trauma to the body.

The amount of storage fat does not differ between men and women except that men tend to store fat around the waist and women more so around the hips and thighs.

● Techniques for Assessing Body Composition

Body composition can be assessed through several procedures. The most common techniques are: (a) hydrostatic or underwater weighing, (b) skinfold thickness, (c) girth measurements, and (d) bioelectrical impedance. Because these procedures yield estimates of body fat, each technique may yield slightly different values. Therefore, when assessing body composition, the same technique should be used for pre- and post-test comparisons.

Hydrostatic Weighing

Hydrostatic weighing has been used as the "standard" of body composition. Almost all other techniques to determine body composition are validated against hydrostatic weighing. It is the most accurate technique if it is done properly and if the individual is able to perform the test adequately. The procedure requires a considerable amount of time, skill, space, and equipment and must be administered by a well-trained technician.

Because each individual assessment can take as long as 30 minutes, hydrostatic weighing is not feasible when testing a lot of people. Furthermore, the person's residual lung volume (amount of air left in the lungs following complete forceful exhalation) has to be measured before testing. If residual volume cannot be measured, as is the case in many laboratories and health/fitness centers, it can be estimated using the predicting equations, which may decrease the

TERMS

Percent body fat Total amount of fat in the body based on the person's weight; includes both essential and storage fat.

Lean body mass Body weight without body fat.

Recommended or healthy body weight Body weight at which there seems to be no harm to human health.

Body composition The fat and nonfat components of the human body; important in assessing recommended body weight.

Essential fat Minimal amount of body fat needed for normal physiological functions; constitutes about 3% of the total weight in men and 12% in women.

Storage fat Body fat in excess of the essential fat; stored in adipose tissue.

Hydrostatic weighing Underwater technique to assess body composition, including percent body fat.

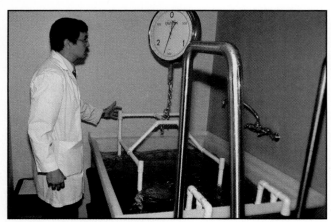

Hydrostatic weighing technique for body composition assessment.

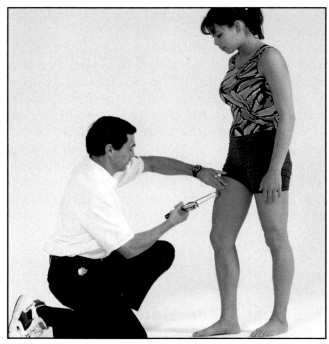

The skinfold thickness test is an anthropometric technique for assessing body composition.

accuracy of hydrostatic weighing. Also, the psychological variables in being weighed while submerged underwater makes hydrostatic weighing difficult to administer to aquaphobic people (those with a fear of water).

Because of the cost, time, and complexity of hydrostatic weighing, most health and fitness programs prefer **anthropometric measurement techniques**, which correlate quite well with hydrostatic weighing. These techniques, primarily skinfold thickness and girth measurements, allow a quick, simple, and inexpensive estimate of body composition.

Skinfold Thickness

Assessing body composition using **skinfold thickness** is based on the principle that approximately half of the body's fatty tissue is directly beneath the skin. Valid and reliable measurements of this tissue give a good indication of percent body fat.

The skinfold test is done with the aid of pressure calipers. Several sites must be measured to reflect the total percentage of fat: triceps, suprailium, and thigh skinfolds for women; and chest, abdomen, and thigh for men (see Figure 6.1). All measurements should be taken on the right side of the body.

Even with the skinfold technique, training is necessary to obtain accurate measurements. Also, different technicians may produce slightly different measurements from the same person. Therefore, the same technician should take pre- and post-measurements.

Measurements should be done at the same time of the day, preferably in the morning, as changes in water hydration from activity and exercise can affect

Various types of skinfold calipers are used to assess skinfold thickness.

skinfold girth. The procedure for assessing percent body fat using skinfold thickness is given in Figure 6.2. If skinfold calipers* are available to you, you may proceed to assess your percent body fat with the help of your instructor or an experienced technician.

---

*This instrument is available at most colleges and universities. If unavailable, you can purchase an inexpensive, yet reliable Skinfold Caliper from: Fat Control Inc., P. O. Box 10117, Towson, MD 21204, Phone (301) 296-1993.

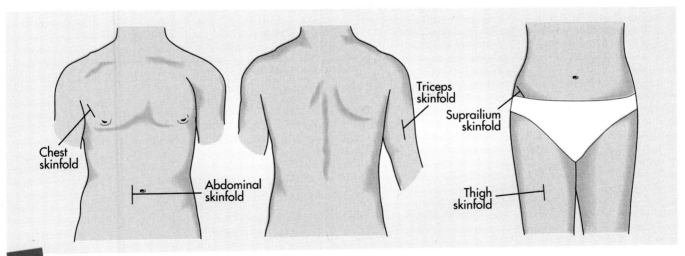

Figure 6.1 ● *Anatomical landmarks for skinfold measurements.*

TERMS

Anthropometric measurement techniques Measurement of body girths at different sites.

Skinfold thickness Technique to assess body composition, including percent body fat, by measuring the thickness of a double fold of skin at different body sites.

BODY FAT ASSESSMENT ACCORDING TO SKINFOLD THICKNESS

1. Select the proper anatomical sites. For men: chest, abdomen, and thigh. For women: triceps, suprailium, and thigh (*see* Figure 6.1). Take all measurements on the right side of the body with the person standing. The correct anatomical landmarks for skinfolds are:

    Chest: a diagonal fold halfway between the shoulder crease and the nipple.

    Abdomen: a vertical fold taken about an inch to the right of the umbilicus.

    Triceps: a vertical fold on the back of the upper arm, halfway between the shoulder and the elbow.

    Thigh: a vertical fold on the front of the thigh, midway between the knee and hip.

    Suprailium: a diagonal fold above the crest of the ilium (on the side of the hip).

2. Measure each site by grasping a double thickness of skin firmly with the thumb and forefinger, pulling the fold slightly away from the muscular tissue. Hold the calipers perpendicular to the fold, and take the measurement ½" below the finger hold. Measure each site three times, and read the values to the nearest .1 to .5 mm. Record the average of the two closest readings as the final value. Take the readings without delay to avoid excessive compression of the skinfold. Releasing and refolding the skinfold is required between readings.

3. When doing pre- and post-assessments, conduct the measurement at the same time of day. The best time is early in the morning to avoid water hydration changes resulting from activity or exercise.

4. Obtain percent fat by adding the three skinfold measurements and looking up the respective values on Table 6.1 for women, Table 6.2 for men under age 40, and Table 6.3 for men over 40.

    For example, if the skinfold measurements for an 18-year-old female are: (a) triceps = 16, (b) suprailium = 4, and (c) thigh = 30 (total = 50), the percent body fat is 20.6%

Figure 6.2 ● *Skinfold thickness procedure for body fat assessment.*

Table 6.1   *Percent Fat Estimates for Women Calculated from Triceps, Suprailium, and Thigh Skinfold Thickness*

Sum of 3 Skinfolds	AGE TO THE LAST YEAR								
	Under 22	23 to 27	28 to 32	33 to 37	38 to 42	43 to 47	48 to 52	53 to 57	Over 58
23- 25	9.7	9.9	10.2	10.4	10.7	10.9	11.2	11.4	11.7
26- 28	11.0	11.2	11.5	11.7	12.0	12.3	12.5	12.7	13.0
29- 31	12.3	12.5	12.8	13.0	13.3	13.5	13.8	14.0	14.3
32- 34	13.6	13.8	14.0	14.3	14.5	14.8	15.0	15.3	15.5
35- 37	14.8	15.0	15.3	15.5	15.8	16.0	16.3	16.5	16.8
38- 40	16.0	16.3	16.5	16.7	17.0	17.2	17.5	17.7	18.0
41- 43	17.2	17.4	17.7	17.9	18.2	18.4	18.7	18.9	19.2
44- 46	18.3	18.6	18.8	19.1	19.3	19.6	19.8	20.1	20.3
47- 49	19.5	19.7	20.0	20.2	20.5	20.7	21.0	21.2	21.5
50- 52	20.6	20.8	21.1	21.3	21.6	21.8	22.1	22.3	22.6
53- 55	21.7	21.9	22.1	22.4	22.6	22.9	23.1	23.4	23.6
56- 58	22.7	23.0	23.2	23.4	23.7	23.9	24.2	24.4	24.7
59- 61	23.7	24.0	24.2	24.5	24.7	25.0	25.2	25.5	25.7
62- 64	24.7	25.0	25.2	25.5	25.7	26.0	26.2	26.4	26.7
65- 67	25.7	25.9	26.2	26.4	26.7	26.9	27.2	27.4	27.7
68- 70	26.6	26.9	27.1	27.4	27.6	27.9	28.1	28.4	28.6
71- 73	27.5	27.8	28.0	28.3	28.5	28.8	29.0	29.3	29.5
74- 76	28.4	28.7	28.9	29.2	29.4	29.7	29.9	30.2	30.4
77- 79	29.3	29.5	29.8	30.0	30.3	30.5	30.8	31.0	31.3
80- 82	30.1	30.4	30.6	30.9	31.1	31.4	31.6	31.9	32.1
83- 85	30.9	31.2	31.4	31.7	31.9	32.2	32.4	32.7	32.9
86- 88	31.7	32.0	32.2	32.5	32.7	32.9	33.2	33.4	33.7
89- 91	32.5	32.7	33.0	33.2	33.5	33.7	33.9	34.2	34.4
92- 94	33.2	33.4	33.7	33.9	34.2	34.4	34.7	34.9	35.2
95- 97	33.9	34.1	34.4	34.6	34.9	35.1	35.4	35.6	35.9
98-100	34.6	34.8	35.1	35.3	35.5	35.8	36.0	36.3	36.5
101-103	35.2	35.4	35.7	35.9	36.2	36.4	36.7	36.9	37.2
104-106	35.8	36.1	36.3	36.6	36.8	37.1	37.3	37.5	37.8
107-109	36.4	36.7	36.9	37.1	37.4	37.6	37.9	38.1	38.4
110-112	37.0	37.2	37.5	37.7	38.0	38.2	38.5	38.7	38.9
113-115	37.5	37.8	38.0	38.2	38.5	38.7	39.0	39.2	39.5
116-118	38.0	38.3	38.5	38.8	39.0	39.3	39.5	39.7	40.0
119-121	38.5	38.7	39.0	39.2	39.5	39.7	40.0	40.2	40.5
122-124	39.0	39.2	39.4	39.7	39.9	40.2	40.4	40.7	40.9
125-127	39.4	39.6	39.9	40.1	40.4	40.6	40.9	41.1	41.4
128-130	39.8	40.0	40.3	40.5	40.8	41.0	41.3	41.5	41.8

Body density is calculated based on the generalized equation for predicting body density of women developed by A. S. Jackson, M. L. Pollock, and A. Ward. *Medicine and Science in Sports and Exercise* 12, (1980), 175–182. Percent body fat is determined from the calculated body density using the Siri formula.

Table 6.2 *Percent Fat Estimates for Men Under Age 40 Calculated from Chest, Abdomen, and Thigh Skinfold Thickness*

Sum of 3 Skinfolds	AGE TO THE LAST YEAR							
	Under 19	20 to 22	23 to 25	26 to 28	29 to 31	32 to 34	35 to 37	38 to 40
8- 10	.9	1.3	1.6	2.0	2.3	2.7	3.0	3.3
11- 13	1.9	2.3	2.6	3.0	3.3	3.7	4.0	4.3
14- 16	2.9	3.3	3.6	3.9	4.3	4.6	5.0	5.3
17- 19	3.9	4.2	4.6	4.9	5.3	5.6	6.0	6.3
20- 22	4.8	5.2	5.5	5.9	6.2	6.6	6.9	7.3
23- 25	5.8	6.2	6.5	6.8	7.2	7.5	7.9	8.2
26- 28	6.8	7.1	7.5	7.8	8.1	8.5	8.8	9.2
29- 31	7.7	8.0	8.4	8.7	9.1	9.4	9.8	10.1
32- 34	8.6	9.0	9.3	9.7	10.0	10.4	10.7	11.1
35- 37	9.5	9.9	10.2	10.6	10.9	11.3	11.6	12.0
38- 40	10.5	10.8	11.2	11.5	11.8	12.2	12.5	12.9
41- 43	11.4	11.7	12.1	12.4	12.7	13.1	13.4	13.8
44- 46	12.2	12.6	12.9	13.3	13.6	14.0	14.3	14.7
47- 49	13.1	13.5	13.8	14.2	14.5	14.9	15.2	15.5
50- 52	14.0	14.3	14.7	15.0	15.4	15.7	16.1	16.4
53- 55	14.8	15.2	15.5	15.9	16.2	16.6	16.9	17.3
56- 58	15.7	16.0	16.4	16.7	17.1	17.4	17.8	18.1
59- 61	16.5	16.9	17.2	17.6	17.9	18.3	18.6	19.0
62- 64	17.4	17.7	18.1	18.4	18.8	19.1	19.4	19.8
65- 67	18.2	18.5	18.9	19.2	19.6	19.9	20.3	20.6
68- 70	19.0	19.3	19.7	20.0	20.4	20.7	21.1	21.4
71- 73	19.8	20.1	20.5	20.8	21.2	21.5	21.9	22.2
74- 76	20.6	20.9	21.3	21.6	22.0	22.2	22.7	23.0
77- 79	21.4	21.7	22.1	22.4	22.8	23.1	23.4	23.8
80- 82	22.1	22.5	22.8	23.2	23.5	23.9	24.2	24.6
83- 85	22.9	23.2	23.6	23.9	24.3	24.6	25.0	25.3
86- 88	23.6	24.0	24.3	24.7	25.0	25.4	25.7	26.1
89- 91	24.4	24.7	25.1	25.4	25.8	26.1	26.5	26.8
92- 94	25.1	25.5	25.8	26.2	26.5	26.9	27.2	27.5
95- 97	25.8	26.2	26.5	26.9	27.2	27.6	27.9	28.3
98-100	26.6	26.9	27.3	27.6	27.9	28.3	28.6	29.0
101-103	27.3	27.6	28.0	28.3	28.6	29.0	29.3	29.7
104-106	27.9	28.3	28.6	29.0	29.3	29.7	30.0	30.4
107-109	28.6	29.0	29.3	29.7	30.0	30.4	30.7	31.1
110-112	29.3	29.6	30.0	30.3	30.7	31.0	31.4	31.7
113-115	30.0	30.3	30.7	31.0	31.3	31.7	32.0	32.4
116-118	30.6	31.0	31.3	31.6	32.0	32.3	32.7	33.0
119-121	31.3	31.6	32.0	32.3	32.6	33.0	33.3	33.7
122-124	31.9	32.2	32.6	32.9	33.3	33.6	34.0	34.3
125-127	32.5	32.9	33.2	33.5	33.9	34.2	34.6	34.9
128-130	33.1	33.5	33.8	34.2	34.5	34.9	35.2	35.5

Body density is calculated based on the generalized equation for predicting body density of men developed by A. S. Jackson and M. L. Pollock, *British Journal of Nutrition* 40, (1978) 497–504. Percent body fat is determined from the calculated body density using the Siri formula.

Table 6.3 *Percent Fat Estimates for Men Over Age 40 Calculated from Chest, Abdomen, and Thigh Skinfold Thickness*

Sum of 3 Skinfolds	AGE TO THE LAST YEAR							
	41 to 43	44 to 46	47 to 49	50 to 52	53 to 55	56 to 58	59 to 61	Over 62
8- 10	3.7	4.0	4.4	4.7	5.1	5.4	5.8	6.1
11- 13	4.7	5.0	5.4	5.7	6.1	6.4	6.8	7.1
14- 16	5.7	6.0	6.4	6.7	7.1	7.4	7.8	8.1
17- 19	6.7	7.0	7.4	7.7	8.1	8.4	8.7	9.1
20- 22	7.6	8.0	8.3	8.7	9.0	9.4	9.7	10.1
23- 25	8.6	8.9	9.3	9.6	10.0	10.3	10.7	11.0
26- 28	9.5	9.9	10.2	10.6	10.9	11.3	11.6	12.0
29- 31	10.5	10.8	11.2	11.5	11.9	12.2	12.6	12.9
32- 34	11.4	11.8	12.1	12.4	12.8	13.1	13.5	13.8
35- 37	12.3	12.7	13.0	13.4	13.7	14.1	14.4	14.8
38- 40	13.2	13.6	13.9	14.3	14.6	15.0	15.3	15.7
41- 43	14.1	14.5	14.8	15.2	15.5	15.9	16.2	16.6
44- 46	15.0	15.4	15.7	16.1	16.4	16.8	17.1	17.5
47- 49	15.9	16.2	16.6	16.9	17.3	17.6	18.0	18.3
50- 52	16.8	17.1	17.5	17.8	18.2	18.5	18.8	19.2
53- 55	17.6	18.0	18.3	18.7	19.0	19.4	19.7	20.1
56- 58	18.5	18.8	19.2	19.5	19.9	20.2	20.6	20.9
59- 61	19.3	19.7	20.0	20.4	20.7	21.0	21.4	21.7
62- 64	20.1	20.5	20.8	21.2	21.5	21.9	22.2	22.6
65- 67	21.0	21.3	21.7	22.0	22.4	22.7	23.0	23.4
68- 70	21.8	22.1	22.5	22.8	23.2	23.5	23.9	24.2
71- 73	22.6	22.9	23.3	23.6	24.0	24.3	24.7	25.0
74- 76	23.4	23.7	24.1	24.4	24.8	25.1	25.4	25.8
77- 79	24.1	24.5	24.8	25.2	25.5	25.9	26.2	26.6
80- 82	24.9	25.3	25.6	26.0	26.3	26.6	27.0	27.3
83- 85	25.7	26.0	26.4	26.7	27.1	27.4	27.8	28.1
86- 88	26.4	26.8	27.1	27.5	27.8	28.2	28.5	28.9
89- 91	27.2	27.5	27.9	28.2	28.6	28.9	29.2	29.6
92- 94	27.9	28.2	28.6	28.9	29.3	29.6	30.0	30.3
95- 97	28.6	29.0	29.3	29.7	30.0	30.4	30.7	31.1
98-100	29.3	29.7	30.0	30.4	30.7	31.1	31.4	31.8
101-103	30.0	30.4	30.7	31.1	31.4	31.8	32.1	32.5
104-106	30.7	31.1	31.4	31.8	32.1	32.5	32.8	33.2
107-109	31.4	31.8	32.1	32.4	32.8	33.1	33.5	33.8
110-112	32.1	32.4	32.8	33.1	33.5	33.8	34.2	34.5
113-115	32.7	33.1	33.4	33.8	34.1	34.5	34.8	35.2
116-118	33.4	33.7	34.1	34.4	34.8	35.1	35.5	35.8
119-121	34.0	34.4	34.7	35.1	35.4	35.8	36.1	36.5
122-124	34.7	35.0	35.4	35.7	36.1	36.4	36.7	37.1
125-127	35.3	35.6	36.0	36.3	36.7	37.0	37.4	37.7
128-130	35.9	36.2	36.6	36.9	37.3	37.6	38.0	38.5

Body density is calculated based on the generalized equation for predicting body density of men developed by A. S. Jackson and M. L. Pollock, *British Journal of Nutrition* 40 (1978), 497–504. Percent body fat is determined from the calculated body density using the Siri formula.

Girth Measurements

A simpler method to determine body fat is by measuring circumferences at various body sites. This technique requires only a standard measuring tape. Good accuracy can be achieved with little practice. The limitation is that it may not be valid for athletic individuals (men or women) who participate actively in strenuous physical activity or for people who can be classified visually as thin or obese.

The required procedure for **girth measurements** is given in Figure 6.3. Measurements for women include the upper arm, hip, and wrist; for men, the waist and wrist.

TERMS

Girth measurements Technique to assess body composition, including percent body fat, by measuring circumferences at various body sites.

BODY FAT ASSESSMENT ACCORDING TO GIRTH MEASUREMENTS

Girth Measurements for Women*

1. Using a regular tape measure, determine the following girth measurements in centimeters (cm):

   Upper Arm: take the measure halfway between the shoulder and the elbow.

   Hip: measure at the point of largest circumference.

   Wrist: take the girth in front of the bones where the wrist bends.

2. Obtain the person's age.

3. Using Table 6.4, find the girth measurement for each site and age in the lefthand columns. Look up the constant values in the righthand columns. These values will allow you to derive body density (BD) by substituting the constants in the following formula:

   BD = A − B − C + D

4. Using the derived body density, calculate percent body fat (%F) according to the following equation:

   %F = (495 ÷ BD) − 450**

   Example: Jane is 20 years old, and the following girth measurements were taken: biceps = 27 cm, hip = 99.5 cm, wrist = 15.4 cm.

Data	Constant
Upper Arm = 27 cm	A = 1.0813
Age = 20	B = .0102
Hip = 99.5 cm	C = .1206
Wrist = 15.4 cm	D = .0971

   BD = A − B − C + D
   BD = 1.0813 − .0102 − .1206 + .0971 = 1.0476

   %F = (495 ÷ BD) − 450
   %F = (495 ÷ 1.0476) − 450 = 22.5%

Girth Measurements for Men***

1. Using a regular tape measure, determine the following girth measurements in inches (the men's measurements are taken in inches as contrasted with centimeters for women):

   Waist: measure at the umbilicus (belly button).

   Wrist: measure in front of the bones where the wrist bends.

2. Subtract the wrist from the waist measurement.

3. Obtain the person's weight in pounds.

4. Look up the percent body fat (%F) in Table 6.5 by using the difference obtained in step 2 above and the person's body weight.

   Example: John weighs 160 pounds, and his waist and wrist girth measurements are 36.5 and 7.5 inches, respectively.

   Waist girth = 36.5 inches
   Wrist girth = 7.5 inches
   Difference = 29.0 inches
   Body weight = 160.0 lbs.
   %F = 22

---

* Reproduced by permission from R. B. Lambson, "Generalized Body Density Prediction Equations for Women Using Simple Anthropometric Measurements," unpublished doctoral dissertation, Brigham Young University, Provo, UT, August 1987.

** From W. E. Siri, *Body Composition From Fluid Spaces and Density* (Berkeley: University of California, Donner Laboratory of Medical Physics, 1956).

*** Table 6.5 reproduced by permission from A. G. Fisher, and P. E. Allsen, *Jogging* (Dubuque, IA: Wm. C. Brown, 1987). This table was developed according to the generalized body composition equation for men using simple measurement techniques by K. W. Penrouse, A. G Nelson, and A G. Fisher, *Medicine and Science in Sports and Exercise* 17(2):189, 1985. © American College of Sports Medicine 1985.

Figure 6.3 ● *Procedure for assessing body fat by girth measurements.*

Table 6.4 *Conversion Constants from Girth Measurements (Centimeters) to Calculate Body Density for Women*

Upper Arm (cm)	Constant A	Age	Constant B	Hip (cm)	Constant C	Hip (cm)	Constant C	Wrist (cm)	Constant D
20.5	1.0966	17	.0086	79	.0957	114.5	.1388	13.0	.0819
21	1.0954	18	.0091	79.5	.0963	115	.1394	13.2	.0832
21.5	1.0942	19	.0096	80	.0970	115.5	.1400	13.4	.0845
22	1.0930	20	.0102	80.5	.0976	116	.1406	13.6	.0857
22.5	1.0919	21	.0107	81	.0982	116.5	.1412	13.8	.0807
23	1.0907	22	.0112	81.5	.0988	117	.1418	14.0	.0882
23.5	1.0895	23	.0117	82	.0994	117.5	.1424	14.2	.0895
24	1.0883	24	.0122	82.5	.1000	118	.1430	14.4	.0908
24.5	1.0871	25	.0127	83	.1006	118.5	.1436	14.6	.0920
25	1.0860	26	.0132	83.5	.1012	119	.1442	14.8	.0933
25.5	1.0848	27	.0137	84	.1018	119.5	.1448	15.0	.0946
26	1.0836	28	.0142	84.5	.1024	120	.1454	15.2	.0958
26.5	1.0824	29	.0147	85	.1030	120.5	.1460	15.4	.0971
27	1.0813	30	.0152	85.5	.1036	121	.1466	15.6	.0983
27.5	1.0801	31	.0157	86	.1042	121.5	.1472	15.8	.0996
28	1.0789	32	.0162	86.5	.1048	122	.1479	16.0	.1009
28.5	1.0777	33	.0168	87	.1054	122.5	.1485	16.2	.1021
29	1.0775	34	.0173	87.5	.1060	123	.1491	16.4	.1034
29.5	1.0754	35	.0178	88	.1066	123.5	.1497	16.6	.1046
30	1.0742	36	.0183	88.5	.1072	124	.1503	16.8	.1059
30.5	1.0730	37	.0188	89	.1079	124.5	.1509	17.0	.1072
31	1.0718	38	.0193	89.5	.1085	125	.1515	17.2	.1084
31.5	1.0707	39	.0198	90	.1091	125.5	.1521	17.4	.1097
32	1.0695	40	,0203	90.5	.1097	126	.1527	17.6	.1109
32.5	1.0683	41	.0208	91	.1103	126.5	.1533	17.8	.1122
33	1.0671	42	.0213	91.5	.1109	127	.1539	18.0	.1135
33.5	1.0666	43	.0218	92	.1115	127.5	.1545	18.2	.1147
34	1.0648	44	.0223	92.5	.1121	128	.1551	18.4	.1160
34.5	1.0636	45	.0228	93	.1127	128.5	.1558	18.6	.1172
35	1.0624	46	.0234	93.5	.1133	129	.1563		
35.5	1.0612	47	.0239	94	.1139	129.5	.1569		
36	1.0601	48	,0244	94.5	.1145	130	.1575		
36.5	1.0589	49	.0249	95	.1151	130.5	.1581		
37	1.0577	50	.0254	95.5	.1157	131	.1587		
37.5	1.0565	51	.0259	96	.1163	131.5	.1593		
38	1.0554	52	.0264	96.5	.1169	132	.1600		
38.5	1.0542	53	.0269	97	.1176	132.5	.1606		
39	1.0530	54	.0274	97.5	.1182	133	.1612		
39.5	1.0518	55	.0279	98	.1188	133.5	.1618		
40	1.0506	56	.0284	98.5	.1194	134	.1624		
40.5	1.0495	57	.0289	99	.1200	134.5	.1630		
41	1.0483	58	.0294	99.5	.1206	135	.1636		
41.5	1.0471	59	.0300	100	.1212	135.5	.1642		
42	1.0459	60	.0305	100.5	.1218	136	.1648		
42.5	1.0448	61	.0310	101	.1224	136.5	.1654		
43	1.0434	62	.0315	101.5	.1230	137	.1660		
43.5	1.0424	63	.0320	102	.1236	137.5	.1666		
44	1.0412	64	.0325	102.5	.1242	138	.1672		
		65	.0330	103	.1248	138.5	.1678		*(Continued)*

Table 6.4 *Conversion Constants from Girth Measurements (Centimeters) to Calculate Body Density for Women (continued)*

Upper Arm (cm)	Constant A	Age	Constant B	Hip (cm)	Constant C	Hip (cm)	Constant C	Wrist (cm)	Constant D
44		66	.0335	103.5	.1254	139	.1685		
		67	.0340	104	.1260	139.5	.1691		
		68	.0345	104.5	.1266	140	.1697		
		69	.0350	105	.1272	140.5	.1703		
		70	.0355	105.5	.1278	141	.1709		
		71	.0360	106	.1285	141.5	.1715		
		72	.0366	106.5	.1291	142	.1721		
		73	.0371	107	.1297	142.5	.1728		
		74	.0376	107.5	.1303	143	.1733		
		75	.0381	108	.1309	143.5	.1739		
				108.5	.1315	144	.1745		
				109	.1321	144.5	.1751		
				109.5	.1327	145	.1757		
				110	.1333	145.5	.1763		
				110.5	.1339	146	.1769		
				111	.1345	146.5	.1775		
				111.5	.1351	147	.1781		
				112	.1357	147.5	.1787		
				112.5	.1363	148	.1794		
				113	.1369	148.5	.1800		
				113.5	.1375	149	.1806		
				114	.1382	149.5	.1812		
						150	.1818		

Bioelectrical Impedance

The **bioelectrical impedance** technique is much simpler to administer, but it does require costly equipment. In this technique the individual is hooked up to a machine and a weak electrical current (totally painless) is run through the body to analyze body composition (body fat, lean body mass, and body water). The technique is based on the principle that fat tissue is not as good a conductor of an electrical current as lean tissue is. The easier the conductance, the leaner the individual.

The accuracy of current equations used to estimate percent body fat with this technique is still questionable. More research is required before the equations approach the accuracy of hydrostatic weighing, skinfolds, or girth measurements.

An advantage of bioelectrical impedance is that results are highly reproducible. Unlike other techniques, in which experienced technicians are necessary to obtain valid results, almost anyone can administer bioelectrical impedance. And, although the test results

may not be completely accurate, this instrument is valuable in assessing body composition changes over time.

If this instrument or some other type of equipment for body composition assessment is available to you, you can use it to determine your percent body fat. You may want to compare the results with other techniques. Following all manufacturer's instructions will ensure the best possible result.

Waist-to-Hip Ratio

Scientific evidence suggests that the way people store fat affects the risk for disease. Some individuals tend to store fat in the abdominal area (called the "apple"

TERMS
Bioelectrical impedance Technique to assess body composition, including percent body fat, by running a weak electrical current through the body.

Table 6.5 Estimated Percent Body Fat for Men Obtained from Waist Minus Wrist Girth Measurements (Inches) and Body Weight shape). Others store it mainly around the hips and thighs (gluteal femoral fat or "pear" shape).

Obese individuals with a lot of abdominal fat clearly are at higher risk for coronary heart disease, congestive heart failure, hypertension, Type II diabetes (adult-onset or non-insulin-dependent diabetes), and strokes than are obese people with similar amounts of total body fat stored primarily in the hips and thighs. Relatively new evidence also indicates that, among individuals with a lot of abdominal fat, those whose fat deposits are around internal organs (visceral fat) have an even greater risk for disease than those whose abdominal fat is mainly beneath the skin (subcutaneous fat).[1]

Individuals with a lot of abdominal fat are at higher risk for coronary heart disease, congestive heart failure, hypertension, Type II diabetes, and strokes.

Because of the higher risk for disease in individuals who tend to store a lot of fat in the abdominal area, as contrasted with the hips and thighs, a **waist-to-hip ratio** test was designed by a panel of scientists appointed by the National Academy of Sciences and the Dietary Guidelines Advisory Council for the U.S. Departments of Agriculture and Health and Human Services. The waist measurement is taken at the point of smallest circumference, and the hip measurement is taken at the point of greatest circumference.

The waist-to-hip ratio differentiates the "apples" from the "pears." Most men are apples, and most women are pears. The panel recommends that men need to lose weight if the waist-to-hip ratio is 1.0 or higher. Women need to lose weight if the ratio is .85 or higher (see Table 6.6). More conservative estimates indicate that the risk starts to increase when the ratio exceeds .95 and .80 for men and women, respectively. For example, the waist-to-hip ratio for a man with a 40-inch waist and a 38-inch hip would be 1.05 (40 ÷ 38). This ratio may indicate higher risk for disease.

Body Mass Index

Another technique scientists use to determine thinness and excessive fatness is the **Body Mass Index (BMI)**. This index incorporates height and weight to estimate critical fat values at which the risk for disease increases.

BMI is calculated by dividing the weight in kilograms by the square of the height in meters or multiplying your weight in pounds by 705, dividing this figure by the square of the height in inches. For example, the BMI for an individual who weighs 172 pounds (78 kg) and is 67 inches (1.7 mts) tall would be 27 [$78 \div (1.7)^2$] or [$172 \times 705 \div (67)^2$].

According to BMI, the lowest risk for chronic disease is in the 22 to 25 range (see Table 6.7). Individuals are classified as overweight between 25 and 30. BMIs above 30 are defined as obese and below 20 as underweight.

BMI is a useful tool to screen the general population, but, similar to height/weight charts, it fails to differentiate fat from lean body mass or where most of the fat is located (waist-to-hip ratio). Using BMI, athletes with a large amount of muscle mass (body builders, football players) easily can fall in the moderate or even high-risk categories. Therefore, body

Table 6.7 *Disease Risk According to Body Mass Index (BMI)*

BMI	Disease Risk
<20.00	Moderate to Very High
20.00 to 21.99	Low
22.00 to 24.99	Very Low
25.00 to 29.99	Low
30.00 to 34.99	Moderate
35.00 to 39.99	High
≥40.00	Very High

Table 6.6 *Disease Risk According to Waist-to-Hip Ratio*

Waist-to-Hip Ratio		
Men	Women	Disease Risk
≤0.95	≤0.80	Very Low
0.96–0.99	0.81–0.84	Low
≥1.00	≥0.85	High

TERMS

Waist-to-hip ratio A test to assess potential risk for diseases associated with obesity.

Body mass index (BMI) Ratio of weight to height, used to determine thinness and fatness.

composition and waist-to-hip ratios are better procedures to determine health risk and recommended body weight.

Determining Recommended Body Weight

After finding out your percent body fat, you can determine your current body composition classification according to Table 6.8. In this table you will find the health fitness and the high physical fitness percent fat standards.

For example, the recommended health fitness fat percentage for a 20-year-old female is 28% or less. The health fitness standard is established at the point at which there seems to be no harm to health in terms of percent body fat. A high physical fitness range for this same woman would be between 18% and 23%.

The high physical fitness standard does not mean you cannot be somewhat below this number. Many highly trained male athletes are as low as 3%, and some female distance runners have been measured at 6% body fat (which may not be healthy).

Although people generally agree that the mortality rate is higher for obese people, some evidence indicates that the same is true for underweight people. "Underweight" and "thin" do not necessarily mean the same thing. The body fat of a healthy thin person

is around the high physical fitness standard, whereas an underweight person has extremely low body fat, even to the point of compromising the essential fat.

The 3% essential fat for men and 12% for women seem to be the lower limits for people to maintain good health. Below these percentages normal physiologic functions can be seriously impaired. Some experts point out that a little storage fat (over the essential fat) is better than none at all. As a result, the health and high fitness standards for percent fat in Table 6.8 are set higher than the minimum essential fat requirements, at a point beneficial to optimal health and well-being. Finally, because lean tissue decreases with age, one extra percentage point is allowed for every additional decade of life.

Your recommended body weight is computed based on the selected health or high fitness fat percentage for your age and sex. Your decision to select a "desired" fat percentage should be based on your current percent body fat and your personal health/fitness objectives. To compute your own recommended body weight:

1. Determine the pounds of body weight in fat (FW). Multiply body weight (BW) by the current percent fat (%F) expressed in decimal form (FW = BW × %F).

2. Determine lean body mass (LBM) by subtracting the weight in fat from the total body weight

Table 6.8 *Body Composition Classification According to Percent Body Fat*

			MEN			
Age	**Excellent**	**Good**		**Moderate**	**Overweight**	**Significantly Overweight**
≤19	12.0	12.1-17.0		17.1-22.0	22.1-27.0	≥27.1
20-29	13.0	13.1-18.0		18.1-23.0	23.1-28.0	≥28.1
30-39	14.0	14.1-19.0		19.1-24.0	24.1-29.0	≥29.1
40-49	15.0	15.1-20.0		20.1-25.0	25.1-30.0	≥30.1
≥50	16.0	16.1-21.5		21.1-26.0	26.1-31.0	≥31.1
			WOMEN			
Age	**Excellent**	**Good**		**Moderate**	**Overweight**	**Significantly Overweight**
≤19	17.0	17.1-22.0		22.1-27.0	27.1-32.0	≥32.1
20-29	18.0	18.1-23.0		23.1-28.0	28.1-33.0	≥33.1
30-39	19.0	19.1-24.0		24.1-29.0	29.1-34.0	≥34.1
40-49	20.0	20.1-25.0		25.1-30.0	30.1-35.0	≥35.1
≥50	21.0	21.1-26.5		26.1-31.0	31.1-36.0	≥36.1

▨ High physical fitness standard   ▨ Health fitness standard

(LBM = BW − FW). (Anything that is not fat must be part of the lean component.)

3. Select a desired body fat percentage (DFP) based on the health or high fitness standards given in Table 6.8.

4. Compute recommended body weight (RBW) according to the formula: RBW = LBM ÷ (1.0 − DFP).

As an example of these computations, a 19-year-old female who weighs 160 pounds and is 30% fat would like to know what her recommended body weight would be at 22%:

Sex: female
Age: 19
BW: 160 lbs
%F: 30% (.30 in decimal form)

1. FW = BW × %F
   FW = 160 × .30 = 48 lbs

2. LBM = BW − FW
   LBM = 160 − 48 = 112 lbs

3. DFP: 22% (.22 in decimal form)

4. RBW = LBM ÷ (1.0 − DFP)
   RBW = 112 ÷ (1.0 − .22)
   RBW = 112 ÷ (.78) = 143.6 lbs

In Figures 6.6 and 6.7 at the end of the chapter you will have the opportunity to determine your own body composition, recommended body weight, and disease risk according to waist-to-hip ratio and BMI.

Other than hydrostatic weighing, skinfold thickness seems to be the most practical and valid technique to estimate body fat. If skinfold calipers are available, use this technique to assess your percent body fat. If calipers are unavailable, estimate your percent fat according to the girth measurements technique or another technique available to you. (You may wish to use several techniques and compare the results.)

● Importance of Regular Body Composition Assessment

Children in the United States do not start with a weight problem. Although a small group struggles with weight throughout life, most are not overweight when they reach age 20.

Current trends indicate that starting at age 25, the average man and woman in the United States gains 1 pound of weight per year. Thus, by age 65,

the average American will have gained 40 pounds of weight. Because of the typical reduction in physical activity in our society, however, each year the average person also loses a half a pound of lean tissue. Therefore, over this span of 40 years there has been an actual fat gain of 60 pounds accompanied by a 20-pound loss of lean body mass[2] (see Figure 6.4). These changes cannot be detected unless body composition is assessed periodically.

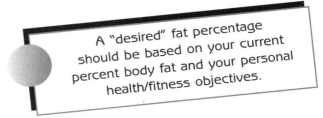

A "desired" fat percentage should be based on your current percent body fat and your personal health/fitness objectives.

If you are on a diet/exercise program, you should repeat your percent body fat assessment and recommended weight computations about once a month. This is important because lean body mass is affected by weight reduction programs and amount of physical activity. As lean body mass changes, so will your recommended body weight. To make valid comparisons, the same technique should be used between pre- and post-assessments.

Changes in body composition resulting from a weight control/exercise program were illustrated in a co-ed aerobics (aerobic dance) course taught during

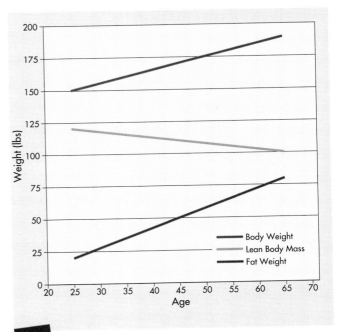

Figure 6.4 ● *Typical body composition changes for adults in the United States.*

a 6-week summer term. Students participated in aerobics routines four times a week, 60 minutes each time. On the first and last days of class, several physiological parameters, including body composition, were assessed. Students also were given information on diet and nutrition, and they basically followed their own dietary program.

At the end of the 6 weeks, the average weight loss for the entire class was 3 pounds (see Figure 6.5). But, because body composition was assessed, class members were surprised to find that the average fat loss was actually 6 pounds, accompanied by a 3-pound increase in lean body mass.

When dieting, body composition should be reassessed periodically because of the effects of negative caloric balance on lean body mass. As discussed in Chapter 8, dieting does decrease lean body mass. The loss of lean body mass can be offset or eliminated by combining a sensible diet with physical exercise.

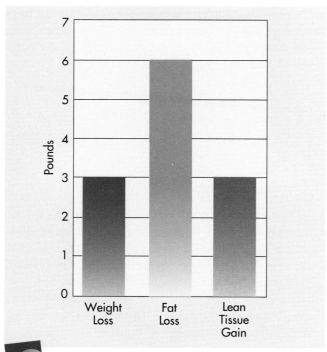

Figure 6.5 ● *Effects of a 6-week aerobics program on body composition.*

Notes

1. C. Bouchard, G. A. Bray, and V. S. Hubbard, "Basic and Clinical Aspects of Regional Fat Distribution," *American Journal of Clinical Nutrition*, 52 (1990), 946-950.
2. J. H. Wilmore, "Exercise and Weight Control: Myths, Misconceptions, and Quackery," lecture given at annual meeting of the American College of Sports Medicine, Indianapolis, June 1994.

Suggested Readings

Bouchard, C., and F. E. Johnson, Editors. *Fat Distribution During Growth and Later Health Outcomes.* New York: Alan R. Liss, 1988.

Bouchard, C., G. A. Bray, and V. S. Hubbard. "Basic and Clinical Aspects of Regional Fat Distribution." *American Journal of Clinical Nutrition*, 52 (1990), 946950.

Bray, G. A. "Pathophysiology of Obesity." *American Journal of Clinical Nutrition*, 55 (1992), 488S-494S.

Fisher, A. G., and P. E. Allsen. *Jogging.* Dubuque, IA: Wm C. Brown, 1987.

Hoeger, W. W. K., and S. A. Hoeger. *Principles and Labs for Physical Fitness & Wellness.* Englewood, CO: Morton Publishing, 1997.

Jackson, A. S., and M. L. Pollock. "Generalized Equations for Predicting Body Density of Men." *British Journal of Nutrition*, 40 (1978), 497504.

Jackson, A. S., M. L. Pollock, and A. Ward. "Generalized Equations for Predicting Body Density of Women." *Medicine and Science in Sports and Exercise*, 3 (1980), 175–182.

Lambson, R. B. *Generalized Body Density Prediction Equations for Women Using Simple Anthropometric Measurements.* Unpublished doctoral dissertation, Brigham Young University, Provo, UT, August 1987.

Penrouse, K. W., A. G. Nelson, and A. G. Fisher. "Generalized Body Composition Equation for Men Using Simple Measurement Techniques." *Medicine and Science in Sports and Exercise*, 17:2 (1985), 189.

Siri, W. E. "Body Composition from Fluid Spaces and Density." Berkeley, CA: Donner Laboratory of Medical Physics, University of California, 1956.

Stensland, S. H., and S. Margolis. "Simplifying the Calculation of Body Mass Index for Quick Reference." *Journal of the American Dietetic Association*, 90 (1990), 856.

I.　Percent Body Fat According to Skinfold Thickness

Men

Date:	_____	_____
Chest (mm):	_____	_____
Abdomen (mm):	_____	_____
Thigh (mm):	_____	_____
Total (mm):	_____	_____
Percent Fat:	_____	_____

Women

Date:	_____	_____
Triceps (mm):	_____	_____
Suprailium (mm):	_____	_____
Thigh (mm):	_____	_____
Total (mm):	_____	_____
Percent Fat:	_____	_____

II.　Percent Body Fat According to Girth Measurements

Men

Date:	_____	_____
Waist (inches):	_____	_____
Wrist (inches):	_____	_____
Difference:	_____	_____
Body Weight:	_____	_____
Percent Fat:	_____	_____

Women

Date:	_____	_____			
Upper Arm (cm):	_____	_____	Constant A =	_____	_____
Age:	_____	_____	Constant B =	_____	_____
Hip (cm):	_____	_____	Constant C =	_____	_____
Wrist (cm):	_____	_____	Constant D =	_____	_____
BD:*	_____	_____			
Percent Fat:**	_____	_____			

*Body density (BD) = A − B − C + D
**Percent Fat = (495 ÷ BD) − 450

III.　Recommended Body Weight Determination

Date:	_____	_____
Body Weight (BW):	_____	_____
Current Percent Fat (%F)*:	_____	_____
Fat Weight (FW) = BW × %F		
FW = _____ × _____ =	_____	_____
Lean Body Mass (LBM) = BW − FW		
LBM = _____ − _____ =	_____	_____
Desired Fat Percent (DFP − see Table 6.8):	_____	_____
Recommended Body Weight (RBW) = LBM ÷ (1.0 − DFP*)		
RBW = _____ ÷ (1.0 − _____) =	_____	_____

*Express percentages in decimal form (e.g., 25% = .25)

Figure 6.6 ● *Percent body fat and recommended body weight assessment (use second column for a retest or post-test).*

Waist-to-Hip Ratio

Date: _____   _____

Waist (inches):   _____   _____

Hip (inches):   _____   _____

Ratio (waist ÷ hip):   _____   _____

Disease risk: _____   _____

Body Mass Index*

Date: _____   _____

Weight (lbs):   _____   _____

Height (inches):   _____   _____

BMI:*   _____   _____

Disease risk: _____   _____

*BMI = [Weight in lbs. × 705 ÷ (Height in inches)²]
*BMI = [Weight in kgs ÷ (Height in meters)²]

Figure 6.7 • *Waist-to-hip ratio and body mass index computation.*

Nutrition for Wellness

7

*S*cientific evidence has long linked good **nutrition** to overall health and well-being. Proper nutrition means that a person's diet supplies all the essential nutrients to carry out tissue growth, repair, and maintenance. The diet also should provide enough **substrates** to produce the energy necessary for work, physical activity, and relaxation. As illustrated in Figure 7.1, the Food Guide Pyramid, these **nutrients** should be obtained from a wide variety of sources. The recommended number of servings from each food group for proper nutrition are also found in the Pyramid.

Too much or too little of any nutrient can precipitate serious health problems. The typical North American diet is too high in calories, sugar, fat, saturated fat, and sodium, and not high enough in fiber — factors that undermine good health. Food availability is not the problem. The problem is overconsumption.

According to a 1988 report on nutrition and health issued by the U. S. Surgeon General[1] — the first ever of

Objectives

- Define nutrition and describe its relationship to health and well-being.
- Become familiar with the Food Guide Pyramid and learn how to use it to achieve a balanced diet.
- Describe the functions of carbohydrates in the human body and be able to differentiate simple from complex carbohydrates.
- Describe the role and health benefits of adequate fiber in the diet.
- Describe the role of fats in the human body and be able to differentiate and characterize saturated, monounsaturated, and polyunsaturated fats.
- Describe the functions of proteins in the human body.
- Describe the role of vitamins and minerals in the human body.
- Learn to conduct a comprehensive nutrient analysis, be capable of recognizing areas of deficiencies, and be able to implement changes to improve overall nutrition.
- Understand the role of antioxidants in preventing disease.
- Be aware of guidelines for nutrient supplementation.
- Become familiar with the National Dietary Guidelines for Americans.
- Identify myths and fallacies regarding nutrition.

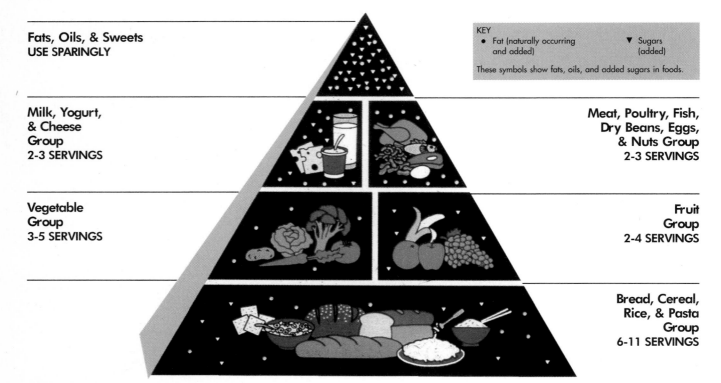

Fats, Oils, & Sweets
USE SPARINGLY

KEY
● Fat (naturally occurring and added)   ▼ Sugars (added)
These symbols show fats, oils, and added sugars in foods.

Milk, Yogurt, & Cheese Group
2-3 SERVINGS

Meat, Poultry, Fish, Dry Beans, Eggs, & Nuts Group
2-3 SERVINGS

Vegetable Group
3-5 SERVINGS

Fruit Group
2-4 SERVINGS

Bread, Cereal, Rice, & Pasta Group
6-11 SERVINGS

What counts as one serving?

Breads, Cereals, Rice, and Pasta
1 slice of bread
1/2 cup of cooked rice or pasta
1/2 cup of cooked cereal
1 ounce of ready-to-eat cereal

Vegetables
1/2 cup of chopped raw or cooked vegetables
1 cup of leafy raw vegetables

Fruits
1 piece of fruit or melon wedge
3/4 cup of juice
1/2 cup of canned fruit
1/4 cup of dried fruit

Milk, Yogurt, and Cheese
1 cup of milk or yogurt
1 1/2 to 2 ounces of cheese

Meat, Poultry, Fish, Dry Beans, Eggs, and Nuts
2 1/2 to 3 ounces of cooked lean meat, poultry, or fish
Count 1/2 cup of cooked beans, or 1 egg, or 2 tablespoons of peanut butter as 1 ounce of lean meat (about 1/3 serving)

Fats, Oils, and Sweets
LIMIT CALORIES FROM THESE especially if you need to lose weight

The amount you eat may be more than one serving. For example, a dinner portion of spaghetti would count as two or three servings of pasta.

A Closer Look at Fat and Added Sugars

The small tip of the Pyramid shows fats, oils, and sweets. These are foods such as salad dressings, cream, butter, margarine, sugars, soft drinks, candies, and sweet desserts. Alcoholic beverages are also part of this group. These foods provide calories but few vitamins and minerals. Most people should go easy on foods from this group.

Some fat or sugar symbols are shown in the other food groups. That's to remind you that some foods in these groups can also be high in fat and added sugars, such as cheese or ice cream from the milk group, or french fries from the vegetable group. When choosing foods for a healthful diet, consider the fat and added sugars in your choices from all the food groups, not just fats, oils, and sweets from the Pyramid tip.

How many servings do you need each day?

	Women & some older adults	Children, teen girls, active women, most men	Teen boys & active men
Calorie level*	about 1,600	about 2,200	about 2,800
Bread group	6	9	11
Vegetable group	3	4	5
Fruit group	2	3	4
Milk group	2–3**	2–3**	**2–3
Meat group	2, for a total of 5 ounces	2, for a total of 6 ounces	3, for a total of 7 ounces

* These are the calorie levels if you choose lowfat, lean foods from the 5 major food groups and use foods from the fats, oils, and sweets group sparingly.

** Women who are pregnant or breastfeeding, teenagers, and young adults to age 24 need 3 servings.

*Developed by the U.S. Department of Agriculture to promote a healthy diet for people in the United States.

Figure 7.1 ● *Food Guide Pyramid: A Guide to Daily Food Choices.*

its kind — diseases of dietary excess and imbalance are among the leading causes of death in the United States. Similar trends are observed in developed countries throughout the world. In the report, based on more than 2,000 scientific studies, the U.S. Surgeon General said dietary changes can bring better health to all Americans. Other surveys reveal that on a given day, nearly half of the American people eat no fruit and almost a fourth eat no vegetables.

Studies also indicate that diet and nutrition often play a crucial role in the development and progression of chronic diseases. A diet high in saturated fat and cholesterol increases the risk for atherosclerosis and coronary heart disease. In sodium-sensitive individuals, high salt intake has been linked to high blood pressure. Some researchers believe that 30% to 50% of all cancers are diet-related. Obesity, diabetes, and osteoporosis also have been associated with faulty nutrition.

An effective wellness program must incorporate current dietary recommendations to lower the risk for chronic disease. For a healthful diet:

- Eat a variety of foods.
- Avoid too much fat, saturated fat, and cholesterol.
- Eat foods with adequate starch and fiber.
- Avoid too much sugar and sodium.
- Maintain adequate calcium intake.
- Maintain recommended body weight.
- Drink alcoholic beverages in moderation, if at all.

These guidelines will be discussed throughout this chapter and in later chapters of this book.

● Nutrients

The essential nutrients the human body requires are carbohydrates, fat, protein, vitamins, minerals, and water. The first three are called fuel nutrients because they are the only substances the body uses to supply the energy (commonly measured in calories) needed for work and normal body functions. Vitamins, minerals, and water have no caloric value but still are necessary for a person to function normally and maintain good health. Many nutritionists add a seventh nutrient to this list, one that has received a great deal of attention recently: dietary fiber.

Carbohydrates, fats, proteins, and water are termed *macronutrients* because proportionately large amounts are needed daily. Vitamins and minerals are required only in small amounts. Therefore, nutritionists refer to them as *micronutrients*.

Depending on the amount of nutrients and calories, foods can be classified according to high nutrient density and low nutrient density. *High nutrient density* refers to foods that contain few or moderate calories but are packed with nutrients. Foods that have a lot of calories but few nutrients are of *low nutrient density* and commonly are called "junk food."

A **calorie** is the unit of measure indicating the energy value of food and the cost of physical activity. Technically, a kilocalorie (kcal) or large calorie is the amount of heat necessary to raise the temperature of 1 kilogram of water 1° Centigrade, but for simplification people call it a calorie rather than kcal. For example, if the caloric value of a food is 100 calories (kcal), the energy in this food would raise the temperature of 100 kilograms of water 1° Centigrade.

Carbohydrates

Carbohydrates constitute the major source of calories the body uses to provide energy for work, maintain cells, and generate heat. They also help regulate fat and metabolize protein. Each gram of carbohydrates provides the human body with 4 calories.

The major sources of carbohydrates are breads, cereals, fruits, vegetables, and milk and other dairy products. Carbohydrates are classified into simple carbohydrates and complex carbohydrates (Figure 7.2).

TERMS

Nutrition Science that studies the relationship of foods to optimal health and performance.

Nutrients Substances found in food that provide energy, regulate metabolism, and help with growth and repair of body tissues.

Substrate Substance acted upon by an enzyme (examples: carbohydrates and fats).

Calorie The amount of heat necessary to raise the temperature of one gram of water one degree Centigrade. Used to measure the energy value of food and cost of physical activity.

Carbohydrates Compounds containing carbon, hydrogen, and oxygen; the major source of energy for the human body.

Figure 7.2 • *Major types of carbohydrates.*

Simple Carbohydrates

Often called sugars, **simple carbohydrates** have little nutritive value (for example, candy, soda, cakes). Simple carbohydrates are divided into monosaccharides and disaccharides. These carbohydrates — with -ose endings — often take the place of more nutritive foods in the diet.

Monosaccharides

The simplest sugars are **monosaccharides**. The three most common monosaccharides are glucose, fructose, and galactose.

1. *Glucose* is a natural sugar found in food, but it also is produced in the body from other simple and complex carbohydrates.
2. *Fructose*, or fruit sugar, occurs naturally in fruits and honey.
3. *Galactose* is produced from milk sugar in the mammary glands of lactating animals.

Both fructose and galactose are converted readily to glucose in the body. Glucose is used as a source of energy, or it may be stored in the muscles and liver in the form of glycogen (a long chain of glucose molecules hooked together). Excess glucose in the blood is converted to fat and stored in **adipose tissue**.

Disaccharides

The three major **disaccharides** are:

1. *Sucrose* or table sugar (glucose + fructose).
2. *Lactose* (glucose + galactose).
3. *Maltose* (glucose + glucose).

Complex Carbohydrates

Complex carbohydrates are also called *polysaccharides*. Anywhere from about 10 to thousands of monosaccharide molecules can unite to form a single polysaccharide. Examples of complex carbohydrates are starches, dextrins, and glycogen.

1. *Starch* is the storage form of glucose in plants, needed to promote the earliest growth. Starch is found commonly in grains, seeds, corn, nuts, roots, potatoes, and legumes. Grains, the richest source of starch, should supply most of the energy in a healthful diet. Once eaten, starch is converted to glucose for the body's own energy use.
2. *Dextrins* are formed from the breakdown of large starch molecules exposed to dry heat, such as in baking bread or producing cold cereals. Complex carbohydrates of plant origin provide many valuable nutrients and can be an excellent source of fiber, or roughage.
3. *Glycogen* is the animal polysaccharide synthesized from glucose and found only in slight amounts in meats. Although it serves a function in humans similar to that of starch in plants, glycogen is not found in plants. Glycogen constitutes the body's reservoirs of glucose. Many hundreds to thousands of glucose molecules are linked together to be stored as glycogen in liver and muscle.

   When a surge of energy is needed, enzymes in the muscle and the liver break down glycogen and thus make glucose readily available for energy transformation. This is discussed later in the chapter, under Nutrition for Athletes.

Dietary Fiber

Dietary fiber is a type of complex carbohydrate present mainly in leaves, skins, roots, and seeds. Processing and refining foods remove almost all of the natural fiber. In our daily diets the main sources of dietary fiber are whole-grain cereals and breads, fruits, and vegetables.

The most common types of fiber are:

1. *Cellulose* and hemicellulose, found in plant cell walls.
2. *Pectins*, found in fruits.
3. *Gums*, also found in small amounts in foods of plant origin.
4. *Macilages*.

Cellulose and hemicellulose are water-insoluble fibers. Pectins and gums are water-soluble fibers.

Fiber is important in the diet because it binds water, causing a softer and bulkier stool that increases peristalsis (involuntary muscle contractions of intestinal walls that force the stool onward) and allows food residues to pass through the intestinal tract more quickly. Many researchers believe that speeding up passage of food residues through the intestines lowers the risk for colon cancer, mainly because cancer-causing agents are not in contact as long with the intestinal wall. Fiber also is thought to bind with carcinogens (cancer-producing substances), and more water in the stool may dilute the cancer-causing agents, lessening their potency.

Increased fiber intake also may lower the risk for coronary heart disease because: (a) saturated fats often take the place of fiber in the diet, increasing

High-fiber foods are essential in a healthy diet.

cholesterol formation or absorption, and (b) specific water-soluble fibers such as pectin and guar gum, found in beans, oat bran, corn, and fruits, seem to bind cholesterol in the intestines, preventing its absorption. In addition to heart disease, several health disorders, including constipation, diverticulitis, hemorrhoids, gallbladder disease, and obesity have been linked to low intake of fiber.

To decrease the risk for certain diseases, a low-fat, high-carbohydrate diet with adequate amounts of fiber is recommended. Although a recommended dietary allowance for fiber has not yet been established, most experts recommend 20 to 35 grams of dietary fiber per day. The fiber content of selected foods is provided in Table 7.1. The main sources of fiber in the diet should be fruits, vegetables, legumes, and whole grain cereals because they provide vitamins and minerals.

This may be surprising, but too much fiber can be detrimental to health. It can produce loss of calcium, phosphorus, and iron, not to mention gastrointestinal discomfort. When eating more fiber, a person also should drink more water, as too little fluid can cause constipation and even dehydration.

Fat

The human body uses **fats** as a source of energy. Fats are the most concentrated energy source. Each gram

TERMS

Simple carbohydrates Formed by simple or double sugar units with little nutritive value; divided into monosaccharides and disaccharides.

Monosaccharides The simplest carbohydrates (sugars) formed by five- or six-carbon skeletons. The three most common monosaccharides are glucose, fructose, and galactose.

Adipose tissue Fat cells.

Disaccharides Simple carbohydrates formed by two monosaccharide units linked together, one of which is glucose. The major disaccharides are sucrose, lactose, and maltose.

Complex carbohydrates Carbohydrates formed by three or more simple sugar molecules linked together; also referred to as polysaccharides.

Dietary fiber A complex carbohydrate in plant foods that cannot be digested by the human body but is essential in the digestion process.

Fats Compounds made of a combination of triglycerides.

Table 7.1	*Dietary Fiber Content of Selected Foods*		

Food	Serving Size	Dietary Fiber (gm)
Almonds	1 oz.	3.0
Apple	1 medium	4.3
Banana	1 medium	3.3
Beans — red, kidney	.5 cup	10.2
Blackberries	.5 cup	4.9
Beets (cooked)	.5 cup	2.0
Brazil nuts	1 oz.	2.5
Broccoli (cooked)	.5 cup	3.3
Brown rice (cooked)	.5 cup	2.0
Carrots (cooked)	.5 cup	2.9
Cauliflower (cooked)	.5 cup	1.7
Cereal		
All Bran	1 oz.	8.5
Cheerios	1 oz.	1.1
Cornflakes	1 oz.	0.5
Fruit and Fibre	1 oz.	4.0
Fruit Wheats	1 oz.	2.0
Just Right	1 oz.	2.0
Wheaties	1 oz.	2.0
Corn (cooked)	.5 cup	3.9
Eggplant (cooked)	.5 cup	3.0
Lettuce (chopped)	.5 cup	0.4
Orange	1 medium	3.0
Parsnips (cooked)	.5 cup	2.1
Pear	1 medium	5.0
Peas (cooked)	.5 cup	3.7
Popcorn (plain)	1 cup	1.5
Potato (baked)	1 medium	3.9
Strawberries	.5 cup	1.6
Summer squash (cooked)	.5 cup	1.6
Watermelon	1 cup	0.8

of fat supplies 9 calories to the body. Fats are a part of the cell structure. They are used as stored energy and as an insulator to preserve body heat. They absorb shock, supply essential fatty acids, and carry the fat-soluble vitamins A, D, E, and K. Fats can be classified into three main groups: simple, compound, and derived (Figure 7.3). The basic sources of fat are milk and other dairy products, and meats and alternatives.

Simple Fats

A simple fat consists of a glyceride molecule linked to one, two, or three units of fatty acids. According to the number of fatty acids attached, simple fats are divided into monoglycerides (one fatty acid), diglycerides (two fatty acids), and triglycerides (three fatty acids). More than 90% of the weight of fat in foods and more than 95% of the stored fat in the human body are in the form of triglycerides.

The length of the carbon atom chain and the amount of hydrogen saturation in fatty acids vary. Based on the extent of saturation, fatty acids are said to be saturated or unsaturated. Unsaturated fatty acids are classified further into monounsaturated and polyunsaturated. Saturated fatty acids are mainly of animal origin. Unsaturated fats are found mostly in plant products.

In saturated fatty acids the carbon atoms are fully saturated with hydrogens; only single bonds link the carbon atoms on the chain (see Figure 7.4). These saturated fatty acids often are called saturated fats. Examples of foods high in saturated fatty acids are meats, meat fat, lard, whole milk, cream, butter, cheese, ice cream, hydrogenated oils (a process that makes oils saturated), coconut oil, and palm oils.

Figure 7.3 • *Major types of fats (lipids).*

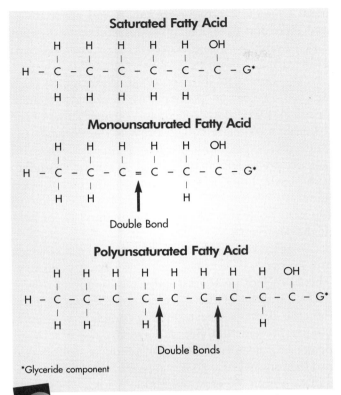

Figure 7.4 • *Chemical structure of saturated and unsaturated fats.*

(HDL) cholesterol. High HDL-cholesterol levels help to decrease the risk of diseases of the cardiovascular system. Additional research, however, does not support these negative effects on HDL-cholesterol.[2] At typical levels found in the diet, both polyunsaturated and monounsaturated fats now appear to have similar effects on blood cholesterol.

Hydrogen often is added to monounsaturated and polyunsaturated fats to increase shelf life and to solidify them so they are more spreadable. During this process of partial hydrogenation, the position of hydrogen atoms may be changed along the chain, transforming the fat into a **transfatty acid**.

Margarine and spreads, crackers, cookies, and french fries often contain transfatty acids. Intake of these types of fats should be minimized. Studies suggest that diets rich in transfatty acids elevate LDL cholesterol and lower HDL cholesterol to the same extent as saturated fats.[3] Paying attention to food labels is important because the words "partially hydrogenated" or "transfatty acids" may indicate that the product carries as high a health risk as consuming saturated fat (eating margarine is still a better choice because its total transfatty acid and saturated fat is about half the saturated fat in butter).

One type of polyunsaturated fatty acids that has gained attention in recent years are **omega-3 fatty acids**. These fatty acids seem to be effective in lowering triglycerides, which are a risk factor for coronary heart disease. Fish, especially fresh or frozen mackerel, herring, tuna, salmon, and lake trout, have omega-3 fatty acids. Canned fish is not recommended for this purpose because the canning process destroys most of the omega-3 oil. These fatty acids also are found, but to a lesser extent, in canola oil, walnuts, soybeans, and wheat germ.

Some data suggest that eating one or two servings of fish weekly lessens the risk for coronary heart disease. People with diabetes, a history of hemorrhaging or strokes, on aspirin, blood-thinning therapy, and presurgical patients should not consume fish oil except under a physician's instruction.

In unsaturated fatty acids (unsaturated fats), double bonds form between the unsaturated carbons. In monounsaturated fatty acids (MUFA), only one double bond is found along the chain. Olive, canola, rapeseed, peanut, and sesame oils are examples of monounsaturated fatty acids. Polyunsaturated fatty acids (PUFA) contain two or more double bonds between unsaturated carbon atoms along the chain. Corn, cottonseed, safflower, walnut, sunflower, and soybean oils are high in polyunsaturated fatty acids.

Saturated fats typically do not melt at room temperature. Unsaturated fats usually are liquid at room temperature. Coconut and palm oils are exceptions, as they are high in saturated fats. Shorter fatty acid chains also tend to be liquid at room temperature.

In general, saturated fats raise the blood cholesterol level, whereas polyunsaturated and monounsaturated fats tend to lower blood cholesterol. When saturated fats are replaced by unsaturated fats in the diet, the latter tend to stimulate the liver to clear cholesterol from the blood.

Earlier studies had suggested that polyunsaturated fats also seemed to cause reduction of "good"

TERMS

Transfatty acid Solidified fat formed by adding hydrogen to monosaturated and polyunsaturated fats to increase shelf life.

Omega-3 fatty acids Polyunsaturated fatty acids found primarily in cold-water seafood; thought to be effective in lowering blood cholesterol and triglycerides.

Compound Fats

Compound fats are a combination of simple fats and other chemicals. Examples are:

1. Phospholipids — similar to triglycerides except that choline (or another compound) and phosphoric acid take the place of one of the fatty acid units.
2. Glucolipids — a combination of carbohydrates, fatty acids, and nitrogen.
3. Lipoproteins — water-soluble aggregates of protein with triglycerides, phospholipids, or cholesterol.

Because lipids do not dissolve in water, lipoproteins transport fats in the blood.

The major forms of **lipoproteins** are high-density (HDL), low-density (LDL), and very-low-density (VLDL) lipoproteins. Lipoproteins play a large role in developing or in preventing heart disease. HDL is more than half protein and contains little cholesterol. High HDL levels have been associated with a lower risk for coronary heart disease. LDL is approximately a fourth protein and nearly half cholesterol. High LDL levels have been linked to increased risk for coronary heart disease. VLDL contains mostly (about half) triglycerides and only about 10% protein and 20% cholesterol.

Derived Fats

Derived fats combine simple and compound fats. **Sterols** are an example. Although sterols contain no fatty acids, they are considered lipids because they do not dissolve in water. The most often mentioned sterol is cholesterol, which is found in many foods or can be manufactured primarily from saturated fats in the body.

Protein

Proteins are the main substances the body uses to build and repair tissues such as muscles, blood, internal organs, skin, hair, nails, and bones. They are a part of hormones, antibodies, and enzymes. **Enzymes** play a key role in all of the body's processes. Because all enzymes are formed by proteins, this nutrient is necessary for normal functioning. Proteins also help maintain the normal balance of body fluids.

Proteins can be used as a source of energy, too, but only if not enough carbohydrates are available. Each gram of protein yields 4 calories of energy. The main sources of protein are meats and alternatives, and milk and other dairy products. Excess proteins may be converted to glucose or fat or even excreted in the urine.

The human body uses 20 **amino acids** to form different types of protein. Amino acids contain nitrogen, carbon, hydrogen, and oxygen. Nine of the 20 amino acids are called *essential amino acids* because the body cannot produce them. The other 11, termed *nonessential amino acids*, can be manufactured in the body if food proteins in the diet provide enough nitrogen (see Table 7.2). For the body to function normally, all amino acids must be present at the same time.

Proteins that contain all the essential amino acids are known as complete or higher-quality protein. These types of proteins usually are of animal origin. If one or more of the essential amino acids is missing, the proteins are termed incomplete or lower-quality protein. Individuals have to take in enough protein to ensure nitrogen for adequate amino acid production and also to get enough high-quality protein to obtain the essential amino acids.

Protein deficiency is not a problem in the usual American diet. Two glasses of skim milk combined with about 4 ounces of poultry or fish meet the daily protein requirement. Protein deficiency, however, could be a concern in some vegetarian diets. **Vegetarians** rely primarily on foods from the bread, cereal, rice, and pasta, and fruit and vegetable groups and avoid most foods from animal sources found in the milk, yogurt, and cheese and meat groups. The

Table 7.2   *Amino Acids*

Essential Amino Acids*	Nonessential Amino Acids
Histidine	Alanine
Isoleucine	Arginine
Leucine	Asparagine
Lysine	Aspartic acid
Methionine	Cysteine
Phenylalanine	Glutamic acid
Threonine	Glutamine
Tryptophan	Glycine
Valine	Proline
	Serine
	Tyrosine

*Must be provided in the diet as the body cannot manufacture them.

four basic types of vegetarians are **vegans, ovovegetarians, lactovegetarians,** and **ovolactovegetarians.**

Vegans in particular must be careful to eat protein foods that provide a balanced distribution of essential amino acids, such as grain products and beans. Strict vegans also need a supplement of vitamin B_{12}. This vitamin is not found in plant foods, and its deficiency may lead to anemia and nerve damage.

Vegetarians who do not select their food combinations properly may develop nutritional deficiencies of protein, vitamins, minerals, and even calories. Vegetarian diets can be balanced, but this is a complicated issue that cannot be covered adequately in a few paragraphs. Those who are interested in vegetarian diets should consult other resources.

Too much animal protein can cause serious health problems as well. Some people eat twice as much protein as they need. Protein foods from animal sources often are high in fat, saturated fat, and cholesterol, which can lead to cardiovascular disease and cancer. Too much animal protein also decreases blood enzymes that prevent precancerous cells from developing into tumors.

As discussed later in this chapter, a well-balanced diet contains a variety of foods from all five basic food groups, including wise selection of foods from animal sources. Based on current nutrition data, meat (poultry and fish included) should be replaced by grains, legumes, vegetables, and fruits as main courses. Meats should be used more for flavoring than for substance. Daily consumption of beef, poultry, or fish should be limited to 3 ounces (about the size of a deck of cards) to 6 ounces.

Vitamins

Vitamins are necessary for normal bodily metabolism, growth, and development. Vitamins are classified into two types based on their solubility: *fat-soluble vitamins* (A, D, E, and K), and *water-soluble vitamins* (B complex and C). In general, the body does not manufacture vitamins. Vitamins can be obtained only through a well-balanced diet. To decrease vitamin losses during cooking, natural foods should be microwaved or steamed rather than boiled in water that later is thrown out.

A few exceptions, such as A, D, and K, are formed in the body. Vitamin A is produced from **beta-carotene,** found in foods such as carrots, pumpkin, and sweet potatoes. Ultraviolet light from the sun

changes a compound in the skin called 7-dehydrocholesterol into vitamin D. Vitamin K is created in the body by intestinal bacteria. The major functions of vitamins are outlined in Table 7.3.

Vitamins C, E, and beta-carotene also function as **antioxidants,** which are thought to play a key role in preventing chronic diseases.[4] The specific function of these antioxidant nutrients, along with the mineral selenium, also an antioxidant, are discussed later in this chapter.

Minerals

Approximately 25 **minerals** have important roles in body functioning. Minerals are contained in all cells, especially those in hard parts of the body (bones, nails, teeth). Minerals are crucial in maintaining water balance and the acid-base balance. They are essential components of respiratory pigments, enzymes, and enzyme systems, and they regulate muscular and nervous tissue excitability, blood clotting, and normal heart rhythm.

TERMS

Lipoproteins Lipids covered by proteins; transport fats in the blood.

Sterols Derived fats, of which cholesterol is the best known example.

Proteins Complex organic compounds containing nitrogen and formed by combinations of amino acids; the main substances used in the body to build and repair tissues.

Enzymes Catalysts that facilitate chemical reactions in the body.

Amino acids Chemical compounds that contain nitrogen, carbon, hydrogen, and oxygen; the basic building blocks the body uses to build different types of protein.

Vegetarians Individuals whose diet is of vegetable or plant origin.

Vegans Vegetarians who eat no animal products at all.

Ovovegetarians Vegetarians who allow eggs in the diet.

Lactovegetarians Vegetarians who eat foods from the milk group.

Ovolactovegetarians Vegetarians who include eggs and milk products in the diet.

Vitamins Organic substances essential for normal metabolism, growth, and development of the body.

Beta-carotene A precursor to vitamin A.

Minerals Inorganic elements found in the body and in food; essential for normal body functions.

Table 7.3 *Major Functions of Vitamins*

Nutrient	Good Sources	Major Functions	Deficiency Symptoms
Vitamin A	Milk, cheese, eggs, liver, and yellow/dark green fruits and vegetables	Required for healthy bones, teeth, skin, gums, and hair; maintenance of inner mucous membranes, thus increasing resistance to infection; adequate vision in dim light.	Night blindness, decreased growth, decreased resistance to infection, rough-dry skin
Vitamin D	Fortified milk, cod liver oil, salmon, tuna, egg yolk	Necessary for bones and teeth; needed for calcium and phosphorus absorption.	Rickets (bone softening), fractures, and muscle spasms
Vitamin E	Vegetable oils, yellow and green leafy vegetables, margarine, wheat germ, whole grain breads and cereals	Related to oxidation and normal muscle and red blood cell chemistry.	Leg cramps, red blood cell breakdown
Vitamin K	Green leafy vegetables, cauliflower, cabbage, eggs, peas, and potatoes	Essential for normal blood clotting.	Hemorrhaging
Vitamin B_1 (Thiamine)	Whole grain or enriched bread, lean meats and poultry, organ fish, liver, pork, poultry, organ meats, legumes, nuts, and dried yeast	Assists in proper use of carbohydrates; normal functioning of nervous system; maintenance of good appetite.	Loss of appetite, nausea, confusion, cardiac abnormalities, muscle spasms
Vitamin B_2 (Riboflavin)	Eggs, milk, leafy green vegetables, whole grains, lean meats, dried beans and peas	Contributes to energy release from carbohydrates, fats, and proteins; needed for normal growth and development, good vision, and healthy skin.	Cracking of the corners of the mouth, inflammation of the skin, impaired vision
Vitamin B_6 (Pyridoxine)	Vegetables, meats, whole grain cereals, soybeans, peanuts, and potatoes	Necessary for protein and fatty acids metabolism, and normal red blood cell formation.	Depression, irritability, muscle spasms, nausea
Vitamin B_{12}	Meat, poultry, fish, liver, organ meats, eggs, shellfish, milk, and cheese	Required for normal growth, red blood cell formation, nervous system and digestive tract functioning.	Impaired balance, weakness, drop in red blood cell count
Niacin	Liver and organ meats, meat, fish, poultry, whole grains, enriched breads, nuts, green leafy vegetables, and dried beans and peas	Contributes to energy release from carbohydrates, fats, and proteins; normal growth and development, and formation of hormones and nerve-regulating substances.	Confusion, depression, weakness, weight loss
Biotin	Liver, kidney, eggs, yeast, legumes, milk, nuts, dark green vegetables	Essential for carbohydrate metabolism and fatty acid synthesis.	Inflamed skin, muscle pain, depression, weight loss
Folic Acid	Leafy green vegetables, organ meats, whole grains and cereals, and dried beans	Needed for cell growth and reproduction and red blood cell formation.	Decreased resistance to infection
Pantothenic Acid	All natural foods, especially liver, kidney, eggs, nuts, yeast, milk, dried peas and beans, and green leafy vegetables	Related to carbohydrate and fat metabolism.	Depression, low blood sugar, leg cramps, nausea, headaches
Vitamin C (Ascorbic Acid)	Fruits and vegetables	Helps protect against infection; formation of collagenous tissue; normal blood vessels, teeth, and bones.	Slow healing wounds, loose teeth, hemorrhaging, rough-scaly skin, irritability

The three minerals mentioned most commonly are calcium, iron, and sodium. As pointed out later in this chapter, calcium deficiency may result in osteoporosis, and low iron intake can induce iron-deficiency anemia. High sodium intake may contribute to high blood pressure. The specific functions of some of the most important minerals are given in Table 7.4.

Water

Approximately 70% of total body weight is water. Water is the most important nutrient, involved in almost every vital body process: in digesting and absorbing food, in the circulatory process, in removing waste products, in building and rebuilding cells, and in transporting other nutrients.

Water is contained in almost all foods, but primarily in liquid foods, fruits, and vegetables. Besides the natural content in foods, every person should drink about eight glasses of fluids a day.

● Energy (ATP) Production

The energy derived from food is not used directly by the cells. It is transferred to form **adenosine triphosphate (ATP)**. The subsequent breakdown of this compound provides the energy used by all energy-requiring processes of the body (also see Figure 7.5). ATP must be recycled continually to sustain life and work. ATP can be resynthesized in three ways:

1. *ATP and ATP-CP system.* The body stores small amounts of ATP and creatine phosphate (CP). These stores are used during all-out activities up to 10 seconds in duration, such as sprinting, long

TERMS

Adenosine triphosphate (ATP) A high-energy chemical compound used for immediate energy by the body.

Table 7.4 *Major Functions of Minerals*

Nutrient	Good Sources	Major Functions	Deficiency Symptoms
Calcium	Milk, yogurt, cheese, green leafy vegetables, dried beans, sardines, and salmon	Required for strong teeth and bone formation; maintenance of good muscle tone, heartbeat, and nerve function.	Bone pain and fractures, periodontal disease, muscle cramps
Iron	Organ meats, lean meats, seafoods, eggs, dried peas and beans, nuts, whole and enriched grains, and green leafy vegetables	Major component of hemoglobin; aids in energy utilization.	Nutritional anemia, and overall weakness
Phosphorus	Meats, fish, milk, eggs, dried beans and peas, whole grains, and processed foods	Required for bone and teeth formation; energy release regulation.	Bone pain and fracture, weight loss, and weakness
Zinc	Milk, meat, seafood, whole grains, nuts, eggs, and dried beans	Essential component of hormones, insulin, and enzymes; used in normal growth and development.	Loss of appetite, slow-healing wounds, and skin problems
Magnesium	Green leafy vegetables, whole grains, nuts, soybeans, seafood, and legumes	Needed for bone growth and maintenance; carbohydrate and protein utilization; nerve function; temperature regulation.	Irregular heartbeat, weakness, muscle spasms, and sleeplessness
Sodium	Table salt, processed foods, and meat	Body fluid regulation; transmission of nerve impulses; heart action.	Rarely seen
Potassium	Legumes, whole grains, bananas, orange juice, dried fruits, and potatoes	Heart action; bone formation and maintenance; regulation of energy release; acid-base regulation.	Irregular heartbeat, nausea, weakness
Selenium	Seafood, meat, whole grains	Component of enzyme; functions in close association with vitamin E.	Muscle pain, possible heart muscle deterioration; possible hair and nail loss

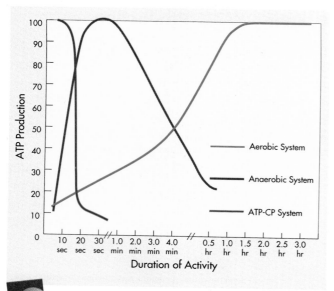

Figure 7.5 • *Contributions of energy formation mechanisms during various forms of physical activity.*

jumping, and power (weight) lifting. The amount of stored ATP provides energy for just a few seconds. With all-out efforts, ATP is resynthesized from CP, another high-energy phosphate compound. This is referred to as the ATP-CP or phosphagen system.

Depending on the amount of physical training, the concentration of CP stored in cells is sufficient to allow maximum exertion for about 10 seconds. Once the CP stores are depleted, the person is forced to slow down or rest to allow ATP to form through anaerobic and aerobic pathways.

2. *Anaerobic or lactic acid system.* During anaerobic exercise that is sustained between 10 and 180 seconds maximum, ATP is replenished from the breakdown of glucose through a series of chemical reactions that do not require oxygen. In the process, though, **lactic acid** is produced, which causes muscular fatigue.

Because of the accumulation of lactic acid with high-intensity exercise, the formation of ATP during anaerobic activities is limited to about 3 minutes. A recovery period then is necessary to allow for the elimination of lactic acid. Formation of ATP through the anaerobic system is possible from glucose (carbohydrates) only.

3. *Aerobic system.* The production of energy during slow-sustained exercise is derived primarily

through aerobic metabolism. Both glucose (carbohydrates) and fatty acids (fat) are used in this process. Oxygen is required to form ATP, and under steady-state exercise conditions lactic acid accumulation is minimal.

Because oxygen is required, a person's capacity to utilize oxygen is crucial for successful athletic performance in aerobic events. The higher the maximal oxygen uptake (VO_{2max}), the greater is the capacity to generate ATP through the aerobic system.

● Balancing the Diet

Most people would like to have good health and live life to its fullest. One of the fundamental ways to accomplish this is through a well-balanced diet. As illustrated in Figure 7.6, the generally recommended guideline states that daily caloric intake should be distributed so 58% of the total calories come from carbohydrates (48% complex carbohydrates and 10% sugar), less than 30% of the total calories from fat (equally divided [10% each] among saturated, monounsaturated, and polyunsaturated fats), and 12% of the total calories from protein (0.8 grams of protein per kilogram [2.2 pounds] of body weight). The diet also must include all of the essential vitamins, minerals, and water. To rate a diet accurately is difficult without a complete nutrient analysis.

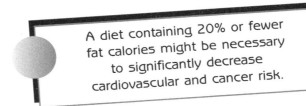

A diet containing 20% or fewer fat calories might be necessary to significantly decrease cardiovascular and cancer risk.

The 30% fat guideline has been widely accepted and endorsed by most health organizations during the last two decades. More recently, however, nutritionists and preventive medicine specialists are beginning to point toward a daily fat intake much lower than the current 30% of total calories. In terms of reducing cardiovascular and cancer risk, limiting fat intake to 20% of calories or less might be necessary. Most scientific studies have shown little or no improvement in lowering cholesterol levels while on a 30%-fat diet.[5] The role of high fat intake in increasing cancer risk is undeniable, and the data suggest that an intake of about 20% is better

Figure 7.6 • *Current and recommended percentages of fat, carbohydrate, and protein intake (expressed as a percent of total daily caloric intake).*

for overall cancer risk reduction.[6] Although the 30% guideline is still valid, a gradual change to a lower value might take effect in the next few years.

Diets in most developed countries have changed significantly since the turn of the century. People in the 1990s eat more fat, fewer carbohydrates, and about the same amount of protein, but fewer calories. At the same time, people weigh more than they did in 1900, an indication that they are not as physically active as their grandparents were.

> The role of high fat intake in increasing cancer risk is undeniable, and the data suggest that an intake of about 20% is better for overall cancer risk reduction.

Diets also were much healthier at the turn of the century. In the United States in 1909, carbohydrates accounted for 57% of the total daily caloric intake, 67% of which were complex carbohydrates. Today, carbohydrate intake has decreased to 51%, and complex carbohydrates account for only 24% of the daily carbohydrate intake. The proportion of fat has risen from 32% to 37%. Protein intake has remained unchanged at about 12% of the total caloric intake.

● Nutrient Analysis

The first step in evaluating your diet is to conduct a nutrient analysis. This can be quite educational because most people do not realize how harmful and non-nutritious many common foods are. The analysis covers calories, carbohydrates, fats, cholesterol, and sodium, as well as eight crucial nutrients: protein, calcium, iron, vitamin A, thiamine, riboflavin, niacin, and vitamin C. If the diet has enough of these eight nutrients, the foods consumed in natural form to provide these nutrients typically contain all the other nutrients the human body needs.

To do the nutrient analysis, keep a 3-day record of everything you eat, using the forms in Appendix B, Figure B.1. At the end of each day, look up the nutrient content for those foods in the list of Nutritive Value of Selected Foods, also in Appendix B. Record this information on your 3-day listing of foods in Figure B.1. If you do not find a food in the list given in Appendix B, the information often is stated on the food container itself, or you might refer to the references at the end of the list.

When you have recorded the nutritive values for each day, add up each column and write the totals at the bottom of the chart. After the third day, use Figure B.2 and compute an average for the 3 days. To rate your diet, compare your figures with those in the **recommended dietary allowances (RDA)** (Table

TERMS

Lactic acid End product of anaerobic glycolysis (metabolism).

Recommended dietary allowances Daily suggested intakes of nutrients for normal, healthy people, as developed by National Academy of Sciences.

7.5). The results give a good indication of areas of strength and deficiency in your current diet.

Every 10 years or so, the National Academy of Sciences issues a new RDA based on a review of the most current research on nutrient needs of healthy people. The RDA provides daily nutrient intake recommendations, usually set high enough to encompass 97.5% of the healthy population in the United States. Stated another way, the RDA recommendation for any nutrient is well above almost everyone's actual requirement.

Between the late 1960s and the early 1990s, nutrient information on labels was expressed in terms of the U. S. RDA — a set of standard values for the average consumer — derived from the 1968 edition of the RDA. In 1993 the Food and Drug Administration (FDA) revised food labeling regulations and has replaced the U.S. RDA with **Daily Values** (see Figure 7.7). These daily values are based on a 2,000-calorie diet and may require adjustments depending on an individual's daily caloric needs.

In setting the Daily Values, the FDA first created two sets of standards: Reference Daily Intakes (RDI) and Daily Reference Values (DRV). For FDA purposes, these two sets of standards serve different functions. To avoid consumer confusion in food labeling, however, the FDA combined the RDI and DRV into the Daily Values.

The RDI are reference values for protein, vitamins, and minerals. These are similar in purpose to the old U.S. RDA, but they reflect average allowances based on the 1989 RDA. The DRV are standards for

TERMS

Daily Values A set of standard nutritive values developed by the FDA (replaces the U.S. RDA).

Table 7.5 *Recommended Dietary Allowances (RDA)*

	Calories	Protein	Fat	Sat. Fat	Choles-terol (mg)	Carbo-hydrates	Calcium (mg)	Iron (mg)	Sodium (mg)	Vit. A (I. U.)	Thiamin (Vit. B₁) (mg)	Riboflavin (Vit. B₂) (mg)	Niacin (mg)	Vit. C (mg)
Men 15–18 years	See below[a]	See below[b]	<30%[c]	<10%[c]	<300	58%>[c]	1,200	12	2,400	5,000	1.5	1.8	20	60
Men 19–24 years			<30%[c]	<10%[c]	<300	58%>[c]	1,200	10	2,400	5,000	1.5	1.7	19	60
Men 25–50 years			<30%[c]	<10%[c]	<300	58%>[c]	800	10	2,400	5,000	1.5	1.7	19	60
Men 51 +			<30%[c]	<10%[c]	<300	58%>[c]	800	10	2,400	5,000	1.2	1.4	15	60
Women 15–18 years			<30%[c]	<10%[c]	<300	58%>[c]	1,200	15	2,400	4,000	1.1	1.3	15	60
Women 19–24 years			<30%[c]	<10%[c]	<300	58%>[c]	1,200	15	2,400	4,000	1.1	1.3	15	60
Women 25–50 years			<30%[c]	<10%[c]	<300	58%>[c]	800	15	2,400	4,000	1.1	1.3	15	60
Women 51 +			<30%[c]	<10%[c]	<300	58%>[c]	800	10	2,400	4,000	1.0	1.2	13	60
Pregnant			<30%[c]	<10%[c]	<300	58%>[c]	1,200	30	2,400	4,000	1.5	1.6	17	70
Lactating	↓	↓	<30%[c]	<10%[c]	<300	58%>[c]	1,200	15	2,400	6,000	1.6	1.8	20	95

[a] Use Table 8.1 in Chapter 8 for all categories.
[b] Protein intake should be .8 grams per kilogram of body weight. Pregnant women should consume an additional 15 grams of daily protein; lactating women should have an extra 20 grams.
[c] Percentage of total calories based on recommendations by nutrition experts.

Adapted from *Recommended Dietary Allowances*, © 1989, by National Academy of Sciences, National Academy Press, Washington DC.

1. Better by Design
How to recognize the new food labels

The new food labels feature a revamped nutrition panel titled "Nutrition Facts," with nutrient listings that reflect current health concerns. Now you'll be able to find information on fat, fiber and other food components fundamental to lowering your risk of cancer and other chronic diseases. Listings for nutrients like thiamin and riboflavin will no longer be required, because Americans generally eat enough of them these days.

2. Size Up the Situation
All serving sizes are created equal

Now you can compare similar products and know that their serving sizes are basically identical. So when you realize how much fat is packed into that carton of double-dutch-chocolate-caramel-chew ice cream you're eyeing, you might opt for lowfat frozen yogurt instead. Serving sizes will also be standardized, so manufacturers can't make nutrition claims for unrealistically small portions. That means a chocolate cake, for example, must be divided into 8 servings sized to satisfy the average person — not 16 servings sized to satisfy the average munchkin.

3. Look Before You Leap
Use the Daily Values

You will find the Daily Values on the bottom half of the "Nutrition Facts" panel. Some represent maximum levels of nutrients that should be consumed each day for a healthful diet (as with fat) while others refer to minimum levels that can be exceeded (as with carbohydrates). They are based on both a 2,000 and 2,500 calorie diet. Your own needs may be more or less, but these figures give you a point from which to compare. For example, the sample label indicates that someone with a 2,000 calorie diet should eat no more than 65 grams of fat per day. This is based on a diet getting 30% of calories as fat. If you normally eat less calories, or want to eat less than 30% of calories as fat, your daily fat consumption will be lower.

4. Rate It Right
Scan the % Daily Values

The % Daily Values make judging the nutritional quality of a food a snap. For instance, you can look at the % Daily Value column and find that a food has 25% of the Daily Value for fiber. This means the product will give you a substantial portion of the recommended amount of fiber for the day. You can also use this column to compare nutrients in similar products. The % Daily Values are based on a 2,000 calorie diet.

5. Trust Adjectives
Descriptors have legal definitions

Terms like "low," "high" and "free" have long been used on food labels. What these words actually mean, however, could vary. Thanks to the new labeling laws, such descriptions must now meet legal definitions. For example, you may be shopping for foods high in vitamin A, which has been linked to lower risk of certain cancers. Under the new label laws, a food described as "high" in a particular nutrient must contain 20% or more of the Daily Value for that nutrient. So if the bottle of juice you're thinking of buying says "high in vitamin A,'" you can now feel confident that it really is a good source of the vitamin.

6. Read Health Claims with Confidence
The nutrient link to disease prevention

You can also expect to see food packages with health claims linking certain nutrients to reduced risk of cancer and other diseases. The federal government has approved three health claims dealing with cancer prevention: a low fat diet may reduce your risk for cancer; high fiber foods may reduce your risk for cancer; and fruits and vegetables may reduce your risk for cancer. A food may not make such a health claim for one nutrient if it contains other nutrients that undermine its health benefits. A high fiber, but high fat, jelly doughnut cannot carry a health claim!

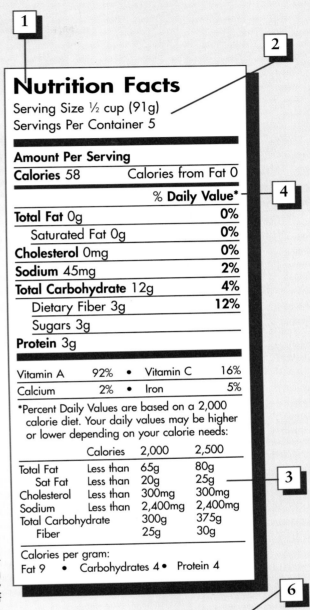

Nutrition Facts		
Serving Size ½ cup (91g)		
Servings Per Container 5		

Amount Per Serving		
Calories 58	Calories from Fat 0	

	% Daily Value*
Total Fat 0g	0%
Saturated Fat 0g	0%
Cholesterol 0mg	0%
Sodium 45mg	2%
Total Carbohydrate 12g	4%
Dietary Fiber 3g	**12%**
Sugars 3g	
Protein 3g	

Vitamin A	92%	Vitamin C	16%
Calcium	2%	Iron	5%

*Percent Daily Values are based on a 2,000 calorie diet. Your daily values may be higher or lower depending on your calorie needs:

		Calories	2,000	2,500
Total Fat	Less than		65g	80g
Sat Fat	Less than		20g	25g
Cholesterol	Less than		300mg	300mg
Sodium	Less than		2,400mg	2,400mg
Total Carbohydrate			300g	375g
Fiber			25g	30g

Calories per gram:
Fat 9 • Carbohydrates 4 • Protein 4

Many factors affect cancer risk. Eating a diet low in fat and high in fiber may lower risk of this disease.

• GOOD SOURCE OF FIBER
• LOWFAT

Figure 7.7 • *Food label with U.S. Recommended Daily Values.*

Fruits and vegetables in general contain large amounts of cancer-fighting phytochemicals.

nutrients and food components that do not have an established RDA. The DRV include carbohydrate, fat, saturated fat, fiber, cholesterol, and sodium. These standards (computed in grams and milligrams based on a 2,000-calorie diet) represent dietary intakes to attain or restrict based on a consensus of critical values associated with health. For example, carbohydrate intake should be about 60% of total daily calories (300 grams), and fat intake should be limited to less than 30% (65 grams).

Both the RDA and the Daily Values apply only to healthy people. They are not intended for people who are ill and may require additional nutrients.

If you are using the software available with this book when conducting a nutrient analysis, you need only record the foods by code and the number of servings based on the standard amounts given in the list of selected foods in Appendix B (the form provided in Figure B.3). Sample nutrient analysis printouts are shown in Figures 7.8 and 7.9.

Some of the most revealing information learned in a nutrient analysis is the source of fat intake in the diet. The average daily fat consumption in the American diet is about 37% of the total caloric intake, which increases the risk for chronic diseases such as cardiovascular disease, cancer, diabetes, and obesity. Less than 30% of total calories should come from fat.

As illustrated in Figure 7.10, each gram of carbohydrates and protein supplies the body with 4 calories, and fat provides 9 calories per gram consumed (alcohol yields 7 calories per gram). In this regard, just looking at the total grams consumed for each type of food can be misleading.

For example, a person who eats 160 grams of carbohydrates, 100 grams of fat, and 70 grams of protein has a total intake of 330 grams of food. This indicates that 30% of the total grams of food is in the form of fat (100 grams of fat ÷ 330 grams of total food × 100). In reality, almost half of that diet is fat calories.

In the sample diet, 640 calories are derived from carbohydrates (160 grams × 4 calories per gram), 280 calories from protein (70 grams × 4 calories per gram), and 900 calories from fat (100 grams × 9 calories per gram), for a total of 1,820 calories. If 900 calories are derived from fat, almost half of the total caloric intake is in the form of fat (900 ÷ 1,820 × 100 = 49.5%).

Each gram of fat provides 9 calories. When figuring out the percent fat calories of individual foods, a useful guideline is given in Figure 7.11. Multiply the grams of fat by 9 and divide by the total calories in that particular food (per serving). You then multiply that number by 100 to get the percentage. For example, if a food label lists a total of 120 calories and 5 grams of fat, the fat content is 38% of total calories. This simple guideline can help you decrease the fat in your diet. The fat content of selected foods, given in grams and as a percent of total calories, is presented in Figure 7.12. The percentage of fat is further subdivided into saturated, monounsaturated, polyunsaturated, and other fatty acids. Beware of products labeled "97% fat-free." These products use weight and not percent of total calories as a measure of fat. Many of these foods still are in the range of 30% fat calories.

An apple a day will not keep the doctor away if most meals are high in fat content.

NUTRIENT ANALYSIS
Fitness & Wellness Series - Ver 3.96
by Werner W.K. Hoeger & Sharon A. Hoeger
Morton Publishing Company -- Englewood, Colorado

Jane R. Moore   Date: 09-12-1996
Age: 20
Body Weight: 141 lbs (64.0 kg)
Activity Rating: Moderate

Food Intake Day One

Food	Amount	Calo-ries	Pro-tein gm	Fat gm	Sat Fat gm	Cho-les-terol mg	Car-bohy-drate gm	Cal-cium mg	Iron mg	Sodium mg	Vit A I.U.	Thi-amin mg	Ribo-fla-vin mg	Nia-cin mg	Vit C mg
Cocoa/hot/with whole milk	1 c	218	9.1	9	6.1	33	26	298	0.8	123	318	0.10	0.44	0.4	2
Egg/scrambled w/milk butter	1 egg(s)	95	6.0	7	3.0	244	1	54	0.9	176	510	0.04	0.18	0.0	0
Bread/white	2 slice(s)	136	4.4	2	0.4	0	26	42	1.2	254	0	0.12	0.10	1.2	0
Butter	2 tsp	72	0.0	8	0.8	24	0	2	0.0	92	320	0.00	0.00	0.0	0
Milk/whole	1 c	159	9.0	9	5.1	34	12	288	0.1	120	350	0.07	0.40	0.2	2
Bread/whole wheat	2 slice(s)	122	5.2	2	1.2	0	24	50	1.6	264	0	0.12	0.06	1.4	0
Tuna/canned/oil/drained	1.5 oz.	84	12.5	4	0.9	30	0	4	0.8	69	35	0.02	0.05	5.1	0
Mayonnaise	2 tsp.	72	0.0	8	1.4	6	0	2	0.0	56	26	0.00	0.00	0.0	0
Pickles/dill	1 large	15	0.9	0	0.0	0	3	35	1.4	1,928	140	0.00	0.03	0.0	8
Potato/French fried	20 strips	428	6.8	20	3.4	0	56	24	2.0	10	0	0.20	0.12	4.8	32
Tomato sauce (catsup)	1 tbsp.	16	0.3	0	0.0	0	4	3	0.1	156	105	0.01	0.01	0.2	2
Apple/raw	1 med	80	0.3	1	0.0	0	20	10	0.4	1	120	0.04	0.03	0.1	6
Soda pop/Root beer	12 oz.	140	0.0	0	0.0	0	36	17	0.2	45	0	0.00	0.00	0.0	0
Coleslaw	1 c	173	1.6	17	1.0	5	6	53	0.5	144	190	0.06	0.06	0.4	35
Spaghetti/meat balls/sauce	1 c	332	18.6	12	3.0	75	39	124	3.7	1,009	1,590	0.25	0.30	4.0	22
Pie/apple	1 pc. (3.5 in.)	302	2.6	13	3.5	120	45	9	0.4	355	40	0.02	0.02	0.5	1
Totals Day One		2,444	77.3	112	29.8	571	298	1,015	14.1	4,802	3,744	1.0	1.8	18.3	110

Figure 7.8 ● *Computerized Nutrient Analysis: Sample food list.*

Jane R. Moore

NUTRIENT ANALYSIS: DAILY ANALYSIS, AVERAGE, AND
RECOMMENDED DIETARY ALLOWANCE (RDA) COMPARISON

	Calories	Protein gm	Fat %	Sat Fat %	Cholesterol mg	Carbohydrate %	Calcium mg	Iron mg	Sodium mg	Vit A I.U.	Thiamin mg	Riboflavin mg	Niacin mg	Vit C mg
Day One	2,444	77.3	40	11	571	48	1,015	14.1	4,802	3,744	1.0	1.8	18.3	110
Day Two	2,139	99.7	43	11	258	38	611	19.7	5,606	1,582	1.1	1.6	21.6	60
Day Three	2,045	86.7	38	15	274	45	885	15.1	3,544	4,791	1.4	2.2	30.8	49
Three Day Average	2,209	87.9	41	12	368	44	837	16.3	4,651	3,372	1.2	1.9	23.6	73
RDA	1,904*	51.2	<30	<10	<300	58>	1,200	15.0	1,904	4,000	1.1	1.3	15.0	60

*Estimated caloric value based on gender, current body weight, and activity rating (does not include additional calories burned through a physical exercise program).

OBSERVATIONS

Daily caloric intake should be distributed in such a way that about 58 percent of the total calories come from carbohydrates and less than 30 percent of the total calories from fat. Protein intake should be about .8 to 1.5 grams per kilogram of body weight or about 12 percent of the total calories. Pregnant women need to consume an additional 15 grams of daily protein, while lactating women should have an extra 20 grams of daily protein (these additional grams of protein are already included in the RDA values for pregnant and lactating women). Saturated fats should constitute less than 10 percent of the total daily caloric intake. Please note that the daily listings of food intake express the amount of carbohydrates, fat, saturated fat, and protein in grams. However, on the daily analysis and the RDA, only the amount of protein is given in grams. The amount of carbohydrates, fat, and saturated fat are expressed in percent of total calories. The final percentages are based on the total grams and total calories for all days analyzed, not from the average of the daily percentages.

If your average intake for protein, fat, saturated fat, cholesterol, or sodium is high, refer to the daily listings and decrease the intake of foods that are high in those nutrients. If your diet is deficient in carbohydrates, calcium, iron, vitamin A, thiamin, riboflavin, niacin, or vitamin C, refer to the statements below and increase your intake of the indicated foods or consult the list of selected foods in your textbook.

Caloric intake may be too high.

Total fat intake is too high.

Saturated fat intake is too high, which increases your risk for coronary heart disease.

Dietary cholesterol intake is too high. An average consumption of dietary cholesterol above 300 mg/day increases the risk for coronary heart disease. Do you know your blood cholesterol level?

Carbohydrate intake is low. Good sources of carbohydrates are whole grain breads and cereals, pasta, rice, fruits, and vegetables such as potatoes and peas.

Calcium intake is low. Good sources of calcium are milk, yogurt, cheese, green leafy vegetables, dried beans, sardines, and salmon.

Sodium intake is too high.

Vitamin A intake is low. Foods high in vitamin A include skim milk fortified with vit. A, cheese, butter, fortified margarine, eggs (yolk), liver, and dark green/yellow fruits and vegetables.

Figure 7.9 • *Computerized Nutritional Analysis: Sample daily analysis, average, and RDA comparison.*

Figure 7.10 • *Caloric value of food (fuel nutrients).*

● Achieving a Balanced Diet

Anyone who has completed a nutrient analysis and has given careful attention to Tables 7.3 (vitamins) and 7.4 (minerals) probably will realize that a well-balanced diet entails eating a variety of foods and reducing daily intake of fats and sweets. The Healthy Eating Pyramid contained in Figure 7.13 provides simple and sound instructions for nutrition. The pyramid contains five major food groups, along with fats, oils, and sweets, which are to be used sparingly. The daily recommended number of servings of the five major food groups are:

1. Six to 11 servings of the bread, cereal, rice, and pasta group.
2. Three to five servings of the vegetable group.
3. Two to four servings of the fruit group.
4. Two to three servings of the milk, yogurt, and cheese group.
5. Two to three servings of the meat, poultry, fish, dry beans, eggs, and nuts group.

As illustrated in the Healthy Eating Pyramid, grains, vegetables, and fruits provide the nutritional base for a healthy diet. Daily fruits and vegetables should include as a minimum, one good source of pro-vitamin A or carotene (apricots, cantaloupe, broccoli, carrots, pumpkin, dark leafy vegetables) and one good source of vitamin C (citrus fruit, kiwi fruit, cantaloupe, strawberries, broccoli, cabbage, cauliflower, green pepper).

An entirely new field of research with promising results in disease prevention, especially in the fight against cancer, is in the area of **phytochemicals**[7]

Nutrition Facts

Serving Size 1 cup (240 ml)
Servings Per Container 4

Amount Per Serving	
Calories 120	Calories from Fat 45

	% Daily Value*
Total Fat 5g	**8%**
Saturated Fat 3g	**15%**
Cholesterol 20mg	**7%**
Sodium 120mg	**5%**
Total Carbohydrate 12g	**4%**
Dietary Fiber 0g	**0%**
Sugars 12g	
Protein 8g	

Vitamin A	10%	Vitamin C	4%
Calcium	30%	Iron	0%

*Percent Daily Values are based on a 2,000 calorie diet. Your daily values may be higher or lower depending on your calorie needs:

	Calories	2,000	2,500
Total Fat	Less than	65g	80g
Sat Fat	Less than	20g	25g
Cholesterol	Less than	300mg	300mg
Sodium	Less than	2,400mg	2,400mg
Total Carbohydrate		300g	375g
Fiber		25g	30g

Calories per gram:
Fat 9 • Carbohydrate 4 • Protein 4

Percent fat calories = (grams of fat × 9) ÷ calories per serving × 100

5 grams of fat × 9 calories per grams of fat = 45 calories from fat

45 calories from fat ÷ 120 calories per serving × 100 = 38% fat

Figure 7.11 • *Determining percent calories from fat in food.*

TERMS
Phytochemicals Compounds, found in fruits and vegetables, that block the formation of cancerous tumors and disrupt the process.

FAT CONTENT OF SELECTED FOODS

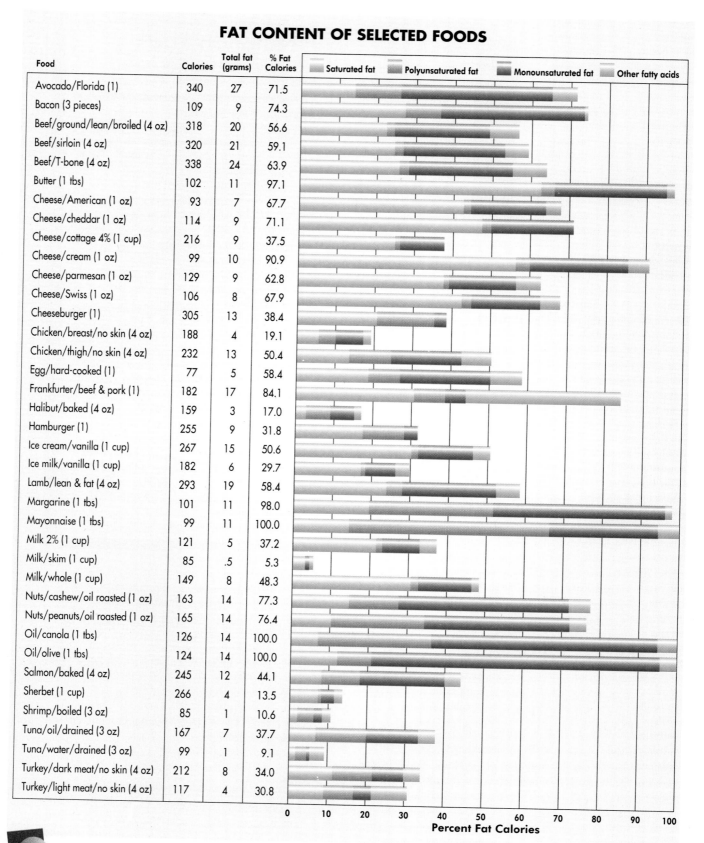

Food	Calories	Total fat (grams)	% Fat Calories
Avocado/Florida (1)	340	27	71.5
Bacon (3 pieces)	109	9	74.3
Beef/ground/lean/broiled (4 oz)	318	20	56.6
Beef/sirloin (4 oz)	320	21	59.1
Beef/T-bone (4 oz)	338	24	63.9
Butter (1 tbs)	102	11	97.1
Cheese/American (1 oz)	93	7	67.7
Cheese/cheddar (1 oz)	114	9	71.1
Cheese/cottage 4% (1 cup)	216	9	37.5
Cheese/cream (1 oz)	99	10	90.9
Cheese/parmesan (1 oz)	129	9	62.8
Cheese/Swiss (1 oz)	106	8	67.9
Cheeseburger (1)	305	13	38.4
Chicken/breast/no skin (4 oz)	188	4	19.1
Chicken/thigh/no skin (4 oz)	232	13	50.4
Egg/hard-cooked (1)	77	5	58.4
Frankfurter/beef & pork (1)	182	17	84.1
Halibut/baked (4 oz)	159	3	17.0
Hamburger (1)	255	9	31.8
Ice cream/vanilla (1 cup)	267	15	50.6
Ice milk/vanilla (1 cup)	182	6	29.7
Lamb/lean & fat (4 oz)	293	19	58.4
Margarine (1 tbs)	101	11	98.0
Mayonnaise (1 tbs)	99	11	100.0
Milk 2% (1 cup)	121	5	37.2
Milk/skim (1 cup)	85	.5	5.3
Milk/whole (1 cup)	149	8	48.3
Nuts/cashew/oil roasted (1 oz)	163	14	77.3
Nuts/peanuts/oil roasted (1 oz)	165	14	76.4
Oil/canola (1 tbs)	126	14	100.0
Oil/olive (1 tbs)	124	14	100.0
Salmon/baked (4 oz)	245	12	44.1
Sherbet (1 cup)	266	4	13.5
Shrimp/boiled (3 oz)	85	1	10.6
Tuna/oil/drained (3 oz)	167	7	37.7
Tuna/water/drained (3 oz)	99	1	9.1
Turkey/dark meat/no skin (4 oz)	212	8	34.0
Turkey/light meat/no skin (4 oz)	117	4	30.8

Legend: Saturated fat | Polyunsaturated fat | Monounsaturated fat | Other fatty acids

Percent Fat Calories (0–100)

Figure 7.12 • *Fat content of selected foods.*

("phyto" comes from the Greek word for plant). These compounds, just recently discovered by scientists, are found in large quantities in fruits and vegetables.

Phytochemicals seem to have a powerful ability to block the formation of cancerous tumors.

The main function of phytochemicals in plants is to protect them from sunlight. In humans, they seem to have a powerful ability to block the formation of cancerous tumors. Their actions are so diverse that, at almost every stage of cancer, phytochemicals have the ability to block, disrupt, slow down, or even reverse the process. These compounds are not found in pills. The message here is to eat a diet with ample fruits and vegetables. The recommendation of five to nine servings of fruits and vegetables daily has absolutely no substitute. People can't expect to eat a poor diet, pop a few pills, and derive the same benefits.

Milk, poultry, fish, and meats are to be consumed in moderation. Milk should be skim, and milk products should be low-fat. Three ounces of poultry, fish, or meat and not to exceed 6 ounces daily is the recommendation. All visible fat and skin should be trimmed off meats and poultry before cooking. Egg consumption should be limited to no more than three eggs per week.

As an aid in balancing your diet, the form given in Figure 7.16 (at the end of the chapter) enables you to record your daily food intake. This record is much easier to keep than the complete dietary analysis. Make as many copies of this lab as the number of days you wish to record. Whenever you have something to eat, record, in Figure 7.16, the food and the amount eaten. Record this information immediately after each meal so you will be able to keep track of your actual food intake more easily.

If you eat twice the amount of a standard serving, double the number of servings. Evaluate your diet by checking whether you ate the minimum required servings for each food group. If you meet the minimum required servings at the end of each day, you are doing well in balancing your diet.

Restructure your meals on the plate so rice, pasta, beans, breads, and vegetables are in the center, meats are on the side and are added primarily for flavoring, and desserts consist of fruits. Substitute

Restructure your meals to emphasize pasta, beans, breads, vegetables, and fruits.

low-fat or nonfat milk and milk products. This is another strategy to help you enjoy a healthy diet, prevent disease, and improve your overall quality of life.

● Nutrient Supplementation

According to the Food and Drug Administration, four of every 10 adults in the United States take nutrient supplements daily, and one in every seven has a nutrient intake almost eight times the RDA. With some exceptions, vitamin and mineral requirements for the body can be met by consuming as few as 1200 calories per day, as long as the diet contains the recommended servings from the five food groups.

Water-soluble vitamins cannot be stored as long as fat-soluble vitamins. The body excretes excessive intakes readily. Small amounts, however, can be retained for weeks or months in various organs and tissues of the body. Fat-soluble vitamins, on the other hand, are stored in fatty tissue. Therefore, daily intake of these vitamins is not as crucial. Too much vitamin A and vitamin D actually can be detrimental to health.

People should not take **megadoses** of vitamins. Mineral doses should not exceed three times the RDA.

Presently, no standard percentage above the RDA is available to guide us in determining the level

Megadoses For most vitamins, 10 times the RDA or more. For A and D, five and two times the RDA, respectively.

Figure 7.13 ● *Healthy Eating Pyramid: A guide to daily food choices (Continued).*

Figure 7.13 ● *(Continued).*

at which a high dose of a given nutrient may cause health problems. For some nutrients, a dose of five times the RDA taken over several months may create problems. For others, it may not pose any threat to human health.

Iron deficiency (determined through blood testing) is common in women. Iron supplementation frequently is recommended for these women who have heavy menstrual flow. Some pregnant and lactating women also may require supplements. According to 1990 guidelines by the National Academy of Science, the average pregnant woman who eats an adequate amount of a variety of foods needs only to take a low dose of iron supplement daily. Women who are pregnant with more than one baby may need additional supplements. In the above instances, supplements should be taken under a physician's supervision.

Other people who may benefit from supplementation are alcoholics and street-drug users who do not have a balanced diet, smokers, strict vegetarians, individuals on extremely low-calorie diets, elderly people who don't eat balanced meals regularly, and newborn infants (usually given a single dose of vitamin K to prevent abnormal bleeding). While some supplements are encouraged (see discussion that follows), for healthy people with a balanced diet, most supplements do not seem to provide additional benefits. They do not help people run faster, jump higher, relieve stress, improve sexual prowess, cure a common cold, or boost energy levels.

Antioxidants: Free Radical Combatants

Much research currently is being done to study the effects of antioxidant supplements in thwarting several chronic diseases. Vitamins C, E, beta-carotene (a precursor to vitamin A), and the mineral selenium serve as **antioxidants**, preventing oxygen from combining with other substances it may damage (see Table 7.6). Oxygen is utilized during metabolism to change carbohydrates and fats into energy. During this process oxygen is transformed into stable forms of water and carbon dioxide. A small amount of oxygen, however, ends up in an unstable form, referred to as **oxygen free radicals**.

A free radical molecule has a normal proton nucleus with a single unpaired electron. Having only one electron makes the free radical extremely reactive, and it constantly looks to pair the electron up with one from another molecule. When a free radical steals the second electron from another molecule, that other molecule in turn becomes a free radical. This chain reaction goes on until two free radicals meet to form a stable molecule. Antioxidants absorb free radicals before they can cause damage, and they interrupt the sequence of reactions once damage has begun.

Free radicals attack and damage proteins and lipids, in particular the cell membrane and DNA. This damage is thought to contribute to the development of conditions such as cardiovascular disease, cancer, emphysema, cataracts, Parkinson's disease, and premature aging. Solar radiation, cigarette smoke, radiation, and other environmental factors also seem to encourage the formation of free radicals. Antioxidants are thought to offer protection by absorbing free radicals before they can cause damage and also by interrupting the sequence of reactions once damage has begun, thwarting certain chronic diseases (see Figure 7.14).

Antioxidants are found abundantly in food, especially in fruits and vegetables. Unfortunately,

Table 7.6   *Antioxidant Nutrients, Sources, and Functions*

Nutrient	Good Sources	Antioxidant Effect
Vitamin C	Citrus fruit, kiwi fruit, cantaloupe, strawberries, broccoli, green or red peppers, cauliflower, cabbage	Appears to inactivate oxygen-free radicals
Vitamin E	Vegetable oils, yellow and green leafy vegetables, margarine, wheat germ, oatmeal, almonds, and whole grain breads, cereals	Protects lipids from oxidation.
Beta-carotene	Carrots, squash, pumpkin, sweet potatoes, broccoli, green leafy vegetables	Soaks up oxygen-free radicals
Selenium	Seafood, meat, whole grains	Helps prevent damage to cell structures

Figure 7.14 ● *Antioxidant protection: blocking and absorbing oxygen-free radicals to prevent chronic diseases.*

only 9% of Americans eat the minimum five daily servings of fruits and vegetables[8] (five to nine are recommended). In a departure from past recommendations, in 1994 the editorial board of the *University of California at Berkeley Wellness Letter* issued the following antioxidant nutrient guidelines for people who eat at least five daily servings of antioxidant-rich fruits and vegetables:[9]

- 250 to 500 mg of vitamin C.
- 200 to 800 **IU** of vitamin E.
- 10,000 to 25,000 IU of beta-carotene.

In a special report, the editorial board also issued the following statement:[10]

> The editorial board of the Wellness Letter has been reluctant to recommend supplementary vitamins on a broad scale for healthy people eating healthy diets. But the accumulation of research in recent years has caused us to change our minds.

Based on these recommendations, people who consume nine ample amounts of fresh fruits and vegetables daily could get their daily beta-carotene and vitamin C requirements through the diet. To obtain the recommended guideline for vitamin E through diet alone, however, is practically impossible. As shown in Table 7.7, vitamin E is not easily found in large quantities in foods typically consumed in the diet. Thus, supplements are encouraged. When supplements (in general) are taken, they should be taken with meals and split in two to three doses per day.[11]

According to further evidence released in 1996, the editorial board of *University of California at Berkeley Wellness Letter* has indicated that it is better to obtain your daily dose of beta-carotene from natural sources (food) and not from supplements (pills).[12]

Two separate clinical trials found that beta-carotene supplements offered no protection against heart disease and cancer. One of these studies actually found a higher lung cancer and mortality rate in smokers who took beta-carotene supplements. For former smokers and nonsmokers, these supplements do not cause any harm but offer no additional health benefits either. It is therefore recommended that you "skip the pill and eat the carrot." One medium raw carrot contains about 20,000 IU of beta-carotene (the recommended daily dose). Supplements of vitamin E and C are still encouraged as they offer several potential health benefits.

Supplements of the mineral selenium are not widely recommended at this point. Research published in 1996, nonetheless, showed that individuals who took 200 mcg of selenium daily decreased the risk of prostate cancer by 63%, colorectal cancer by 58%, and lung cancer by 46%.[13] Other evidence suggests that taking 100 mcg of selenium supplements daily increases energy levels, decreases anxiety, and improves immune function.[14]

TERMS

Antioxidants Compounds such as vitamins C, E, beta-carotene, and selenium that prevent oxygen from combining with other substances to which it may cause damage.

Oxygen free radicals Substances formed during metabolism that attack and damage proteins and lipids, in particular the cell membrane and DNA, leading to the development of diseases such as heart disease, cancer, and emphysema.

IU International units, for measuring nutrients.

One unshelled Brazil nut (which you may crack yourself) provides about 100 mcg of selenium. Shelled nuts found in supermarkets average only about 20 mcg each. Toxic levels of selenium are thought to be around 2,500 mcg per day. Based on the current body of research, 100 to 200 mcg per day seem to provide the necessary amount of antioxidant for this nutrient. There is no reason to take more than 200 mcg daily.

Although not an antioxidant, folacin (a B vitamin) also is recommended (400 mcg) for all premenopausal women.[15] Folacin helps prevent certain birth defects and seems to offer protection against colon and cervical cancers.

Toxic effects with antioxidant supplementation are rare when taken in the previously recommended amounts. Generally, up to 4,000 mg of vitamin C, 3,200 IU of vitamin E, and 50,000 IU of beta-carotene seem safe. If any of the following side effects arise, stop supplementation and check with your physician:

- Vitamin E: gastrointestinal disturbances; increase in blood lipids (determined through blood tests).
- Vitamin C: nausea, diarrhea, abdominal cramps, kidney stones, liver problems.
- Beta-carotene: although not harmful, yellow pigmentation of the skin.
- Selenium: nausea, vomiting, diarrhea, irritability, fatigue, flulike symptoms, lesions of the skin and nervous tissue, loss of hair and nails, respiratory failure, and liver damage.

Large supplements of vitamin E are not recommended for individuals on **anticoagulant** therapy. Vitamin E is an anticoagulant in itself. If you are on such therapy, check with your physician. Pregnant women need a physician's approval prior to beta-carotene supplementation. It also may be unsafe if taken with alcohol and by people who drink more than 4 ounces of pure alcohol per day (the equivalent of eight beers).

A few researchers are expressing concern for people who participate regularly in high-intensity exercise (above 70% of heart rate reserve — see Chapter 3) or prolonged exercise (more than 5 hours per week). Overtraining increases the production of free radicals and well may exceed the body's antioxidant defense mechanism. This high amount of free radicals may increase the risk for chronic diseases, including cancer.[16]

Scientists, therefore, are examining a possible link between "heavy" exercise and disease in people who otherwise lead a healthy lifestyle. Although the research is scarce, Dr. Kenneth Cooper, in his book *Antioxidant Revolution*, recommends higher doses

Table 7.7 Antioxidant Content of Selected Foods

Beta-Carotene	IU
Apricot (1 medium)	675
Broccoli (½ cup, frozen)	1,740
Broccoli (½ cup, raw)	680
Cantaloupe (1 cup)	5,160
Carrot (1 medium, raw)	20,255
Green peas (½ cup, frozen)	535
Mango (1 medium)	8,060
Mustard greens (½ cup, frozen)	3,350
Papaya (1 medium)	6,120
Spinach (½ cup, frozen)	7,395
Sweet potato (1 medium, baked)	24,875
Tomato (1 medium)	1,395
Turnip greens (½ cup, boiled)	3,960

Vitamin C	mg
Acerola (1 cup, raw)	1,640
Acerola juice (8 oz)	3,864
Cantaloupe (½ melon, medium)	90
Cranberry juice (8 oz)	90
Grapefruit (½, medium, white)	52
Grapefruit juice (8 oz)	92
Guava (1 medium)	165
Kiwi (1 medium)	75
Lemon juice (8 oz)	110
Orange (1 medium)	66
Orange juice (8 oz)	120
Papaya (1 medium)	85
Pepper (½ cup, red, chopped, raw)	95
Strawberries (1 cup, raw)	88

Vitamin E	IU	mg*
Almond oil (1 tbsp)		5.3
Almonds (1 oz)	10.1	
Canola oil (1 tbsp)		9.0
Cottonseed oil (1 tbsp)		5.2
Hazelnuts (1 oz)	4.4	
Kale (1 cup)	15.0	
Margarine (1 tbsp)		2.0
Peanuts (1 oz)	3.0	
Shrimp (3 oz, boiled)	3.1	
Sunflower seeds (1 oz, dry)	14.2	
Sunflower seed oil (1 tbsp)		6.9
Sweet potato (1 medium, baked)	7.2	
Wheat germ oil (1 tbsp)		20.0

* Vitamin E values for oils are commonly expressed in milligrams (mg). One mg is almost equal to 1 IU (international unit).

of antioxidants for athletes and heavy exercisers: 3000 mg of vitamin C, 1200 IU of vitamin E, and 50,000 IU of beta-carotene.[17] Awareness of side effects is important if these higher amounts are taken.

While supplements are encouraged, fruits and vegetables are the richest sources of antioxidants and phytochemicals. In 1996, researchers at the U.S. Department of Agriculture compared the antioxidant effects of vitamins C and E with those of various common fruits and vegetables.[18] The results indicated that ¾ cup of cooked kale neutralized as many free radicals as approximately 800 IU of vitamin E or 600 mg of vitamin C. Three-fourths cup of cooked kale contains only 11 IU of vitamin E and 76 mg of vitamin C. Other excellent sources investigated by these researchers included blueberries, strawberries, spinach, Brussels sprouts, plums, broccoli, beets, oranges, and grapes. Further, red bell peppers, pink grapefruit, onions, white grapes, corn, eggplant, cauliflower, potatoes, cabbage, leaf lettuce, bananas, apples, green beans, carrots, tomatoes, and pears are recommended as good sources of antioxidants.

Many people who regularly eat foods high in fat content or too many sweets think they need supplementation to balance their diet. This is another fallacy about nutrition. The problem in these cases is not necessarily a lack of vitamins and minerals but, instead, a diet too high in calories, fat, and sodium. Vitamin, mineral, and fiber supplements do not supply all of the nutrients and other beneficial substances present in food and needed for good health. Supplements are no substitute for a well-balanced diet.

Wholesome foods contain vitamins, minerals, carbohydrates, fiber, proteins, fats, phytochemicals, and others not yet discovered. Researchers do not know if the protective effects are caused by the antioxidants themselves, in combination with other nutrients (such as phytochemicals), or actually by some other nutrients in food that have not been investigated yet. Many nutrients work in **synergy**, enhancing chemical processes in the body. Supplementation will not offset poor eating habits. Pills are no substitute for common sense.

If you think your diet is not balanced, you first need to conduct a nutrient analysis to determine which nutrients are missing. Use the Healthy Eating Pyramid and the vitamin and mineral tables in this chapter, and eat more of the foods high in antioxidants and phytochemicals, and those with nutrients that are deficient in your diet.

● Specific Nutrition Considerations

Nutrition for Athletes

The two main fuels that supply energy for physical activity are glucose and fat (fatty acids). The body uses amino acids, derived from proteins, as an energy substrate when glucose is low, such as during fasting, prolonged aerobic exercise, or a low carbohydrate diet.

Glucose is derived from foods high in carbohydrates such as breads, cereals, grains, pasta, beans, fruits, vegetables, and sweets in general. Glucose is stored as **glycogen** in muscles and the liver. As noted earlier in the chapter, fatty acids are derived from the breakdown of fats. Unlike glucose, an almost unlimited supply of fatty acids, stored as fat in the body, can be used during exercise.

During resting conditions fat supplies about two-thirds of the energy to sustain the vital processes. During exercise the body uses both glucose and fat in combination to supply the energy demands. The proportion of fat to glucose changes with the intensity of exercise. When exercising below 60% to 70% of the individual's maximal work capacity, fat is used as the primary energy substrate. As the intensity of exercise increases, so does the percentage of glucose utilization, up to 100% during maximal work sustained for 2 to 3 minutes.

In general, athletes do not require special supplementation or any other special type of diet. Unless the diet is deficient in basic nutrients, no special, secret, or magic diet will help people perform better or develop faster as a result of what they eat. As long as the diet is balanced, based on a large variety of nutrients from the basic food groups, athletes do not require supplements. Even in strength training and body building, protein in excess of 20% of total daily caloric intake is not necessary.

The main difference between a sedentary person and a highly active individual is in the total number of calories required daily and the amount of carbohydrate intake during bouts of prolonged physical

TERMS

Anticoagulant Any substance that inhibits blood clotting.

Synergy A reaction in which the result is greater than the sum of its two parts.

Glycogen Form in which glucose is stored in muscle.

activity. During training, people consume more calories because of the greater energy expenditure required as a result of intense physical training.

Carbohydrate Loading

While on a regular diet, the body is able to store between 1,500 and 2,000 calories in the form of glycogen. About 75% of this glycogen is stored in muscle tissue. This amount, however, can be increased greatly through **carbohydrate loading.**

A regular diet should be altered during several days of heavy aerobic training or when a person is going to participate in a long-distance event of more than 90 minutes (for example, marathon, triathlon, road cycling). For events shorter than 90 minutes, carbohydrate loading does not seem to enhance performance.

During prolonged exercise, glycogen is broken down into glucose, which then is readily available to the muscle for energy production. In comparison to fat, glucose frequently is referred to as the "high-octane fuel" because it provides about 6% more energy per unit of oxygen consumed.

Heavy training over several consecutive days leads to glycogen depletion faster than it can be replaced through the diet. Glycogen depletion with heavy training is common in athletes. Signs of depletion include chronic fatigue, difficulty in maintaining accustomed exercise intensity, and lower performance.

On consecutive days of exhaustive physical training (several hours daily), a carbohydrate-rich diet, 70% of total daily caloric intake or 8 grams of carbohydrate per 2.2 pounds of body weight, is recommended. This diet often restores glycogen levels in 24 hours. Along with the high-carbohydrate diet, a day of rest often is needed to allow the muscles to recover from glycogen depletion following days of intense training. For people who exercise less than an hour a day, a 60% carbohydrate diet or 6 grams of carbohydrate per 2.2 pounds (1 kilogram) of body weight is enough to restore glycogen stores.

Following an exhaustive workout, eating a combination of carbohydrates and protein (tuna sandwich) within 30 minutes of exercise seems to speed up glycogen storage at an even faster rate.[19] Protein intake increases insulin activity, thus enhancing glycogen replenishment. A 70% carbohydrate intake then should be maintained throughout the rest of the day.

By following a special diet/exercise regimen 5 days before a long-distance event, highly trained (aerobically) individuals are capable of storing two to three times the amount of glycogen found in the average person. Athletic performance may be enhanced for long-distance events of more than 90 minutes by eating a regular balanced diet along with intensive physical training the fifth and fourth days before the event, followed by a diet high in carbohydrates (about 70%) and a gradual decrease in training intensity the 3 days before the event.

The amount of glycogen stored as a result of a carbohydrate-rich diet does not seem to be related to the proportion of complex and simple carbohydrates. Intake of simple carbohydrate (sugar) can be raised while on a 70% carbohydrate diet, as long as 48% of the total calories are derived from complex carbohydrates. The latter provide more nutrients and fiber, making them a better choice for a healthier diet.

On the day of the long-distance event, high carbohydrates are still the recommended choice of substrate. But high sugar intake 30 minutes prior to the event might be counterproductive. A "sugar shock" shortly before the event may cause **hypoglycemia.** The pancreas responds to high sugar intake with a large production of insulin. **Insulin** in turn lowers blood glucose. Further, the muscles draw glucose from the blood at the start of exercise, exacerbating the condition.

As a rule of thumb, individuals should consume 1 gram of carbohydrate for each 2.2 pounds of body weight 1 hour prior to exercise. The amount of carbohydrate can be increased to 2, 3, or 4 grams per 2.2 pounds of weight 2, 3, or 4 hours, respectively, before exercise.

During the long-distance event, researchers recommend that 50 to 60 grams of carbohydrate (200 to 240 calories) be consumed every hour. This is best accomplished by drinking 8 ounces of a 6% to 8% carbohydrate sports drink every 15 minutes. This also lessens the chance of dehydration during exercise, which hinders performance and endangers health. The percentage of the carbohydrate drink is determined by dividing the amount of carbohydrate in grams by the amount of fluid, in ml, and multiplying by 100. For example, 18 grams of carbohydrate in 240 ml (8 oz) of fluid yields a drink at 7.5% ($18 \div 240 \times 100$).

Amino Acid Supplements

A myth regarding athletic performance is that protein (amino acid) supplements will increase muscle mass. The claims and safety of these products have not been proven scientifically. The RDA for protein is .8 grams per kilogram of body weight.

Most athletes, including weight lifters and body builders, increase their caloric intake automatically during intense training. As caloric intake increases, so does the intake of protein, approaching in many instances 2 or more grams per kilogram of body weight. This amount is more than enough to build and repair muscle tissue. Athletes in strength training typically consume between 3 and 4 grams per kilogram of body weight.

People who take costly free-amino acid supplements are led to believe that this contributes to the development of muscle mass. The human body cannot distinguish between amino acids obtained from food or through supplements. Excess protein either is used for energy or is turned into fat. With amino acid supplements, each capsule provides up to 500 milligrams of amino acids and no additional nutrients. Three ounces of meat or fish provide more than 20,000 milligrams of amino acids, along with other essential nutrients such as iron, niacin, and thiamin.

Proponents of free-amino acid supplements further claim that only a small amount of amino acids in food is absorbed and that free-amino acids are absorbed more readily than protein food. Neither claim is correct. The human body absorbs and utilizes between 85% and 99% of all protein from food intake. The body handles whole proteins better than single amino acids predigested in the laboratory setting.

Amino acid supplementation can even be dangerous to the body. Supplementation of a group of chemically similar amino acids often prevents the absorption of other amino acids, potentially causing critical imbalances and toxicities. Long-term risks associated with amino acid supplementation have not been determined.

The rate of absorption provides no additional benefit because building muscle takes hours, not minutes. Muscle overload through heavy training, not supplementation, builds muscle. Expensive protein supplements benefit only those who stand to gain financial benefits from selling them.

Bone Health and Osteoporosis

In **osteoporosis**, bones, primarily of the hip, wrist, and spine, become so weak and brittle that they fracture readily. Osteoporosis is preventable. The process begins slowly in the third and fourth decades of life. Women are especially susceptible after menopause because of the accompanying **estrogen** loss, which increases the rate at which bone mass is broken down.

Approximately 15 to 20 million women in the United States have osteoporosis, and about 1.5 million fractures are attributed to this condition each year. An estimated 30,000 to 60,000 of the 200,000 women with hip fractures die of complications resulting from these fractures. According to Dr. Barbara Drinkwater, a leading researcher in this area, "Shocking as these figures are, they cannot adequately convey the pain and deterioration in the quality of life of women who suffer the crippling effects of osteoporotic fractures."[20]

Estrogen is the most important factor in preventing bone loss.

In maximizing bone density in young women and decreasing the rate of bone loss later in life, the importance of normal estrogen levels, adequate calcium intake, and physical activity cannot be overemphasized (see Figure 7.15). All three factors are crucial in preventing osteoporosis. The absence of any one of these three factors leads to bone loss for which the other two factors never completely compensate.

Prevention of osteoporosis begins early in life by having enough calcium in the diet (the RDA is 800 to 1200 mg per day) and by participating in exercise. The calcium RDA can be met easily through diet alone. Some experts, however, recommend calcium supplements for children before puberty. Along with adequate calcium intake, an additional amount

TERMS

Carbohydrate loading Increasing intake of carbohydrates during heavy aerobic training or prior to aerobic endurance events lasting longer than 90 minutes.

Hypoglycemia Low blood sugar (glucose).

Insulin Hormone secreted by the pancreas used in the absorption and utilization of glucose by the body.

Osteoporosis The softening, deterioration, or loss of total body bone.

Estrogen Female sex hormone; essential for bone formation and bone density conservation.

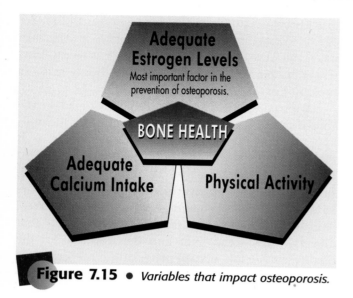

Figure 7.15 • *Variables that impact osteoporosis.*

The key role of exercise in preventing osteoporosis seems to be related to the decrease in rate of bone density loss following menopause. Active people are able to maintain bone density much more effectively than their inactive counterparts, helping to prevent osteoporosis. A combination of weight-bearing exercises, such as walking or jogging and weight training, is especially helpful. The benefits of exercise go beyond maintaining bone density. Exercise strengthens muscles, ligaments, and tendons — all of which provide support to the bones (skeleton). Exercise also improves balance and coordination, which can help prevent falls and injuries.

Current studies indicate that people who are active have denser bone mineral than inactive people do. Similar to other benefits of participating in exercise, there is no such thing as "bone in the bank." To have good bone health, people need to participate in a regular lifetime exercise program.

Prevailing research also tells us that estrogen is the most important factor in preventing bone loss. In one study, lumbar bone density in women who had always had regular menstrual cycles exceeded that of women with a history of oligomenorrhea (irregular cycles) and amenorrhea (cessation of menstruation) interspaced with regular cycles. Furthermore, the lumbar density of these two groups of women was higher than that of women who had never had regular menstrual cycles.

of vitamin D may be needed for optimal calcium absorption. Table 7.8 provides a list of selected foods with their calcium content. A common recommendation is that women after age 45 get 1,500 mg of calcium per day and men, 1,000 mg.

Also, high protein intake may affect calcium absorption by the body. The more protein eaten, the higher the calcium content in the urine. This might be the reason why countries with a high protein intake, including the United States, also have the highest rates of osteoporosis.

Table 7.8   *Low-Fat Calcium-Rich Foods*

Food	Amount	Calcium (mg)	Calories	Calories From Fat
Beans, red kidney, cooked	1 cup	70	218	4%
Beet, greens, cooked	1/2 cup	72	13	—
Broccoli, cooked, drained	1 sm stalk	123	36	—
Burrito, bean	1	173	307	28%
Cottage cheese, 2% low-fat	1/2 cup	78	103	18%
Milk, nonfat, powdered	1 tbsp	52	27	1%
Milk, skim	1 cup	296	88	3%
Ice milk (vanilla)	1/2 cup	102	100	27%
Instant breakfast, whole milk	1 cup	301	280	26%
Kale, cooked, drained	1/2 cup	103	22	—
Okra, cooked, drained	1/2 cup	74	23	—
Shrimp, boiled	3 oz.	99	99	9%
Spinach, raw	1 cup	51	14	—
Yogurt, fruit	1 cup	345	231	8%
Yogurt, low-fat, plain	1 cup	271	160	20%

Following menopause, every woman should consider hormone replacement therapy and discuss it with her physician. Women who have estrogen therapy do not lose bone mineral density at the rate of women who do not have estrogen therapy. Neither exercise nor calcium supplementation will offset the damaging effects of lower estrogen levels. Hormone replacement therapy seems to be the only reasonable therapy that post-menopausal women have to prevent osteoporosis in future years.

For instance, athletes with **amenorrhea** (who have lower estrogen levels) have lower bone mineral density than even nonathletes with normal estrogen levels. One study[21] showed that amenorrheic athletes at age 25 have the bones of 52-year-old women. Other research[22] showed four amenorrheic athletes with a bone density equivalent to that of 70- to 80-year-old women. Over the last few years, it has become clear that sedentary women with normal estrogen levels have better bone mineral density than active amenorrheic athletes. Many experts believe the best predictor of bone mineral content is the history of menstrual regularity.

Iron Deficiency

Iron is a key element of **hemoglobin** in blood. The RDA of iron for adult women is 15 mg per day (10 mg for men). According to a survey by the U.S. Department of Agriculture, 19- to 50-year-old women in the United States consumed only 60% of the RDA for iron. People who do not have enough iron in the body can develop iron-deficiency anemia, in which the concentration of hemoglobin in the red blood cells is less than it should be.

Physically active women also may have a greater than average need for iron. Heavy training creates a demand for iron that is higher than the recommended intake because small amounts of iron are lost through sweat, urine, and stools. Mechanical trauma, caused by the pounding of the feet on the pavement during extensive jogging, also may lead to the destruction of iron-containing red blood cells.

A large percentage of female endurance athletes is reported to have iron deficiency. Blood **ferritin** levels should be checked frequently in women who participate in intense physical training.

The rates of iron absorption and iron loss vary from person to person. In most cases, though, people can get enough iron by eating more iron-rich foods such as beans, peas, green leafy vegetables, enriched grain products, egg yolk, fish, and lean meats. Although organ meats, such as liver, are especially good sources, they also are high in cholesterol. A list of foods high in iron content is given in Table 7.9.

● Dietary Guidelines for North Americans

Based on the available scientific research on nutrition and health and the current dietary habits of the American people, in 1995 the Scientific Committee of the U. S. Department of Health and Human Services and the U.S. Department of Agriculture on diet and health issued the fourth edition of the Dietary Guidelines for healthy American adults and children. These guidelines potentially can reduce the risk of developing certain chronic diseases. The committee's recommendations are:[23]

- Eat a variety of food. No single food can provide all of the necessary nutrients and other beneficial substances in the amounts the body needs. For good nutrition, you should meet the recommended number of daily servings from each of the five food groups in the Food Guide Pyramid. Within each food group, choose a variety of foods. Food items vary, and each item provides different combinations of nutrients and other substances needed for good health.

- Balance the food you eat with physical activity to maintain or improve your weight. Excessive body weight increases the risk for diseases including heart disease, stroke, diabetes, high blood pressure, and certain cancers. Many people gain weight as adults, and this does not have to be the case. To maintain body weight, you need to balance food intake with the amount of calories the body uses. In ensuing chapters you will find extensive information on weight management and exercise programs to help you balance your energy requirements according to your personal needs.

TERMS

Amenorrhea Cessation of regular menstrual flow.

Hemoglobin Protein-iron compound in red blood cells that transports oxygen in the blood.

Ferritin Iron stored in the body.

Table 7.9   *Iron-Rich Foods*

Food	Amount	Iron (mg)	Calories	Cholesterol	Calories From Fat
Beans, red kidney, cooked	1 cup	4.4	218	0	4%
Beef, ground lean	3 oz.	3.0	186	81	48%
Beef, sirloin	3 oz.	2.5	329	77	74%
Beef, liver, fried	3 oz.	7.5	195	345	42%
Beet, greens, cooked	1/2 cup	1.4	13	0	—
Broccoli, cooked, drained	1 sm stalk	1.1	36	0	—
Burrito, bean	1	2.4	307	14	28%
Egg, hard-cooked	1	1.0	72	250	63%
Farina (Cream of Wheat), cooked	1/2 cup	6.0	51	0	—
Instant breakfast, whole milk	1 cup	8.0	280	33	26%
Peas, frozen, cooked, drained	1/2 cup	1.5	55	0	—
Shrimp, boiled	3 oz.	2.7	99	128	9%
Spinach, raw	1 cup	1.7	14	0	—
Vegetables, mixed, cooked	1 cup	2.4	116	0	—

- Choose a diet with plenty of grain products, vegetables, and fruits. Most of your daily calories should come from these food products. They contain ample amounts of vitamins, minerals, complex carbohydrates, and other substances important for good health.

- Choose a diet low in fat, saturated fat, and cholesterol. Reduce fat intake to 30% or less of total calories. Reduce saturated fatty acid intake to less than 10% of total calories and intake of cholesterol to no more than 300 mg daily. Intake of fat and cholesterol can be lowered by substituting fish, poultry without skin, lean meats, and low or nonfat dairy products for fatty meats and whole-milk dairy products; by choosing more vegetables, fruits, cereals, and legumes; and by limiting oils, fats, egg yolks, and fried and other fatty foods.

- Choose a diet moderate in sugars. Excessive sugar and starch intake can contribute to weight gain and tooth decay. This guideline advises against frequent and large consumption of food items and snacks high in sugar that provide unnecessary calories and few nutrients. The more often that high sugar foods are consumed, and the longer before brushing the teeth following their consumption, the greater is the risk for tooth decay.

- Choose a diet moderate in salt and sodium. Limit total daily intake of salt (sodium chloride) to 6 grams or less. This amount represents the equivalent of 2,400 mg of sodium listed in the Daily Value of the Nutrition Label. To decrease your daily sodium intake, limit the use of salt in cooking and do not add it to food at the table. Sparingly consume salty, highly processed salty, salt- preserved, and salt-pickled foods.

- If you drink alcoholic beverages, do so in moderation. Alcoholic beverages provide calories but few or no nutrients. Moderate drinking has been linked to a decreased risk for coronary heart disease in some people. High levels of alcohol consumption lead to an increased risk for heart disease, stroke, high blood pressure, certain cancers, cirrhosis of the liver, inflammation of the pancreas, brain damage, birth defects, accidents, violence, suicides, and malnutrition. Limit consumption to the equivalent of less than an ounce of pure alcohol in a single day. This translates into two cans of beer, two small glasses of wine, or two average cocktails. If pregnant, avoid alcoholic beverages altogether.

● Proper Nutrition: A Lifetime Prescription for Healthy Living

Proper nutrition, a sound exercise program, and quitting smoking (for those who smoke) are the three factors that do the most for health, longevity, and quality of life. Achieving and maintaining a balanced diet is not as difficult as most people would think. If parents were to do a better job of teaching and reinforcing proper nutrition habits in early youth, we would not have the magnitude of nutrition-related health problems that we do. Although the treatment of obesity is important, we should place far greater emphasis in preventing obesity in youth and adults alike.

Children tend to eat the way their parents do. If parents adopt a healthy diet, children most likely will follow. The difficult part for most people is retraining themselves to follow a lifetime healthy nutrition plan — a diet that includes lots of grains, legumes, fruits, vegetables, and low-fat dairy products, with moderate use of animal protein, junk food, sodium, and alcohol.

In spite of the ample scientific evidence linking poor dietary habits to early disease and mortality rates, most people are not willing to change their eating patterns. Even when faced with obesity, elevated blood lipids, hypertension, and other nutrition-related conditions, people do not change. The motivating factor to change one's eating habits seems to be a major health breakdown, such as a

Positive nutrition habits should be taught and reinforced in early youth.

heart attack, a stroke, or cancer. By this time the damage already has been done. In many cases it is irreversible and, for some, fatal.

An ounce of prevention is worth a pound of cure. The sooner you implement the dietary guidelines presented in this chapter, the better will be your chances of preventing chronic diseases and reaching a higher state of wellness.

Notes

1. *Surgeon General's Report on Nutrition and Health: Summary and Recommendations*, DHHS (PHS) publication no. 88-50211 (Washington, D.C.: U.S. Government Printing Office, 1988).
2. "The Facts About Fats," Consumer Reports on Health (Boulder, CO: The Editors, March, 1997).
3. D. J. Mela and D. A. Sacchetti, "Sensory Preferences for Fat: Relationships with Diet and Body Composition," *American Journal of Clinical Nutrition*, 53 (1991), 908–915.
4. J. M. Gaziano and C. H. Hennekens. "A New Look at What Can Unclog Your Arteries." *Executive Health Report*, 27:8 (1991), 16.

5. R. J. Barnard, "Effects of Lifestyle Modification on Serum Lipids," *Archives of Internal Medicine*, 151 (1991), 1389–1394.
6. J. H. Weisburger and G. M. Williams, "Causes of Cancer," in *Textbook of Clinical Oncology* (Atlanta: American Cancer Society, 1995).
7. S. Begley. "Beyond Vitamins," *Newsweek*, April 25, 1994, pp. 45–49.
8. "Vitamin Report," *University of California at Berkeley Wellness Letter* (Palm Coast, FL: The Editors, October, 1994).
9. "Antioxidants: Never Too Late," *University of California at Berkeley Wellness Letter*, 10:8 (1994), 2.
10. "Vitamin Report."

11. S. Kalish, "The Free Radical Radical: Kenneth Cooper, M.D., on Antioxidants and the Dangers of Hard Running," *Running Times*, March 1995, pp. 16–17.
12. "Beta Carotene Pills: Should You Take Them?" *University of California at Berkeley Wellness Letter*, 12:7 (1996), 1–2.
13. L. C. Clark, et al., "Effects of Selenium Supplementation for Cancer Prevention in Patients with Carcinoma of the Skin: A Randomized Controlled Trial," *Journal of the American Medical Association*, 276 (1996), 1957–1963.
14. J. Carper, "Selenium: A Cancer Knockout?" *USA Weekend*, October 2–4, 1996, p. 8.
15. "Vitamin Report."
16. K. H. Cooper, *Antioxidant Revolution* (Nashville, TN: Thomas Nelson Publishers, 1994).

Notes *Continued*

17. Cooper.
18. "The Antioxidant All-Stars," *University of California at Berkeley Wellness Letter* (Palm Coast, FL: The Editors, March 1997).
19. K. M. Zawadzki, B. B. Yaspelkis III, and J. L. Ivy, "Carbohydrate-Protein Complex Increases the Rate of Muscle Glycogen Storage After Exercise," *Journal of Applied Physiology*, 72 (1992), 1854–1859.
20. "Nutrition, Exercise, and Bone Health" (Seattle: Pacific Medical Center, 1990).

21. B. L. Drinkwater, "Osteoporosis and the Female Masters Athlete," *Sports Medicine for the Mature Athlete*, edited by J. R. Sutton and R. M. Brock (Benchmark Press, 1986), pp. 353–359.
22. K. H. Myburgh, L. K. Bachrach, B. Lewis, K. Kent, and R. Marcus, "Low Bone Mineral Density at Axial and Appendicular Sites in Amenorrheic Athletes," *Medicine and Science in Sports and Exercise*, 25:11(1993), 1197–1202.

23. U. S. Department of Agriculture and U. S. Department of Health and Human Services, "Nutrition and Your Health: Dietary Guidelines for Americans," *Home and Garden Bulletin No. 232*, December 1995.

Suggested Readings

American Medical Association: Council on Scientific Affairs. "Dietary Fiber and Health." *Journal of the American Medical Association*, 262 (1989), 542–546.

Brownell, K., and J. P. Forey. *Handbook of Eating Disorders*. New York: Basic Books, 1986.

Cristian, J. L., and J. L. Greger. *Nutrition for Living*. Menlo Park, CA: Benjamin/Cummings Publishing, 1991.

Coleman, E. *Eating for Endurance*. Palo Alto, CA: Bull Publishing, 1992.

Drinkwater, B. L.. "Does Physical Activity Play a Role in Preventing Osteoporosis?" *Research Quarterly for Exercise and Sport*, 65 (1994), 197–206.

Drinkwater, B. L., B. Bruemner, and C. H. III Chestnut. "Menstrual History as a Determinant of Current Bone Density in Young Athletes." *Journal of the American Medical Association*, 263 (1990), 545–548.

Girdano, D. A., D. Dusek, and G. S. Everly. *Experiencing Health*. Englewood Cliffs, NJ: Prentice Hall, 1985.

"How to Balance Your Diet." *Fitness*: April 1983, pp. 46–47.

Hoeger, W. W. K., and S. A. Hoeger. *Principles and Labs for Fitness and Wellness*. Englewood, CO: Morton Publishing, 1997.

Kanders, B., D. W. Demster, and R. Lindsay. "Interaction of Calcium Nutrition and Physical Activity on Bone Mass in Young Women." *Journal of Bone Mineral Research*, 3 (1988), 145–149.

Kirschmann, J. D. *Nutrition Almanac*. New York: McGraw-Hill, 1989.

Kleiner, S. M. "Seafood and Your Heart." *Physician and Sportsmedicine*, 18:4 (1990), 19–20.

Morgan, B. L. G. *The Lifelong Nutrition Guide*. Englewood Cliffs, NJ: Prentice Hall, 1983.

National Academy of Sciences, Institute of Medicine. *Eat for Life: the Food and Nutrition Board's Guide to Reducing Your Risk of Chronic Disease*, edited by C. E. Woteki and P. R. Thomas. Washington, DC: National Academy Press, 1992.

Thornton, J. S. "Feast or Famine: Eating Disorders in Athletes." *Physician and Sportsmedicine*, 18:4 (1990), 116–122.

Whitney, E. N., and S. R. Rolfes. *Understanding Nutrition*. St. Paul: West Publishing, 1996.

Name: _____

No.	Code*	Food	Amount	Calories	Fat (gm)	Food Groups (servings)				
						Bread, Cereal, Rice & Pasta	Vegetable	Fruit	Milk, Yogurt & Cheese	Meat, Poultry, Fish, Dry Beans, Eggs, & Nuts
1										
2										
3										
4										
5										
6										
7										
8										
9										
10										
11										
12										
13										
14										
15										
16										
17										
18										
19										
20										
21										
22										
23										
24										
25										
26										
27										
28										
29										
30										
Totals				**	***					
Recommended Amount						6–11	3–5	2–4	2–3	2–3
Deficiencies										

*See list of nutritive value of selected foods in Appendix B.

**Compute using Table 8.1 in Chapter 8.

***Multiply the recommended amount of calories by .30 (30%) and divide by 9 to obtain the recommended amount of grams of fat (if on a diet, multiply by .20 or .10 — see Table 8.3 in Chapter 8).

Figure 7.16 ● *Daily diet record form.*

Name: _____

No.	Code*	Food	Amount	Calories	Fat (gm)	Bread, Cereal, Rice & Pasta	Vegetable	Fruit	Milk, Yogurt & Cheese	Meat, Poultry, Fish, Dry Beans, Eggs, & Nuts
										Food Groups (servings) →
1										
2										
3										
4										
5										
6										
7										
8										
9										
10										
11										
12										
13										
14										
15										
16										
17										
18										
19										
20										
21										
22										
23										
24										
25										
26										
27										
28										
29										
30										
Totals										
Recommended Amount				**	***	6-11	3-5	2-4	2-3	2-3
Deficiencies										

*See list of nutritive value of selected foods in Appendix B.
**Compute using Table 8.1 in Chapter 8.
***Multiply the recommended amount of calories by .30 (30%) and divide by 9 to obtain the recommended amount of grams of fat (if on a diet, multiply by .20 or .10 — see Table 8.3 in Chapter 8).

Figure 7.16 • *Daily diet record form.*

Principles of Weight Management

8

*A*chieving and maintaining recommended body weight is a major objective of a good physical fitness and wellness program. Next to poor cardiorespiratory fitness, excessive body weight is the problem encountered most commonly in fitness and wellness assessments.

Patty Neavill is a typical example of someone who often tried to change her life around but was unable to do so because she did not know how to implement a sound exercise and weight control program. At age 24 and at 240 pounds, she was discouraged with her weight, level of fitness, self-image, and quality of life in general. She had struggled with her weight most of her life. Like thousands of other people, she had made many unsuccessful attempts to lose weight.

Objectives

- Understand the health consequences of obesity.
- Learn about fad diets and other myths and fallacies regarding weight control.
- Become familiar with eating disorders, their associated medical problems and behavior patterns, and understand the need for professional help in treating these conditions.
- Understand the physiology of weight loss, including setpoint theory and the effects of diet on basal metabolic rate.
- Recognize the role of a lifetime exercise program as the key to a successful weight loss and maintenance program.
- Learn how to implement a physiologically sound weight reduction and weight maintenance program.
- Learn behavior modification techniques that help a person adhere to a lifetime weight maintenance program.

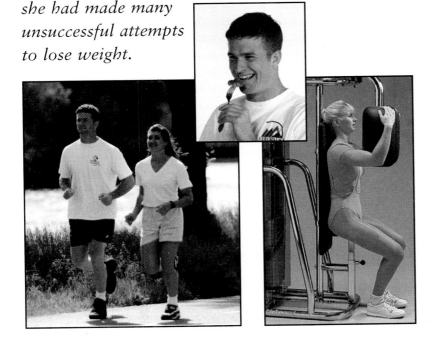

Patty put her fears aside and decided to enroll in a fitness course. As part of the course requirement, a battery of fitness tests was administered at the beginning of the semester. Patty's cardiorespiratory fitness and strength ratings were poor, her flexibility classification was average, and her percent body fat was 41.

Following the initial fitness assessment, Patty met with her course instructor, who prescribed an exercise and nutrition program like the one in this book. Patty fully committed to carry out the prescription. She walked/jogged five times a week. She enrolled in a weight training course that met twice a week. Her daily caloric intake was set in the range of 1,500 to 1,700 calories.

Determined to further increase her level of activity, Patty also signed up for recreational volleyball and basketball courses. Besides fun, these classes provided four additional hours of activity per week.

She took care to meet the minimum required servings from the basic food groups each day, which contributed about 1,200 calories to her diet. The remainder of the calories came primarily from complex carbohydrates.

At the end of the 16-week semester, Patty's cardiorespiratory fitness, strength, and flexibility ratings had all improved to the good category, she lost 50 pounds, and her percent body fat had decreased to 22.5!

Patty was tall. At 190 pounds, most people would have thought she was too heavy. Her percent body fat, however, was lower than the average for college female physical education major students (about 23% body fat).

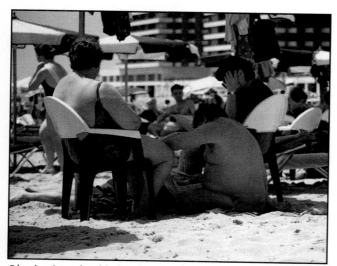

Obesity is a health hazard of epidemic proportions among physically inactive individuals with unhealthy eating practices.

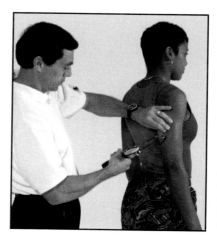

Recommended body weight is best determined through the assessment of body composition.

A thank-you note from Patty to the course instructor at the end of the semester read:

Thank you for making me a new person. I truly appreciate the time you spent with me. Without your kindness and motivation, I would have never made it. It is great to be fit and trim. I've never had this feeling before, and I wish everyone could feel like this once in their life.

Thank you,
Your trim Patty!

Patty never had been taught the principles governing a sound weight loss program. In Patty's case, not only did she need this knowledge, but, like most Americans who never have experienced the process of becoming physically fit, she needed to be in a structured exercise setting to truly feel the joy of fitness.

Even more significant, Patty maintained her aerobic and strength-training programs. A year after ending her calorie-restricted diet, her weight increased by 10 pounds, but her body fat decreased from 22.5% to 21.2%. As you will see later in this chapter, this weight increase is related mostly to changes in lean tissue, lost during the weight reduction phase.

In spite of only a slight drop in weight during the second year following the calorie-restricted diet, the 2-year follow-up revealed a further decrease in body fat, to 19.5%. Patty understood the new quality of life reaped through a sound fitness program, and, at the same time, she finally learned how to apply the principles that regulate weight maintenance.

● Obesity and Overweight

Two terms frequently are used in reference to people who weigh more than recommended: overweight and obesity. **Overweight** indicates an excess amount of weight against a given standard such as height or recommended percent body fat. **Obesity** is characterized by an excessively high amount of body fat in relation to lean body mass. Obesity levels are established at a point at which the excess body fat can lead to health problems.

On the other hand, extreme thinness can also lead to life-threatening medical conditions. About 14% of the American people are underweight. Social pressures to attain model-like thinness have contributed to a gradual increase in the number of people who develop eating disorders. Anorexia nervosa and bulimia are discussed later in this chapter.

Approximately 65 million Americans are overweight or consider themselves to be overweight. Of these, 30 million are obese. About 50% of all women and 25% of all men are on a diet at any given moment. People spend about $40 billion yearly attempting to lose weight. More than $10 billion goes to memberships in weight-reduction centers and another $30 billion to diet food sales.

Overweight and obesity are not the same thing. Most overweight people (an excess of 10 to 20 pounds) are not obese. Although research findings from studies are inconsistent, the health consequences of excessive body weight appear to be exaggerated and may apply primarily to severely overweight individuals.

Traditionally, obesity has been associated with several serious health problems and is thought to account for 15% to 20% of the annual mortality rate in the United States. Obesity has been viewed as a major risk factor for diseases of the cardiovascular system, including coronary heart disease, hypertension, congestive heart failure, high levels of blood lipids, atherosclerosis, strokes, thromboembolitic disease, osteoarthritis, varicose veins, and intermittent claudication.

Data from the Aerobics Research Institute in Dallas confirm that as body fat increases, so does blood cholesterol and triglycerides. As illustrated in Figure 8.1, however, the data also showed that the higher the fitness level, the lower the mortality rate, regardless of body weight.[1] This finding is of significance, because fit/obese men had a lower risk of death than unfit men of average weight and as low as fit men of average weight. Thus, it appears that lack of physical activity and not the weight problem itself, is the cause of premature death rates associated with obesity.

Granted, genetic differences exist. Some moderately overweight people do have health problems,

Based on data from "Physical Fitness, Mortality and Obesity," by C. E. Barlow, H. W. Kohl, III, L. W. Gibbons, and S. N. Blair, *International Journal of Obesity*, 19 (1996), S42.

Figure 8.1 ● *Relationship between body weight, fitness, and mortality.*

but this is not the case for most. Overweight people with diabetes and other cardiovascular risk factors (elevated blood lipids, high blood pressure, physical inactivity, and poor eating habits) benefit from weight loss. Overweight people who are otherwise healthy and are physically active, exercise regularly, and eat a healthy diet do not appear to be at greater risk for early death.

Recommended body composition, nonetheless, is a primary objective of overall physical fitness and enhanced quality of life. Individuals at recommended body weight are able to participate in a wide variety of moderate to vigorous activities without functional limitations. These people have the freedom to enjoy most of life's recreational activities to their fullest potential. Excessive body weight does not provide an individual with the fitness level to enjoy vigorous lifetime activities such as basketball, soccer, racquetball, surfing, mountain cycling, and mountain climbing. Maintaining high fitness and recommended body weight gives a person a degree of independence

TERMS

Overweight An excess amount of weight against a given standard such as height or recommended percent body fat.

Obesity A chronic disease characterized by an excessively high amount of body fat in relation to lean body mass.

throughout life that the great majority of people in developed nations no longer enjoy.

● Tolerable Weight

Many people want to lose weight so they will look better. That's a noteworthy goal. The problem, however, is that they have a distorted image of what they would really look like if they were to reduce to what they think is their ideal weight. Hereditary factors play a big role, and only a small fraction of the population has the genes for a "perfect body."

As people set their own target weight, they should be realistic. Attaining the excellent percent body fat figure in Table 6.8, is extremely difficult for some. It is even more difficult to maintain, unless they are willing to make a commitment to a vigorous lifetime exercise program and permanent dietary changes. Few people are willing to do that. The moderate percent body fat category may be more realistic for many people.

A question you should ask yourself is: Are you happy with your weight? Part of enjoying a higher quality of life is being happy with yourself. If you are not, you either need to do something about it or learn to live with it.

If you are above the moderate percent body fat category, you should try to come down and stay in this category, for health reasons. This is the category in which there appears to be no detriment to health.

If you are in the moderate category but would like to be lower, you need to ask yourself a second question: How badly do I want it? Do I want it badly enough to implement lifetime exercise and dietary changes? If you are not willing to change, you should stop worrying about your weight and deem the moderate category as "tolerable" for you.

● The Weight Loss Dilemma

Yo-yo dieting carries as great a health risk as being overweight and remaining overweight in the first place. Epidemiological data are beginning to show that frequent fluctuations in weight (up or down) markedly increase the risk of dying of cardiovascular disease.

Based on the findings that constant losses and regains can be hazardous to health, quick-fix diets should be replaced by a slow but permanent weight loss program, as described in this chapter. Individuals reap the benefits of recommended body weight when they get to their recommended body weight and stay there throughout life.

Unfortunately, only about 10% of all people who begin a traditional weight loss program without exercise are able to lose the desired weight. Worse, only five in 100 are able to keep the weight off. The body is highly resistant to permanent weight changes through caloric restrictions alone.

Traditional diets have failed because few of them incorporate lifetime changes in food selection and exercise as fundamental to successful weight loss. When the diet stops, weight gain begins. The $40 billion diet industry tries to capitalize on the idea that weight can be lost quickly without taking into consideration the consequences of fast weight loss or the importance of lifetime behavioral changes to ensure proper weight loss and maintenance.

In addition, various studies indicate that most people, especially obese people, underestimate their energy intake. Those who try to lose weight but apparently fail to do so are often described as "diet-resistant." A study published by Dr. Steven Lichtman and colleagues[2] found that, while on a "diet," a group of obese individuals with a self-reported

Achieving and maintaining a high physical fitness percent body fat standard requires a lifetime commitment to regular physical activity and proper nutrition.

history of diet resistance underreported their average daily caloric intake by almost 50% (1028 self-reported versus 2081 actual — see Figure 8.2). These individuals also overestimated their amount of daily physical activity by about 25% (1022 calories self-reported versus 771 actual calories). These differences represent an additional 1304 calories of energy unaccounted for by the subjects in the study. These findings indicate that failing to lose weight often is related to misreports of actual food intake and level of physical activity.

Fad diets continue to appeal to people. These diets deceive people and claim the person will lose weight by following all instructions. Most fad diets are very low in calories and deprive the body of certain nutrients, generating a metabolic imbalance. Under these conditions, a lot of the weight lost is in the form of water and protein, and not fat.

On a crash diet, close to half the weight loss is in lean (protein) tissue. When the body uses protein instead of a combination of fats and carbohydrates as a source of energy, weight is lost as much as 10 times faster.[3] A gram of protein produces half the amount of energy that fat does. In the case of muscle protein, one-fifth of protein is mixed with four-fifths

WHAT IS REDUX (FEN-PHEN)? SHOULD YOU USE IT?

For the first time in almost a quarter of a century, the U.S. Food and Drug Administration recently approved a new anti-obesity drug — dexfenfluramine (Redux or fen-phen). The drug works by raising levels of serotonin and promoting feelings of satiety. Unlike other weight-loss pills, Redux is not an amphetamine and does not appear to cause addiction. Redux is a distant cousin of Prozac, a drug used for the treatment of depression; therefore, it cannot be used in combination with antidepressants. The safety and effectiveness beyond one year's use also remains unknown.

The average cost of Redux is about $2.50 per day. It is not a magic pill and to be effective it must be used in combination with a sensible diet and regular physical activity. The drug only regulates hunger and it will not work for people who eat for reasons other than hunger. The use of Redux is recommended primarily for clinically obese people (20% to 30% overweight). Individuals who don't respond in the first month of use will most likely never respond.

Most health experts, nonetheless, do not recommend the use of Redux because of potential side effects — most notably, an increase in the risk for primary pulmonary hypertension, a rare lung disease that kills half the people who get it. Other side effects include lethargy, drowsiness, and in high doses, brain damage. Because of these harmful side effects, several states have already outlawed the use of Redux.

water. Each pound of muscle yields only one-tenth the amount of energy of a pound of fat. As a result, most of the weight loss is in the form of water, which on the scale, of course, looks good.

Some diets allow only certain specialized foods. If people would realize that no magic foods will provide all of the necessary nutrients, and that a person has to eat a variety of foods to be well-nourished, the diet industry would not be as successful. Most of these diets create a nutritional deficiency, which at times can be fatal.

The reason some of these diets succeed is that people eventually get tired of eating the same thing

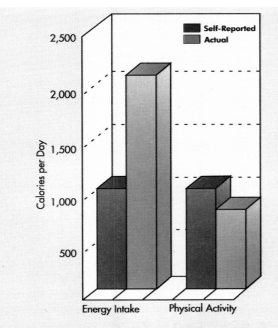

Source: "Discrepancy Between Self-Reported and Actual Caloric Intake and Exercise in Obese Subjects" by S. W. Lichtman et al., in *New England Journal of Medicine*, 327 (1992), 1893-1898.

Figure 8.2 ● *Differences between self-reported and actual daily caloric intake and exercise in obese individuals attempting to lose weight.*

Yo-yo dieting Constantly losing and gaining weight.

day in and day out and start eating less. If they happen to achieve the lower weight but do not make permanent dietary changes, they regain the weight quickly once they go back to their old eating habits.

A few diets recommend exercise along with caloric restrictions — the best method for weight reduction, of course. A lot of the weight lost is because of the exercise, so the diet has achieved its purpose. Unfortunately, if the people do not change their food selection and activity level permanently, they gain back the weight once they discontinue dieting and exercise.

● Eating Disorders

Anorexia nervosa and bulimia are physical and emotional problems, thought to develop from individual, family, or social pressures, characterized by an intense fear of becoming fat, which does not disappear even when losing extreme amounts of weight. These medical disorders are increasing steadily in most industrialized nations where society encourages low-calorie diets and thinness.

Anorexia Nervosa

Anorexia nervosa is a condition of self-imposed starvation to lose and then maintain very low body weight. Approximately 19 of every 20 anorexics are young women. An estimated 1% of the female population in the United States is anorexic. Anorexic individuals seem to fear weight gain more than death from starvation. Furthermore, they have a distorted image of their body and think of themselves as being fat even when they are emaciated.

Although a genetic predisposition may contribute, the anorexic person often comes from a mother-dominated home, with possible drug addictions in the family. The syndrome may emerge following a stressful life event and uncertainty about the ability to cope efficiently.

Because the female role in society is changing more rapidly, women seem to be especially susceptible. Life experiences such as gaining weight, starting menstrual periods, beginning college, losing a boyfriend, having poor self-esteem, being socially rejected, starting a professional career, or becoming a wife or mother may trigger the syndrome.

These individuals typically begin a diet and at first feel in control and happy about the weight loss, even if they are not overweight. To speed up the weight loss, they frequently combine extreme dieting with exhaustive exercise and overuse of laxatives and diuretics.

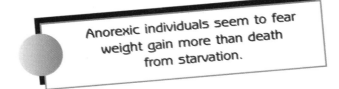
Anorexic individuals seem to fear weight gain more than death from starvation.

Anorexics commonly develop obsessive and compulsive behaviors and emphatically deny their condition. They are preoccupied with food, meal planning, grocery shopping, and unusual eating habits. As they lose weight and their health begins to deteriorate, anorexics feel weak and tired and may realize they have a problem but will not stop the starvation and refuse to consider the behavior as abnormal.

Once they have lost a lot of weight and malnutrition sets in, physical changes become more visible. Some typical changes are amenorrhea (stopping menstruation), digestive problems, extreme sensitivity to cold, hair and skin problems, fluid and electrolyte

DIAGNOSTIC CRITERIA FOR ANOREXIA NERVOSA

- Refusal to maintain body weight over a minimal normal weight for age and height, e.g., weight loss leading to maintenance of body weight 15% below that expected; or failure to make expected weight gain during period of growth, leading to body weight 15% below that expected.

- Intense fear of gaining weight or becoming fat, even though underweight.

- Disturbance in the way in which one's body weight, size, or shape is experienced; e.g., the person claims to "feel fat" even when emaciated or believes that one area of the body is "too fat" even when obviously underweight.

- In females, absence of at least three consecutive menstrual cycles when otherwise expected to occur (primary or secondary amenorrhea). (A woman is considered to have amenorrhea if her periods occur only following hormone, e.g., estrogen, administration.)

Source: American Psychiatric Association, *Diagnostic and Statistical Manual of Mental Disorders* (Washington, DC, Association, 1987), p. 67.

abnormalities (which may lead to an irregular heartbeat and sudden stopping of the heart), injuries to nerves and tendons, abnormalities of immune function, anemia, growth of fine body hair, mental confusion, inability to concentrate, lethargy, depression, skin dryness, lower skin and body temperature, and osteoporosis.

Many of the changes of anorexia nervosa can be reversed, but treatment almost always requires professional help. The sooner it is started, the better the chances for reversibility and cure. Therapy consists of a combination of medical and psychological techniques to restore proper nutrition, prevent medical complications, and modify the environment or events that triggered the syndrome.

Unfortunately, anorexics strongly deny their condition. They are able to hide it and deceive friends and relatives quite effectively. Based on their behavior, many of them meet all of the characteristics of anorexia nervosa, but it goes undetected because both thinness and dieting are socially acceptable. Only a well-trained clinician is able to make a positive diagnosis.

Bulimia

A pattern of binge eating and purging, **bulimia** is more prevalent than anorexia nervosa. For many years it was thought to be a variant of anorexia nervosa, but now it is identified as a separate condition. It afflicts mainly young people. As many as one in every five women on college campuses may be bulimic, according to some estimates. Bulimia also is more prevalent than anorexia nervosa in males.

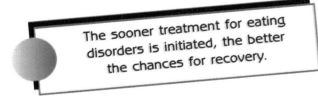

The sooner treatment for eating disorders is initiated, the better the chances for recovery.

Bulimics usually are healthy-looking people, well-educated, near recommended body weight, who enjoy food and often socialize around it. In actuality, they are emotionally insecure, rely on others, and lack self-confidence and esteem. Recommended weight and food are important to them.

The binge-purge cycle usually occurs in stages. As a result of stressful life events or the simple compulsion to eat, bulimics periodically engage in binge eating that may last an hour or longer.

DIAGNOSTIC CRITERIA FOR BULIMIA

- Recurrent episodes of binge eating (rapid consumption of a large amount of food in a discrete period of time).
- A feeling of lack of control over eating behavior during the eating binges.
- Regular practice of either self-induced vomiting, use of laxatives or diuretics, strict dieting or fasting, or vigorous exercise to prevent weight gain.
- A minimum average of two binge eating episodes a week for at least three months.
- Persistent overconcern with body shape and weight.

Source: American Psychiatric Association, *Diagnostic and Statistical Manual of Mental Disorders* (Washington, DC, Association, 1987), p. 68-69.

With some apprehension, bulimics anticipate and plan the cycle. Then they feel an urgency to begin. First they consume a large amount of food — several thousand calories and up to 10,000 calories in extreme cases — in a short amount of time. A brief period of relief and satisfaction is followed by feelings of deep guilt, shame, and intense fear of gaining weight. Purging seems to be an easy answer, as the binging cycle can continue without fear of gaining weight.

The most common form of purging is self-induced vomiting. Bulimics might ingest strong laxatives and emetics. They often go on near-fasting diets and strenuous bouts of exercise. Medical problems associated with bulimia include cardiac arrhythmias, amenorrhea, kidney and bladder damage, ulcers, colitis, tearing of the esophagus or stomach, tooth erosion, gum damage, and general muscular weakness.

Unlike anorexics, bulimics realize their behavior is abnormal and feel great shame about it. Fearing social rejection, they pursue the binge-purge cycle in secrecy and at unusual times of the day.

TERMS

Anorexia nervosa An eating disorder characterized by self-imposed starvation to lose and maintain very low body weight.

Bulimia An eating disorder characterized by a pattern of binge eating and purging to attempt to lose and maintain low body weight.

Bulimia can be treated successfully when the person realizes this destructive behavior is not the solution to life's problems. A change in attitude can prevent permanent damage or death. Treatment is available on most school campuses through the school's counseling center or the health center. Local hospitals also offer treatment for eating disorders. Many communities have support groups, frequently led by professional personnel and usually free of charge.

● Physiology of Weight Loss

Only a few years ago the principles governing a weight loss and maintenance program seemed to be fairly clear, but now we know the final answers are not yet in. Traditional concepts related to weight control have centered on three assumptions: (a) that balancing food intake against output allows a person to achieve recommended weight, (b) that all fat people just eat too much, and (c) that the human body doesn't care how much (or little) fat it stores. Although these statements have some truth, they still are open to much debate and research.

Energy-Balancing Equation

The principle embodied in the **energy-balancing equation** is simple: If daily energy requirements could be determined accurately, caloric intake could be balanced against output. This is not always the case, though, because genetic and lifestyle-related individual differences determine the number of calories required to maintain or lose body weight.

Table 8.1 offers some general guidelines for estimating daily caloric intake according to lifestyle

Table 8.1	*Average Caloric Requirement Per Pound of Body Weight Based on Lifestyle Patterns and Gender*	
	Calories Per Pound	
	Men	**Women***
Sedentary — limited physical activity	13.0	12.0
Moderate physical activity	15.0	13.5
Hard Labor — strenuous physical effort	17.0	15.0

*Pregnant or lactating women add 3 calories to these values.

patterns. This is only an estimated figure and, as discussed later in the chapter, it serves only as a starting point from which individual adjustments have to be made.

One pound of fat represents 3,500 calories. Assuming that a person's basic daily caloric expenditure is 2,500 calories, if this person were to decrease the daily intake by 500 calories per day, it should result in a loss of one pound of fat in 7 days (500 × 7 = 3,500). But research has shown — and many dieters probably have experienced — that even when they carefully balance caloric input against caloric output, weight loss does not always happen as predicted. Furthermore, two people with similar measured caloric intake and output seldom lose weight at the same rate.

The most common explanation regarding individual differences in weight loss and weight gain has been the variation in human metabolism from one person to another. We are all familiar with people who can eat "all day long" and not gain an ounce of weight, while others cannot even "dream about food" without gaining weight. Because experts did not believe that human metabolism alone could account for such extreme differences, they developed several theories that may better explain these individual variations.

Setpoint Theory

Results of several research studies point toward a **weight-regulating mechanism** (WRM) that has a **setpoint** for controlling both appetite and the amount of fat stored. Setpoint is hypothesized to work like a thermostat for body fat, maintaining fairly constant body weight, because it knows at all times the exact amount of adipose tissue stored in the fat cells. Some people have high settings; others have low settings.

If body weight decreases (as in dieting), the setpoint senses this change and triggers the WRM to increase the person's appetite or make the body conserve energy to maintain the "set" weight. The opposite also may be true. Some people have a hard time gaining weight. In this case, the WRM decreases appetite or causes the body to waste energy to maintain the lower weight.

Setpoint and Caloric Input

Every person has his or her own certain body fat percentage (as established by the setpoint) that the body attempts to maintain. The genetic instinct to survive tells the body that fat storage is vital, and therefore it sets an acceptable fat level. This level remains somewhat constant or may climb gradually because of poor lifestyle habits.

For instance, under strict calorie reduction, the body may make extreme metabolic adjustments in an effort to maintain its setpoint for fat. The **basal metabolic rate** may drop dramatically against a consistent negative caloric balance, and a person may be on a plateau for days or even weeks without losing much weight. A low metabolic rate compounds a person's problems in maintaining recommended body weight.

These findings were substantiated by research conducted at Rockefeller University in New York.[4] The authors showed that the body resists maintaining altered weight. Obese and lifetime nonobese individuals were used in the investigation. Following a 10% weight loss, in an attempt to regain the lost weight, the body compensated by burning up to 15% fewer calories than were expected for the new reduced weight (after accounting for the 10% loss). The effects were similar in the obese and nonobese participants. These results imply that after a 10% weight loss, a person would have to eat less or exercise more to account for the estimated deficit of about 200 to 300 calories.

In this same study, when the participants were allowed to increase their weight to 10% above their "normal" body weight (pre-weight loss), the body burned 10% to 15% more calories than expected — an attempt by the body to waste energy and return to the pre-set weight. This is another indication that the body is highly resistant to weight changes unless additional lifestyle changes are incorporated to ensure successful weight management. These methods will be discussed in this chapter.

Dietary restriction alone will not lower the setpoint, even though the person may lose weight and fat. When the dieter goes back to the normal or even below-normal caloric intake, at which the weight may have been stable for a long time, he or she quickly regains the fat loss as the body strives to regain a comfortable fat store.

Let's use a practical illustration. A person would like to lose some body fat and assumes that a stable body weight has been reached at an average daily caloric intake of 1,800 calories (no weight gain or loss occurs at this daily intake). In an attempt to lose weight rapidly, this person now goes on a strict low-calorie diet, or even worse, a near-fasting diet. Immediately the body activates its survival mechanism

and readjusts its metabolism to a lower caloric balance. After a few weeks of dieting at fewer than 400 to 600 calories per day, the body now can maintain its normal functions at 1,000 calories per day.

Having lost the desired weight, the person terminates the diet but realizes the original intake of 1,800 calories per day will have to be lower to maintain the new lower weight. To adjust to the new lower body weight, the intake is restricted to about 1,500 calories per day. The individual is surprised to find that, even at this lower daily intake (300 fewer calories), weight comes back at a rate of one pound every one to two weeks. After ending the diet, this new lowered metabolic rate may take several months to kick back up to its normal level.

From this explanation, individuals clearly should never go on very low-calorie diets. Not only will this slow down resting metabolic rate, but it also will deprive the body of basic daily nutrients required for normal function.

Daily caloric intakes of 1,200 to 1,500 calories provide the necessary nutrients if they are distributed properly over the five basic food groups (meeting the daily required servings from each group). Of course, the individual will have to learn which foods meet the requirements and yet are low in fat and sugar.

Under no circumstances should a person go on a diet that calls for below 1,200 and 1,500 calories for women and men, respectively. Weight (fat) is gained over months and years, not overnight. Likewise, weight loss should be gradual, not abrupt.

A second way in which the setpoint may work is by keeping track of the nutrients and calories consumed daily. It is thought that the body, like a cash register, records the daily food intake and the brain

TERMS

Energy-balancing equation A principle holding that as long as caloric input equals caloric output, the person will not gain or lose weight. If caloric intake exceeds output, the person gains weight; when output exceeds input, the person loses weight.

Weight-regulating mechanism (WRM) Physiologic mechanism located in the hypothalamus of the brain that controls how much the body should weigh.

Setpoint The weight control theory that indicates the body has an established weight and strongly attempts to maintain that weight.

Basal metabolic rate The lowest level of oxygen consumption necessary to sustain life.

will not feel satisfied until the calories and nutrients have been "registered."

This setpoint for calories and nutrients seems to work for some people, even when they participate in moderately intense exercise. Some evidence suggests that people do not become hungrier with moderate physical activity. Therefore, people can choose to lose weight either by going hungry or by stepping up their daily physical activity. A greater number of calories burned through physical activity helps to lower body fat.

Lowering the Setpoint

The most common question regarding the setpoint is how it can be lowered so the body will feel comfortable at a lesser fat percentage. Several factors seem to affect the setpoint directly by lowering the fat thermostat:

1. Aerobic exercise.
2. A diet high in complex carbohydrates.
3. Nicotine.
4. Amphetamines.

The last two are more destructive than the overfatness, so they are not reasonable alternatives (as far as the extra strain on the heart is concerned, smoking one pack of cigarettes per day is said to be the equivalent of carrying 50 to 75 pounds of excess body fat).

On the other hand, a diet high in fats and refined carbohydrates, near-fasting diets, and perhaps even artificial sweeteners seem to raise the setpoint. Therefore, the only practical and sensible way to lower the setpoint and lose fat weight is a combination of aerobic exercise and a diet high in complex carbohydrates and low in fat.

Because of the effects of proper food management on the body's setpoint, many nutritionists believe the total number of calories should not be the main concern in a weight-control program. Rather, it should be the source of those calories. In this regard, most of the effort is spent in retraining eating habits, increasing the intake of complex carbohydrates and high-fiber foods, and decreasing the consumption of refined carbohydrates (sugars) and fats. In most cases, this change in eating habits will bring about a decrease in total daily caloric intake.

In 1996 a new fat substitute, **olestra**, was approved by the FDA for use in "savory snacks." According to the University of California at Berkeley *Wellness Letter,*[5] consumers should "just say no" to

olestra and not buy products that contain this fat substitute.

Olestra can cause diarrhea and cramping, and it can deplete the body of fat-soluble vitamins, including A, D, E, and K. Vitamin E is a strong antioxidant, and low levels of vitamin K pose a risk for people with bleeding disorders and those on blood-thinning medication. In addition, potential cancer-causing liver-cell changes have been found in animal studies. Although the fat and caloric content of olestra-containing foods is lower than that of foods cooked with natural fats, consuming snacks using this fat substitute may not only pose a risk to good health but also may reinforce unhealthy eating habits.

A "diet" no longer is viewed as a temporary tool to aid in weight loss but, instead, as a permanent change in eating behaviors to ensure weight management and better health. The role of increased physical activity also must be considered, because successful weight loss, maintenance, and recommended body composition seldom are attained without a moderate reduction in caloric intake combined with a regular exercise program.

Diet and Metabolism

Fat can be lost by selecting the proper foods, exercising, or restricting calories. When a person tries to lose weight by dietary restrictions alone, lean body mass (muscle protein, along with vital organ protein) always decreases. The amount of lean body mass lost depends entirely on caloric limitation.

When people go on a near-fasting diet, up to half of the weight loss is lean body mass and the other half is actual fat loss (see Figure 8.3).[6] When diet is combined with exercise, close to 100% of the weight loss is in the form of fat, and lean tissue actually may increase.

Loss of lean body mass is never good, because it weakens the organs and muscles and slows down metabolism. Large losses in lean tissue can cause disturbances in heart function and damage to other organs. Equally important is not to overindulge (binge) following very-low-calorie diets. This may cause changes in metabolic rate and electrolyte balance, which could trigger fatal cardiac arrhythmias.

Contrary to some beliefs, aging is not the main reason for the lower metabolic rate. It is not so much that metabolism slows down as that people slow down. As people age, they tend to rely more on the amenities of life (remote controls, cellular

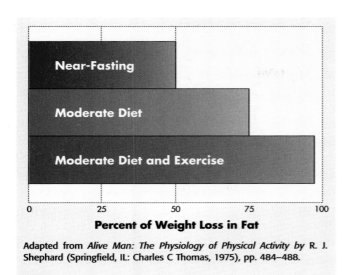

Adapted from *Alive Man: The Physiology of Physical Activity* by R. J. Shephard (Springfield, IL: Charles C Thomas, 1975), pp. 484–488.

Figure 8.3 ● *Effects of three forms of diet on fat loss.*

telephones, intercoms, single-level homes, riding lawnmowers) that lull a person into sedentary living.

Basal metabolism is related directly to lean body weight. The more the lean tissue, the higher the metabolic rate. As a consequence of sedentary living and less physical activity, the lean component decreases and fat tissue increases. The human body requires a certain amount of oxygen per pound of lean body mass. As fat is considered metabolically inert from the point of view of caloric use, the lean tissue uses most of the oxygen, even at rest. As muscle and organ mass (lean body mass) decreases, so do the energy requirements at rest.

Reductions in lean body mass are common in aging people (because of physical inactivity) and those on severely restricted diets. The loss of lean body mass also may account for a lower metabolic rate (described earlier) and the longer time it takes to kick back up.

Diets with caloric intakes below 1,200 to 1,500 calories cannot guarantee the retention of lean body mass. Even at this intake level, some loss is inevitable unless the diet is combined with exercise. Despite the claims of many diets that they do not alter the lean component, the simple truth is that, regardless of what nutrients may be added to the diet, severe caloric restrictions always prompt a loss of lean tissue. Too many people go on low-calorie diets constantly. Every time they do, the metabolic rate slows down as more lean tissue is lost.

Many people in their 40s or older who weigh the same as they did when they were 20 think they are at recommended body weight. During this span of 20 years or more, these people may have dieted many times without participating in an exercise program. They regain the weight shortly after they terminate each diet, but most of that gain is in fat. Maybe at age 20 they weighed 150 pounds, of which only 15% was fat. Now at age 40, even though they still weigh 150 pounds, they might be 30% fat (see Figure 8.4). At recommended body weight, they wonder why they are eating very little and still having trouble staying at that weight.

● Exercise: The Key to Weight Loss and Weight Maintenance

A more effective way to tilt the energy-balancing equation in your favor is by burning calories through physical activity. Exercise also appears to exert control over how much a person weighs.

Starting at age 25, the typical American gains 1 pound of weight per year. This weight gain represents a simple energy surplus of under 10 calories per day. In most cases, the additional weight accumulated in middle age comes from people becoming less physically active and not as a result of increases in caloric intake. Dr. Jack Wilmore, a leading exercise physiologist and expert weight management researcher, stated:[7]

> *Physical inactivity is certainly a major, if not the primary, cause of obesity in the United States today. A certain minimal level of activity might be necessary for us to accurately balance our caloric intake to our caloric expenditure. With too little activity, we appear to lose the fine control we normally have to maintain this incredible balance. This fine balance amounts to less than 10 calories per day, or the equivalent of one potato chip.*

Exercise is crucial to losing weight and maintaining weight. Not only will exercise maintain lean tissue, but advocates of the setpoint theory say that

TERMS

Olestra Fat substitute made from sugar and fatty acids; provides no calories to the body because it passes through the digestive system without being absorbed.

exercise resets the fat thermostat to a new, lower level. This change may be rapid, or it may take time. A few overweight individuals have exercised faithfully almost daily, 60 minutes at a time, for a whole year before seeing significant weight change. People with a "sticky" setpoint have to be patient and persistent.

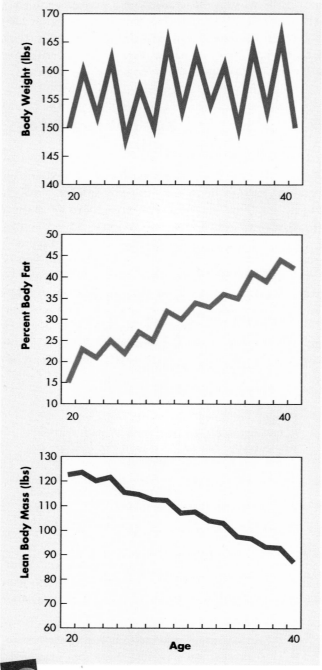

Figure 8.4 ● *Effects of frequent dieting without exercise on lean body mass, percent body fat, and body weight.*

If a person is trying to lose weight, a combination of aerobic and strength-training exercises works best. Aerobic exercise is the best to offset the setpoint, and the continuity and duration of these types of activities cause many calories to be burned in the process. The role of aerobic exercise in successful lifetime weight management cannot be overestimated.

As illustrated in Figure 8.5, greater weight loss is achieved by combining a diet with an aerobic exercise program.[8] Of even greater significance, only the individuals who participated in an 18-month post-diet aerobic exercise program were able to keep the weight off. Those who discontinued exercise gained weight. Furthermore, all those who initiated or resumed exercise during the 18-month follow-up were able to lose weight again. Individuals who only dieted and never exercised regained 60% and 92% of their weight loss at the 6- and 18-month follow-up, respectively.

Weight loss may come more rapidly when aerobic exercise is combined with a strength-training program.[9] Two exercise groups — a 30-minute aerobic group and a 15-minute aerobic plus 15-minute strength-training (30-minutes total) group — participated in an 8-week, 3-days-per-week study. Both groups followed a dietary plan consisting of approximately 60% carbohydrates, 20% fats, and 20% proteins.

The aerobic group lost an average of 3½ pounds, 3 of which were fat and the remaining half-pound lean tissue. The combined aerobic and strength-training group lost an average of 8 pounds. Changes in body composition, however, indicated that the latter group actually lost 10 pounds of fat and gained 2 pounds of lean tissue (see Figure 8.6). These findings suggest that a sensible strength-training program is better to lose weight and to maintain or increase muscle mass and metabolic rate.

Another point of interest is that each additional pound of muscle tissue can raise the basal metabolic rate by about 35 calories per day.[10] Thus, an individual who adds 5 pounds of muscle tissue as a result of strength training increases the basal metabolic rate by 175 calories per day (35 × 5), which equals 63,875 calories per year (175 × 365) or the equivalent of 18.25 pounds of fat (63,875 ÷ 3,500).

Strength training is suggested especially for people who think they are at their recommended body weight, yet their body fat percentage is higher than recommended. The number of calories burned

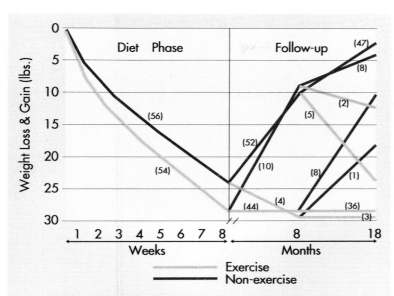

Figure 8.5 • *Aerobic exercise and weight loss and maintenance in moderately obese individuals.*

Note: Numbers in parenthesis indicate number of participants.

Source: "Exercise as an Adjunct to Weight Loss and Maintenance in Moderately Obese Subjects," K. N., Pavlou, S. Krey, and W. P. Steffe, *American Journal of Clinical Nutrition*, 49 (1989), 1115-1123.

during a typical hour-long strength-training session is much less than during an hour of aerobic exercise. Because of the high intensity of strength training, the person needs frequent rest intervals to recover from each set of exercise. The average person actually lifts weights only 10 to 12 minutes in each hour of exercise. In the long run, however, the person enjoys the benefits of gains in lean tissue. Guidelines for developing aerobic and strength-training programs are given in Chapters 3 and 4.

Because exercise results in more lean body mass, body weight often remains the same or even increases after beginning an exercise program, while inches and percent body fat decrease. More lean tissue means a higher functional capacity of the human body. With exercise, most of the weight loss becomes apparent after a few weeks of training, after the lean component has stabilized.

Although we now know that a negative caloric balance of 3,500 calories does not always result in a loss of exactly one pound of fat, the role of exer-

cise in achieving a negative balance by burning additional calories is significant in weight reduction and maintenance programs.

Sadly, some individuals claim that the amount of calories burned during exercise is hardly worth the effort. They think that cutting their daily intake by some 300 calories is easier than participating in some sort of exercise that would burn the same amount of calories. The problem is that the willpower to cut those 300 calories lasts only a few weeks, and then the person goes right back to the old eating patterns.

If a person gets into the habit of exercising regularly, say three times a week, running 3 miles per exercise session (about 300 calories burned), this represents 900 calories in one week, about 3,600 in one month, or 46,800 calories per year. This minimal amount of exercise could mean as many as 13.5 extra pounds of fat in one year, 27 in two, and so on.

We tend to forget that our weight creeps up gradually over the years, not just overnight. Hardly worth the effort? And we have not even taken into consideration the increase in lean tissue, possible resetting of the setpoint, the benefits to the cardiovascular system, and most important, the improved quality of life. The fundamental reasons for overfatness and obesity, few

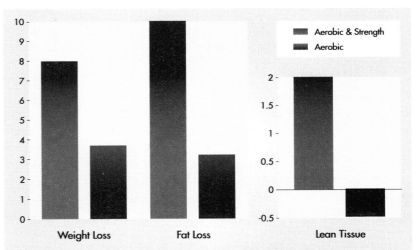

Source: "You Can Sell Exercise for Weight Loss," by W. L. Wescott, *Fitness Management*, 7:12 (1991), 33–34.

Figure 8.6 • *Changes in body composition through aerobic exercise and aerobic/strength-training exercise.*

Regular participation in a combined aerobic and strength-training exercise program is the key to successful weight management.

could argue, are lack of physical activity and sedentary living.

In terms of preventing disease, many of the health benefits people try to achieve by losing weight are reaped through exercise alone, even without weight loss. Exercise offers protection against premature morbidity and mortality for everyone, including people who already have risk factors for disease (see Chapter 9). The lack of exercise, not the weight problem itself, possibly is the cause of many of the health risks associated with obesity.

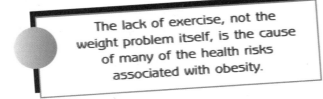

The lack of exercise, not the weight problem itself, is the cause of many of the health risks associated with obesity.

Healthy Weight Gain

"Skinny" people, too, should realize that the only healthy way to gain weight is through exercise (mainly strength-training exercises) and a slight increase in caloric intake. Attempting to gain weight just by overeating will raise the fat component and not the lean component — which is not the path to better health. Exercise is the best solution to weight (fat) reduction and weight (lean) gain.

A strength-training program such as the one outlined in Chapter 4 is the best approach to add body weight. The training program should include at least two exercises of three sets for each major body part. Each set should consist of about 10 repetitions maximum.

Even though the metabolic cost of synthesizing a pound of muscle tissue is still unclear, an estimated 500 additional calories daily, including 15 grams of protein above the RDA, are recommended to gain an average of 1 pound of muscle tissue per week. Based on the typical American diet, the extra 15 grams of protein are not necessary. Each day, the average American already consumes 30 to 60 grams of protein above the RDA. The extra 500 calories should be primarily in the form of complex carbohydrates. If the higher caloric intake is not accompanied by a strength-training program, the increase in body weight will be in the form of fat and not muscle tissue.

Weight-Loss Myths

Cellulite and **spot reducing** are mythical concepts. **Cellulite** is nothing but enlarged fat cells that bulge out from accumulated body fat.

Doing several sets of daily sit-ups will not get rid of fat in the midsection of the body. When fat comes off, it does so throughout the entire body, not just the exercised area. The greatest proportion of fat may come off the biggest fat deposits, but the caloric output of a few sets of sit-ups has practically no effect on reducing total body fat. A person has to exercise much longer to really see results.

Other touted means toward quick weight loss — rubberized sweatsuits, steam baths, mechanical vibrators — are misleading. When a person wears a sweatsuit or steps into a sauna, the weight lost is not fat but merely a significant amount of water. Sure, it looks nice when you step on the scale immediately afterward, but this represents a false loss of weight.

As soon as you replace body fluids, you gain back the weight quickly.

Wearing rubberized sweatsuits not only hastens the rate of body fluid loss — fluid that is vital during prolonged exercise — but it raises core temperature at the same time. This combination puts a person in danger of dehydration, which impairs cellular function and in extreme cases can even cause death.

Similarly, mechanical vibrators are worthless in a weight-control program. Vibrating belts and turning rollers may feel good, but they require no effort whatsoever. Fat cannot be shaken off; it is lost primarily by burning it in muscle tissue.

● Losing Weight the Sound and Sensible Way

Dieting never has been fun and never will be. People who are overweight and are serious about losing weight, however, have to include regular exercise in their life along with proper food management and a sensible reduction in caloric intake.

Some precautions are in order, as excessive body fat is a risk factor for cardiovascular disease. Depending on the extent of the weight problem, a medical examination and possibly a stress ECG (see abnormal electrocardiogram in Chapter 9) may be a good idea before undertaking the exercise program. A physician should be consulted in this regard.

Significantly overweight individuals also may have to choose activities in which they will not have to support their own body weight but that still will be effective in burning calories. Joint and muscle injuries are common in overweight individuals who participate in weight-bearing exercises such as walking, jogging, and aerobics.

Swimming may not be a good exercise either. More body fat makes a person more buoyant, and most people are not at the skill level to swim fast enough to get the best training effect. They tend to just float along, limiting the amount of calories burned as well as the benefits to the cardiovascular system.

Some better alternatives are riding a bicycle (either road or stationary), walking in a shallow pool, doing water aerobics,[11] or running in place in deep water (treading water). The latter forms of water exercise are gaining popularity and have proven to be effective in weight reduction without the "pain" and fear of injuries. Through the caloric

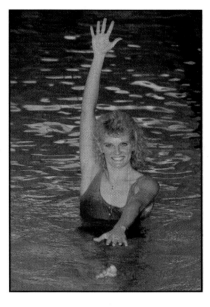

Body fat can be lost through water aerobics.

expenditure of selected physical activities given in Table 8.2, you will be able to determine your own daily caloric requirement using Figure 8.7 at the end of this chapter.

How long should each exercise session last? To develop and maintain cardiorespiratory fitness, 20 to 30 minutes of exercise at the recommended target rate, three to five times per week, is suggested (see Chapter 3). For weight-loss purposes, many experts recommend exercising at least 45 minutes at a time, five to six times a week.

A person should not try to do too much too fast. Unconditioned beginners should start with about 15 minutes of aerobic exercise three times a week, gradually increasing the duration by approximately 5 minutes per week and the frequency by one day per week during the next three to four weeks.

One final benefit of exercise for weight control is that it allows fat to be burned more efficiently. Both carbohydrates and fats are sources of energy. When the glucose levels begin to drop during prolonged exercise, more fat is used as energy substrate.

Equally important is that fat-burning enzymes increase with aerobic training. Fat is lost primarily

TERMS

Spot reducing Fallacious theory that claims that exercising a specific body part will result in significant fat reduction in that area.

Cellulite Term frequently used in reference to fat deposits that "bulge out"; these deposits are just enlarged fat cells from excessive accumulation of body fat.

by burning it in muscle. Therefore, as the concentration of the enzymes increases, so does the ability to burn fat.[12]

In addition to exercise and adequate food management, sensible adjustments in caloric intake are recommended. Most research finds that a negative caloric balance is required to lose weight. Perhaps the only exception is in people who are eating too few calories. A nutrient analysis (see Chapter 7) often reveals that faithful dieters are not consuming enough calories. These people actually need to increase their daily caloric intake (combined with an exercise program) to get their metabolism to kick back up to a normal level.

The reasons for prescribing a lower caloric figure to lose weight are:

1. Most people underestimate their caloric intake and are eating more than they should be eating.

2. Developing new behaviors takes time, and some people have trouble changing and adjusting to new eating habits.

3. Many individuals are in such poor physical condition that they take a long time to increase their activity level enough to offset the setpoint and burn enough calories to aid in loss of body fat.

4. Some dieters have difficulty succeeding unless they can count calories.

Table 8.2   *Caloric Expenditure of Selected Physical Activities*

Activity*	Cal/lb/min	Activity*	Cal/lb/min	Activity*	Cal/lb/min
Aero-belt Exercise		Dance		Stairmaster	
Aero-belt Jogging/6 mph	0.098	Moderate	0.030	Moderate	0.070
Aero-belt Step-Aerobics/8"	0.105	Vigorous	0.055	Vigorous	0.090
Aero-belt Walking/4 mph	0.073	Golf	0.030	Stationary Cycling	
Aerobics		Gymnastics		Moderate	0.055
Moderate	0.065	Light	0.030	Vigorous	0.070
Vigorous	0.095	Heavy	0.056	Strength Training	0.050
Step-Aerobics	0.070	Handball	0.064	Swimming (crawl)	
Archery	0.030	Hiking	0.040	20 yds/min	0.031
Badminton		Judo/Karate	0.086	25 yds/min	0.040
Recreation	0.038	Racquetball	0.065	45 yds/min	0.057
Competition	0.065	Rope Jumping	0.060	50 yds/min	0.070
Baseball	0.031	Rowing (vigorous)	0.090	Table Tennis	0.030
Basketball		Running		Tennis	
Moderate	0.046	11.0 min/mile	0.070	Moderate	0.045
Competition	0.063	8.5 min/mile	0.090	Competition	0.064
Bowling	0.030	7.0 min/mile	0.102	Volleyball	0.030
Calisthenics	0.033	6.0 min/mile	0.114	Walking	
Cycling (level)		Deep water**	0.100	4.5 mph	0.045
5.5 mph	0.033	Skating (moderate)	0.038	Shallow pool	0.090
10.0 mph	0.050	Skiing		Water Aerobics	
13.0 mph	0.071	Downhill	0.060	Moderate	0.050
		Level (5 mph)	0.078	Vigorous	0.070
		Soccer	0.059	Wrestling	0.085

*Values are for actual time engaged in the activity.   **Treading water

Adapted from:

Allsen, P. E., J. M. Harrison, and B. Vance. *Fitness for Life: An Individualized Approach* (Dubuque, IA: Wm. C. Brown, 1989).

Bucher, C. A., and W. E. Prentice, *Fitness for College and Life* (St. Louis: Times Mirror/Mosby College Publishing, 1989).

Consolazio, C. F., R. E. Johnson, and L. J. Pecora. *Physiological Measurements of Metabolic Functions in Man* (New York: McGraw-Hill, 1963).

Hockey, R. V. *Physical Fitness: The Pathway to Healthful Living* (St. Louis: Times Mirror/Mosby College Publishing, 1989).

Hoeger, W. W. K., et al. Research conducted at Boise State University, 1986-1993.

5. A few people simply will not alter their food selection. For those who will not change their food selection (which will still increase the risk for chronic diseases), a large increase in physical activity, a negative caloric balance, or a combination of the two is the only solution to lose weight successfully.

The daily caloric requirement can be estimated by consulting Tables 8.1 and 8.2 and Figure 8.7. As this is only an estimated value, individual adjustments related to many of the factors discussed in this chapter may be necessary to establish a more precise value. Nevertheless, the estimated value does offer a beginning guideline for weight control or reduction.

The average daily caloric requirement without exercise is based on typical lifestyle patterns, total body weight, and gender. Individuals who hold jobs that require heavy manual labor burn more calories during the day than those who have sedentary jobs such as working behind a desk. To find your activity level, refer to Table 8.1 and rate yourself accordingly. The number given in Table 8.1 is per pound of body weight, so you should multiply your current weight by that number. For example, the typical caloric requirement to maintain body weight for a moderately active male who weighs 160 pounds is 2,400 calories (160 lbs $\times$ 15 calories per pound).

The second step is to determine the average number of calories you use daily as a result of exercise. To get this number, figure out the total number of minutes you exercise weekly, and then figure the daily average exercise time. For instance, a person cycling at 13 miles per hour, five times a week, 30 minutes each time, exercises 150 minutes per week (5 $\times$ 30). The average daily exercise time is 21 minutes (150 $\div$ 7). Round off to the lowest unit.

Next, from Table 8.2, find the energy requirement for the activity (or activities) chosen for the exercise program. In the case of cycling (13 miles per hour), the requirement is .071 calories per pound of body weight per minute of activity (cal/lb/min). With a body weight of 160 pounds, this man uses 11.4 calories each minute (body weight $\times$ .071, or 160 $\times$ .071). In 21 minutes, he uses approximately 240 calories (21 $\times$ 11.4).

The fourth step is to obtain the estimated total caloric requirement, with exercise, needed to maintain body weight. To do this, add the typical daily requirement (without exercise) and the average calories used through exercise. In our example, it is 2,640 calories (2,400 + 240).

If a negative caloric balance is recommended to lose weight, this person has to consume fewer than 2,640 daily calories to achieve the objective. Because of the many factors that play a role in weight control, the previous value is only an estimated daily requirement. Furthermore, to lose weight, a person can't predict that exactly one pound of fat will be lost in one week by reducing daily intake by 500 calories (500 $\times$ 7 = 3,500 calories, or the equivalent of one pound of fat).

The estimated daily caloric figure provides only a target guideline for weight control. Periodic readjustments are necessary because individuals differ, and the estimated daily cost changes as you lose weight and modify your exercise habits.

The recommended number of calories to be subtracted from the daily intake to obtain a negative caloric balance depends on the typical daily requirement. The best recommendation is to decrease the daily intake moderately, never below 1,200 calories for women and 1,500 for men.

A good rule to follow is to restrict the intake by no more than 500 calories if the daily requirement is below 3,000 calories. For caloric requirements in excess of 3,000, as many as 1,000 calories per day may be subtracted from the total intake. The daily distribution should be approximately 60% carbohydrates (mostly complex carbohydrates), less than 30% fat, and about 12% protein.

Many experts believe a person may take off weight more efficiently by reducing the amount of daily fat intake to 10% to 20% of the total daily caloric intake. Because 1 gram of fat supplies more than twice the amount of calories that carbohydrates

The establishment of healthy eating patterns start at a young age.

and protein do, the general tendency is not to overeat.

Further, it takes only 3% to 5% of ingested calories to store fat as fat, whereas it takes approximately 25% of ingested calories to convert carbohydrates to fat. Other research appears to indicate that if people eat the same amount of calories as carbohydrate or fat, those on the fat diet will store more fat. Successful weight-loss programs allow only small amounts of fat in the diet.

Many people have trouble adhering to a 10%- to 20%-fat-calorie diet. During weight loss periods, however, you are strongly encouraged to do so. Start with a 20% fat-calorie diet. Refer to Table 8.3 to aid you in determining the grams of fat at 10%, 20%, and 30% of the total calories for selected energy intakes. Also, use the form provided in Figure 7.16, Chapter 7 to monitor your daily fat intake.

The time of day when food is consumed also may play a part in weight reduction. A study conducted at the Aerobics Research Center in Dallas, Texas, indicated that, when a person is on a diet, weight is lost most effectively if most of the calories are consumed before one o'clock and not during the evening meal. This center recommends that, when a

person is attempting to lose weight, intake should consist of a minimum of 25% of the total daily calories for breakfast, 50% for lunch, and 25% or less at dinner.

Other experts have reported that if most of the daily calories are consumed during one meal, the body may perceive that something is wrong and will slow down the metabolism so it can store a greater amount of calories in the form of fat. Eating most of the calories in one meal also causes a person to go hungry the rest of the day, making the diet more difficult to follow.

Consuming most of the calories earlier in the day seems helpful in losing weight, and also in managing atherosclerosis. The time of day when most of the fats and cholesterol are consumed can influence blood lipids and coronary heart disease. Peak digestion time following a heavy meal is about 7 hours after that meal. If most lipids are consumed during the evening meal, digestion peaks while the person is sound asleep, when the metabolism is at its lowest rate. Consequently, the body may not metabolize fats and cholesterol as well, leading to a higher blood lipid count and increasing the risk for atherosclerosis and coronary heart disease.

Table 8.3	Grams of Fat as a Percentage of Total Calories for Selected Energy Intakes		

| Caloric Intake | Grams of Fat | | |
	10%	20%	30%
1,200	13	27	40
1,300	14	29	43
1,400	16	31	47
1,500	17	33	50
1,600	18	36	53
1,700	19	38	57
1,800	20	40	60
1,900	21	42	63
2,000	22	44	67
2,100	23	47	70
2,200	24	49	73
2,300	26	51	77
2,400	27	53	80
2,500	28	56	83
2,600	29	58	87
2,700	30	60	90
2,800	31	62	93
2,900	32	64	97
3,000	33	67	100

Successful weight management is accomplished by making a lifetime commitment to physical activity and proper food selection.

To monitor daily progress, you may use a form such as the one given in Figure 7.16. Meeting the basic requirements from each food group should get top priority. The caloric content for each food is given in the Nutritive Value of Selected Foods list, Appendix B. For a more precise record, the information should be recorded immediately after each meal. According to the person's progress, adjustments can be made in the typical daily requirement or the exercise program, or both.

• Tips for Behavior Modification and Adherence to a Weight Management Program

Achieving and maintaining recommended body composition is by no means impossible, but this does require desire and commitment. If weight management is to become a priority in life, people must realize they have to retrain behavior to some extent.

Modifying old habits and developing new positive behaviors take time. Individuals have applied the following management techniques to change detrimental behavior successfully and adhere to a positive lifetime weight-control program. In developing a retraining program, people are not expected to incorporate all of the strategies listed but should note the ones that apply to them. The form provided in Figure 8.8 will allow you to evaluate and monitor your own weight-management behaviors.

1. *Make a commitment to change.* The first ingredient to modify behavior is the desire to do so. The reasons for change must be more compelling than those for continuing present lifestyle patterns. You must accept the fact that you have a problem and decide by yourself whether you really want to change. If you have a sincere commitment, your chances for success are enhanced already.

2. *Set realistic goals.* Most people with a weight problem would like to lose weight in a relatively short time but fail to realize that the weight problem developed over a span of several years. A sound weight reduction and maintenance program can be accomplished only by establishing new lifetime eating and exercise habits, both of which take time to develop. In setting a realistic long-term goal, you should also plan short-term objectives. The long-term goal may be to decrease body fat to 20% of total body weight. The short-term objective may be to decrease body fat 1% each month. Objectives like these allow for regular evaluation and help maintain motivation and renewed commitment to attain the long-term goal.

3. *Incorporate exercise into the program.* Choose enjoyable activities, places, times, equipment, and people to exercise with. This will help you adhere to an exercise program. Details on developing a complete exercise program are found in Chapters 3 (cardiorespiratory), 4 (strength), and 5 (flexibility).

4. *Develop healthy eating patterns.* Plan to eat three regular meals per day consistent with the body's nutritional requirements. Learn to differentiate hunger from appetite. Hunger is the actual physical need for food. Appetite is a desire for food, usually triggered by factors such as stress, habit, boredom, depression, food availability, or just the thought of food itself. Eat only when you have a physical need. In this regard, developing and sticking to a regular meal pattern helps control hunger.

5. *Avoid automatic eating.* Many people associate certain daily activities with eating. For example, people eat while cooking, watching television, reading, talking on the telephone, or visiting with neighbors. Most of the time, the foods consumed in these situations lack nutritional value or are high in sugar and fat.

6. *Stay busy.* People tend to eat more when they sit around and do nothing. Occupying the mind and body with activities not associated with eating helps take away the desire to eat. Try walking, cycling, playing sports, gardening, sewing, or visiting a library, a museum, a park. Develop other skills and interests, or try something new and exciting to break the routine.

7. *Plan your meals ahead of time.* Sensible shopping is required to accomplish this objective (by the way, shop on a full stomach, because hungry shoppers tend to buy unhealthy foods impulsively, and then snack on the way home). Include whole-grain breads and cereals, fruits and vegetables, low-fat milk and dairy products, lean meats, fish, and poultry.

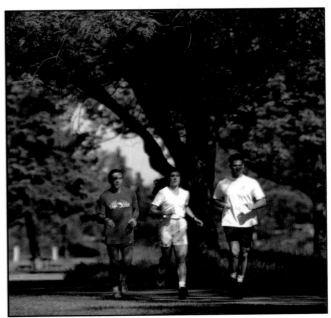

Exercising with other people and in different places helps maintain adherence to exercise.

8. *Cook wisely.* Use less fat and refined foods in food preparation. Trim all visible fat off meats, and remove skin from poultry before cooking. Skim the fat off gravies and soups. Bake, broil, and boil instead of frying. Sparingly use butter, cream, mayonnaise, and salad dressings. Avoid coconut oil, palm oil, and cocoa butter. Prepare plenty of bulky foods. Add whole-grain breads and cereals, vegetables, and legumes to most meals. Try fruits for dessert. Beware of soda pop, fruit juices, and fruit-flavored drinks. In addition to sugar, cut down on other refined carbohydrates such as corn syrup, malt sugar, dextrose, and fructose. Drink plenty of water — at least eight glasses a day.

9. *Do not serve more food than you should eat.* Measure the food portions and keep serving dishes away from the table. This means you will eat less, have a harder time getting seconds, and have less appetite because food is not visible. People should not be forced to eat when they are satisfied (including children after they have already had a healthy, nutritious serving).

10. *Learn to eat slowly and at the table only.* Eating is one of the pleasures of life, and we need to take time to enjoy it. Eating on the run is not good because the body doesn't have enough time to "register" nutritive and caloric consumption and people overeat before the body perceives the signal of fullness. Always eating at the table also forces people to take time out to eat, and it deters snacking between meals, primarily because of the extra time and effort required to sit down and eat. When done eating, do not sit around the table. Clean up and put away the food to keep from unnecessary snacking.

11. *Avoid social binges.* Social gatherings commonly entice self-defeating behavior. Plan ahead and visualize yourself in that gathering. Do not feel pressured to eat or drink, and don't rationalize in these situations. Choose low-calorie foods, and entertain yourself with other activities such as dancing and talking.

12. *Beware of raids on the refrigerator and the cookie jar.* When you find yourself in these tempting situations, take control. Stop and think what is happening. If you have the propensity for raids, try environmental management. Do not bring high-calorie, high-sugar, or high-fat foods into the house. If they are already in the house, store them where they are hard to get to or see. If they are out of sight or not readily available, the temptation is less. Keeping food in places such as the garage and the basement tends to discourage people from taking the time and effort to get them. By no means should you have to eliminate treats completely. Do all things in moderation.

13. *Avoid eating out.* Most meals served at restaurants (especially fast-food restaurants) are high in calories and fat. People who eat out regularly often have a difficult time managing their weight. When eating out, plan your choices by selecting low-fat and low-calorie meals, or go to a restaurant noted for healthful menus.

14. *Practice stress management techniques.* Many people snack and increase food consumption in stressful situations. Eating is not a stress-releasing activity and actually can aggravate the problem if weight control is an issue. Several stress-management techniques are set forth in Chapter 11.

15. *Monitor changes and reward accomplishments.* Feedback on fat loss, lean tissue gain, and weight loss is a reward in itself. Awareness of changes in body composition also helps reinforce new behaviors. Being able to exercise without interruption for 15, 20, 30, 60 minutes, cycling a certain distance, running a mile — all these accomplishments deserve recognition. Meeting objectives calls for rewards, but not related to eating. Buy new clothing, a tennis racquet, a bicycle, exercise shoes, or something else that is special and you would not have acquired otherwise.

16. *Think positive.* Avoid negative thoughts on how difficult changing your past behaviors might be. Instead, think of the benefits you will reap, such as feeling, looking, and functioning better, plus enjoying better health and improving your quality of life. Attempt to stay away from negative environments and people who will not be supportive. Avoid those who do not have the same desires and who encourage self-defeating behaviors.

● In Conclusion

There is no simple and quick way to take off excessive body fat and keep it off for good. Weight management is accomplished by making a lifetime

A. Current body weight   _____

B. Caloric requirement per pound of body weight (use Table 8.1)   _____

C. Typical daily caloric requirement without exercise to maintain body weight
   (A × B)   _____

D. Selected physical activity (e.g., jogging)*   _____

E. Number of exercise sessions per week   _____

F. Duration of exercise session (in minutes)   _____

G. Total weekly exercise time in minutes (E × F)   _____

H. Average daily exercise time in minutes (G ÷ 7)   _____

I. Caloric expenditure per pound per minute (cal/lb/min) of physical activity
   (use Table 8.2)   _____

J. Total calories burned per minute of physical activity (A × I)   _____

K. Average daily calories burned as a result of the exercise program (H × J)   _____

L. Total daily caloric requirement with exercise to maintain body weight (C + K)   _____

M. Number of calories to subtract from daily requirement to achieve
   a negative caloric balance**   _____

N. Target caloric intake to lose weight (L − M)   _____

*If more than one physical activity is selected, you will need to estimate the average daily calories burned as a result of each additional activity (steps D through K) and add all of these figures to L above.

**Subtract 500 calories if the total daily requirement with exercise (L) is below 3,000 calories. As many as 1,000 calories may be subtracted for daily requirements above 3,000 calories.

Figure 8.7 ● *Computation form for daily caloric requirement.*

Name: _____

Strategy / Date:																	
1. I made a commitment to change																	
2. I set realistic goals																	
3. I exercise regularly																	
4. I have healthy eating patterns																	
5. I avoid automatic eating																	
6. I stay busy																	
7. I plan meals ahead of time																	
8. I cook wisely																	
9. I do not serve more food than I should eat																	
10. I eat slowly and at the table only																	
11. I avoid social binges																	
12. I avoid refrigerator and cookie-jar raids																	
13. I avoid eating out. If I do, I eat low fat meals																	
14. I practice stress management																	
15. I monitor behavior changes																	
16. I reward my accomplishments																	
17. I think positive																	

Figure 8.8 ● *Behavioral modification progress form for weight management.*

Preventing Cardiovascular Disease

9

*T*he leading cause of death in the United States, **cardiovascular disease** accounts for nearly half of the total mortality rate in 1990. Some examples of cardiovascular disease are coronary heart disease, **peripheral vascular disease**, congenital heart disease, rheumatic heart disease, strokes, high blood pressure, congestive heart failure, and atherosclerosis.

Although heart and blood vessel disease is still the number-one health problem in the United States, the incidence has declined by 36% in the last two decades (see Figure 9.1), in large part because of health education. More people now are aware of the risk factors for cardiovascular disease and are changing their lifestyles to lower their own potential risk for this disease.

The major form of cardiovascular disease is **coronary heart disease (CHD)**. Narrowing of the coronary arteries diminishes the blood supply to the

Objectives

- Define cardiovascular disease and coronary heart disease.
- Understand the importance of a healthy lifestyle in preventing cardiovascular disease.
- Assess your own risk for developing coronary heart disease.
- Understand the major risk factors that lead to the development of coronary heart disease, including physical inactivity, hypertension, smoking, and abnormal cholesterol profile.
- Become acquainted with a comprehensive program for reducing coronary heart disease risk and managing overall risk for cardiovascular disease.

Figure 9.1 • *Incidence of death from cardio-vascular disease in the United States for selected years: 1900–1990.*

heart muscle, which can precipitate a heart attack (see Figure 9.2).

CHD is the single leading cause of death in the United States, accounting for approximately a third of all deaths and more than half of all cardiovascular deaths. Almost all of the risk factors for CHD are preventable and reversible, and the individual can reduce that risk.

Each year, more than 330,000 coronary by-pass operations and 190,000 coronary **angioplasty**

procedures are performed in the United States. Health care costs for coronary bypass average more than $44,000 and for an angioplasty procedure over $21,000 — or about $11 billion per year for coronary heart disease surgery.

● Coronary Heart Disease Risk Profile

Although genetic inheritance plays a role in CHD, the most important determinant is personal lifestyle. CHD risk factor analyses are administered to evaluate the impact of a person's lifestyle and genetic endowment as potential factors contributing to the development of coronary disease. The specific objectives of a CHD risk factor analysis are:

● To screen individuals who may be at high risk for the disease.
● To educate regarding the leading risk factors for developing CHD.
● To implement programs aimed at risk reduction.
● To use the analysis as a starting point from which to compare changes induced by the intervention program.

The leading risk factors contributing to CHD are listed in Table 9.1. A self-assessment CHD risk factor analysis is given in Figure 9.3. This CHD risk

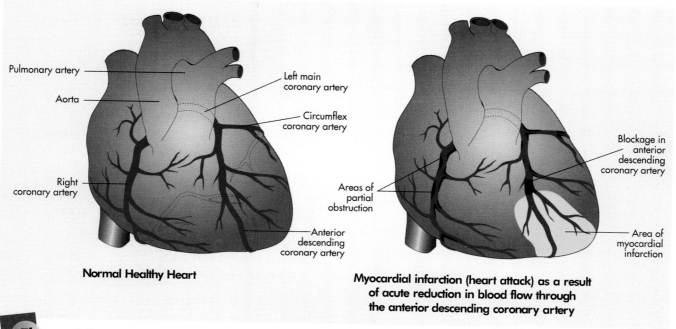

Figure 9.2 • *The heart and its blood vessels.*

factor analysis can be done by people with little or no medical information about their cardiovascular health, as well as by those who have had a thorough medical examination. The guidelines for zero risk are outlined for each factor, making this self-assessment analysis a valuable tool in managing CHD risk factors.

Almost all of the risk factors for coronary heart disease are preventable and reversible, and the individual can reduce risks for acquiring CHD.

For example, a person who fills out the form knows that the ideal blood pressure is around 120/80 or lower, that risk is reduced by smoking less or quitting altogether, that HDL-cholesterol should be 45 mg/dl (milligrams per deciliter) or higher for men and 55 mg/dl or higher for women, and that LDL-cholesterol should be less than 170 mg/dl (if unknown, basic nutritional guidelines also are given). The role of HDL- and LDL-cholesterol in protecting and causing heart disease is discussed later in this chapter.

To provide a meaningful CHD risk score, a weighing system was developed to show the impact of each risk factor on developing the disease. This weighing system is based on the latest research and on the work done at leading preventive medicine facilities in the United States. The most significant risk factors are given the heaviest numeric weight.

For example, a poor cholesterol profile seems to be the best predictor for developing CHD. Up to 12 risk points are assigned to individuals with "very high" LDL-cholesterol levels and "very low" HDL-cholesterol levels. On the other hand, the least heavily weighted risk factor is triglycerides. A maximum of only 2 risk points is assigned to this factor. Each risk factor also is assigned a zero risk level, the level at which it does not appear to increase the risk for disease at all.

Based on actual test results, a person receives a score anywhere from zero to the maximum number of points for each factor. When the risk points from all of the risk factors are totaled, the final number is used to rate an individual in one of five overall risk categories for potential development of CHD.

A risk factor analysis helps to determine the potential effect of lifestyle in the development of coronary heart disease.

A "very low" CHD risk category designates the group at lowest risk for developing heart disease based on age and gender. "Low" CHD suggests that even though people in this category are taking good care of their cardiovascular health, they can still improve it (unless all of the risk points come from age and family history). "Moderate" CHD risk means the person can definitely improve lifestyle to lower

Table 9.1	*Coronary Heart Disease Risk Factors*

Risk Factors		Maximal Risk Points
Abnormal cholesterol profile		12
Low HDL-cholesterol	6	
High LDL-cholesterol	6	
Physical inactivity		8
Smoking		8
Hypertension		8
Systolic blood pressure	4	
Diastolic blood pressure	4	
Personal history of heart disease		8
Abnormal stress electrocardiogram		8
Diabetes		6
High blood glucose	3	
Known diabetes	3	
Family history of heart disease		6
Age		4
Excessive body fat		3
Tension and stress		3
Abnormal resting electrocardiogram		3
Elevated triglycerides		2

TERMS

Cardiovascular disease　The array of conditions that affect the heart and the blood vessels.

Peripheral vascular disease　Narrowing of the peripheral blood vessels (excludes the cerebral and coronary arteries).

Coronary heart disease (CHD)　Condition in which the arteries that supply the heart muscle with oxygen and nutrients are narrowed by fatty deposits such as cholesterol and triglycerides.

Angioplasty　A procedure in which a balloon-tipped catheter is inserted to widen the inner lumen of one or more arteries.

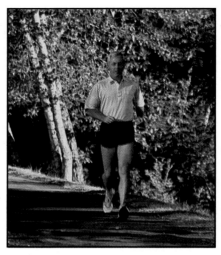

Lifetime participation in aerobic activities is one of the most important ways to prevent cardiovascular disease.

the risk for disease, or medical treatment may be required. A score in the "high" or "very high" CHD risk category points to a strong probability of developing heart disease within the next few years and calls for immediate implementation of a personal risk-reduction program, including medical, nutritional, and exercise intervention by professional staff.

With the exception of age, family history of heart disease, and certain **electrocardiogram (ECG)** abnormalities, the risk factors are preventable and reversible. The leading risk factors for CHD are discussed next, along with the general recommendations for risk reduction.

● Physical Inactivity

Physical inactivity is responsible for low levels of cardiorespiratory endurance (the ability of the heart, lungs, and blood vessels to deliver enough oxygen to the cells to meet the demands of prolonged physical activity). The level of cardiorespiratory endurance (or fitness) is given most commonly by the maximal amount of oxygen (in milliliters) that every kilogram (2.2 pounds) of body weight is able to utilize per minute of physical activity (ml/kg/min). As maximal oxygen uptake increases, so does the efficiency of the cardiorespiratory system.

Even though physical inactivity has not been assigned the most risk points (8 points for a poor level of fitness, as compared to 12 for a poor cholesterol profile — see Table 9.1), improving cardiorespiratory endurance through daily physical activity and aerobic exercise has a great impact in reducing the overall risk for heart disease.

Although specific recommendations can be followed to improve each risk factor, daily physical activity and a regular aerobic exercise program help to control most of the major risk factors that lead to heart disease. Physical activity and aerobic exercise will:

● Increase cardiorespiratory endurance.
● Decrease and control blood pressure.
● Reduce body fat.
● Lower blood lipids (cholesterol and triglycerides).
● Improve HDL-cholesterol.
● Help control diabetes.
● Increase and maintain good heart function, sometimes improving certain ECG abnormalities.
● Motivate toward smoking cessation.
● Alleviate tension and stress.
● Counteract a personal history of heart disease.

The significance of physical inactivity in contributing to cardiovascular risk was clearly shown in 1992, when the American Heart Association added physical inactivity as one of the four major risk factors for cardiovascular disease. (The other three factors are smoking, a poor cholesterol profile, and high blood pressure.) Based on the overwhelming amount of scientific data in this area, evidence of the benefits of aerobic exercise in reducing heart disease is far too impressive to be ignored.

TERMS

Electrocardiogram (ECG) A recording of the electrical activity of the heart.

CORONARY HEART DISEASE RISK FACTOR ANALYSIS

Score

1. Physical Activity	Do you participate in a regular aerobic exercise program (brisk walking, jogging, swimming, bicycling, aerobics, etc.) for more than 30 minutes:	
	Once a week or less 8	
	Two times per week 3	
	Three or more times per week 0	☐

2. Resting and Stress Electrocardiograms (ECG)	Add scores for both ECGs			
	ECG	Resting	Stress	
	Normal	(0)	(0)	 0
	Equivocal	(1)	(4)	 1–5
	Abnormal	(3)	(8)	 3–11

3. HDL-Cholesterol (If unknown, answer question 6)	Men	Women	
	≥ 45	≥ 55	 0
	36–44	46–54	 3
	≤ 35	≤ 45	 6

4. LDL-Cholesterol (If unknown, answer question 6)	≤ 129	 0
	130-159	 3
	≥ 160	 6

5. Triglycerides (If unknown, answer question 6)	≤ 125	 0
	126-499	 1
	≥ 500	 2

6. Diet (Do not answer if questions 3, 4 and 5 have been answered)	Does your regular diet include (high score if all apply): One or more daily servings of red meat; 7 or more eggs/week; daily butter, cheese, whole milk, sweets and alcohol ....10–14 Four to six servings of red meat/week, 4-6 eggs per week, margarine, 1% or 2% milk, some cheese, sweets, and alcohol ....4–10 Fish, poultry, red meat less than three times/week, less than 3 eggs/week, skim milk and skim milk products, moderate sweets and alcohol 0–3

7. Diabetes/Glucose	≤120 0
	121-128 1
	129-136 .... 1.5
	137-144 2
	145-149 .... 2.5
	>150 3
	Diabetics add another 3 points 3

8. Blood Pressure	Score applies to each reading (e.g. 144/88 score = 4)				
		Systolic		Diastolic	
		≤120	(0)	≤80	(0) 0
		121–130	(1)	81–90	(1) 1–2
		131–140	(2)	91–98	(2) 2–4
		141–150	(3)	99–106	(3) 3–6
		≥151	(4)	≥107	(4) 4–8

Subtotal Risk Score: ☐

Figure 9.3 ● *Self-assessment: Coronary heart disease risk factor analysis.*

Score

9. Percent Body Fat

	Men	Women	
	12–17%	18–22%	0
	18–22%	23–27%	1
	23–27%	28–32%	2
	≥28%	≥33%	3

10. Smoking

Lifetime nonsmoker	0
Ex-smoker over one year	0
Ex-smoker less than one year	1
Smoke less than 1 cigarette/day	1
Nonsmoker, but live or work in smoking environment	2
Pipe, cigar smoker, or chew tobacco	2
Smoke 1–9 cigarettes/day	3
Smoke 10–19 cigarettes/day	4
Smoke 20–29 cigarettes/day	5
Smoke 30–39 cigarettes/day	6
Smoke 40 or more cigarettes/day	8

11. Tension and Stress

Are you:

Sometimes tense	0
Often tense	1
Nearly always tense	2
Always tense	3

12. Personal History

Have you ever had a heart attack, stroke, coronary disease, or any known heart problem:

During the last year	8
1–2 years ago	5
2–5 years ago	3
More than 5 years ago	2
Never suffered from heart disease	0

13. Family History

Have any of your blood relatives (parents, uncles, brothers, sisters, grandparents) suffered from cardiovascular disease (heart attack, strokes, bypass surgery):

One or more before age 51	6
One or more between 51 and 60	3
One or more after age 60	1
None have suffered from cardiovascular disease	0

14. Age

29 or younger	0
30–39	1
40–49	2
50–59	3
≥60	4

Total Risk Score:

Risk Categories

Very Low	5 or less points
Low	Between 6 and 15 points
Moderate	Between 16 and 25 points
High	Between 26 and 35 points
Very High	36 or more points

Figure 9.3 ● *Self-assessment: Coronary heart disease risk factor analysis (continued).*

Table 9.4 *Cholesterol and Saturated Fat Content of Selected Foods*

Food	Serving Size	Cholesterol (mg.)	Sat. Fat (gr.)
Avocado	1/8 med.	—	3.2
Bacon	2 slc.	30	2.7
Beans (all types)	any	—	—
Beef — Lean, fat trimmed off	3 oz.	75	6.0
Beef — Heart (cooked)	3 oz.	150	1.6
Beef — Liver (cooked)	3 oz.	255	1.3
Butter	1 tsp.	12	0.4
Caviar	1 oz.	85	—
Cheese — American	2 oz.	54	11.2
Cheese — Cheddar	2 oz.	60	12.0
Cheese — Cottage (1% fat)	1 cup	10	0.4
Cheese — Cottage (4% fat)	1 cup	31	6.0
Cheese — Cream	2 oz.	62	6.0
Cheese — Muenster	2 oz.	54	10.8
Cheese — Parmesan	2 oz.	38	9.3
Cheese — Swiss	2 oz.	52	10.0
Chicken (no skin)	3 oz.	45	0.4
Chicken — Liver	3 oz.	472	1.1
Chicken — Thigh, Wing	3 oz.	69	3.3
Egg (yolk)	1	250	1.8
Frankfurter	2	90	11.2
Fruits	any	—	—
Grains (all types)	any	—	—
Halibut, Flounder	3 oz.	43	0.7
Ice Cream	1/2 cup	27	4.4
Lamb	3 oz.	60	7.2
Lard	1 tsp.	5	1.9
Lobster	3 oz.	170	0.5
Margarine (all vegetable)	1 tsp.	—	0.7
Mayonnaise	1 tbsp.	10	2.1
Milk — Skim	1 cup	5	0.3
Milk — Low Fat (2%)	1 cup	18	2.9
Milk — Whole	1 cup	34	5.1
Nuts	1 oz.	—	1.0
Oysters	3 oz.	42	—
Salmon	3 oz.	30	0.8
Scallops	3 oz.	29	—
Sherbet	1/2 cup	7	1.2
Shrimp	3 oz.	128	0.1
Trout	3 oz.	45	2.1
Tuna (canned — drained)	3 oz.	55	—
Turkey — Dark Meat	3 oz.	60	0.6
Turkey — Light Meat	3 oz.	50	0.4
Vegetables (except avocado)	any	—	—

Substituting low-fat for high-fat products in the diet decreases the risk for disease.

A daily 10%-total-fat diet requires the person to limit fat intake to an absolute minimum. Some health care professionals contend that a diet like this is difficult to follow indefinitely. People with high cholesterol levels, however, may not need to follow that diet indefinitely but should adopt the 10%-fat diet while attempting to lower cholesterol. Thereafter, eating a 20 to 30% fat diet may be adequate to maintain recommended cholesterol levels (1991 national data indicate that current fat consumption in the United States averages 37% of total calories; see Chapter 7, Figure 7.6).

A drawback of very low fat diets (less than 25% fat) is that they tend to lower HDL-cholesterol and increase **triglycerides**. If HDL-cholesterol is already low, monounsaturated and polyunsaturated fats should be added to the diet. Olive, canola, corn, and soybean oils and nuts are sample food items that are high in monounsaturated fats and polyunsaturated fats. A specialized nutrition book should be consulted to determine food items that are high in monounsaturated and polyunsaturated fats (also see Figure 7.12 in Chapter 7).

To lower LDL-cholesterol levels, the following general dietary guidelines are recommended:

1. Consume fewer than three eggs per week.
2. Eat red meats (3 ounces per serving) fewer than three times per week, and no organ meats (such as liver and kidneys).
3. Do not eat commercially baked foods.
4. Drink low-fat milk (1% or less fat, preferably) and eat low-fat dairy products.
5. Do not use coconut oil, palm oil, or cocoa butter.

TERMS

Triglycerides Fats formed by glycerol and three fatty acids.

6. Eat fish instead of red meat.

7. Bake, broil, grill, poach, or steam food instead of frying.

8. Refrigerate cooked meat before adding to other dishes. Remove fat hardened in the refrigerator before mixing the meat with other foods.

9. Avoid fatty sauces made with butter, cream, or cheese.

10. Maintain recommended body weight.

The combination of a healthy diet, a sound aerobic exercise program, and weight control is the best prescription for controlling blood lipids. If this does not work, a physician can administer a blood test to break down the lipoproteins into their various subcategories. Most U.S. laboratories do not conduct these tests. The American Heart Association, however, has established six Lipid Disorder Training Centers that administer comprehensive blood tests. Your local American Heart Association can provide further information.

The NCEP guidelines recommend that people consider drug therapy if, after 6 months on a low-cholesterol, low-fat diet, cholesterol remains unacceptably high. An unacceptable level is an LDL-cholesterol above 190 mg/dl for people with fewer than two risk factors and no signs of heart disease. For people with more than two risk factors and with a history of heart disease, LDL-cholesterol above 160 mg/dl is unacceptable.

BLOOD CHEMISTRY TEST GUIDELINES

People who have never had a blood chemistry test should do so, to establish a baseline for future reference. The blood test should include total cholesterol and the HDL-cholesterol component.

Following an initial normal baseline test no later than age 20, for a person who adheres to the recommended dietary and exercise guidelines, a blood analysis at least every 5 years prior to age 40 should suffice. Thereafter, a blood lipid test is recommended every year, in conjunction with a regular preventive medicine physical examination.

A single baseline test is not necessarily a valid measure. Cholesterol levels vary from month to month and sometimes even from day to day. If the initial test reveals cholesterol abnormalities, the test should be repeated within a few weeks to confirm the results.

● Elevated Triglycerides

Triglycerides are also known as *free fatty acids*. In combination with cholesterol, triglycerides speed up formation of plaque in the arteries. Triglycerides are carried in the bloodstream primarily by **very low-density lipoproteins (VLDLs)** and chylomicrons.

Although they are found in poultry skin, lunch meats, and shellfish, these fatty acids are manufactured mainly in the liver, from refined sugars, starches, and alcohol. High intake of alcohol and sugars (honey included) significantly raises triglyceride levels. Triglycerides can be lowered by cutting down on these foods along with reducing weight (if overweight) and doing aerobic exercise. An optimal blood triglyceride level is less than 125 mg/dl (see Table 9.5).

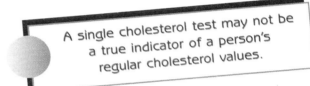

A single cholesterol test may not be a true indicator of a person's regular cholesterol values.

Some people consistently have slightly elevated triglyceride levels (above 140 mg/dl) and HDL-cholesterol levels below 35 mg/dl. About 80% of these people have a genetic condition called LDL phenotype B (approximately 40% of the U.S. population falls in this category). Although the blood lipids may not be notably high, these people are at higher risk for atherosclerosis and CHD.[10]

● Diabetes

Diabetes mellitus is a condition in which the blood glucose is unable to enter the cells because the pancreas either totally stops producing **insulin,** does not produce enough to meet the body's needs, or the body cannot properly use insulin. As a result, glucose (sugar) absorption by the cells and the liver is low, leading to high glucose levels in the blood. The incidence of cardiovascular disease and death in the

Table 9.5   *Triglycerides Guidelines*

Amount	Rating
≤125 mg/dl	Desirable
126–499 mg/dl	Borderline high
≥500 mg/dl	High risk

diabetic population is quite high. Over 80% of people with diabetes mellitus die from cardiovascular disease. People with chronically high blood glucose levels also may have problems metabolizing fats, making them more susceptible to atherosclerosis, increasing the risk for coronary disease, and contributing to other conditions such as loss of vision and kidney damage.

Fasting blood glucose levels above 120 mg/dl may be an early sign of diabetes and should be brought to the attention of a physician. Many health care practitioners consider blood glucose levels around 150 to 160 mg/dl as borderline diabetes (see Table 9.6).

> Adult-onset diabetes is related closely to overeating, obesity, and lack of physical activity.

Diabetes is of two types: Type I, or insulin-dependent diabetes, and Type II, or non-insulin-dependent diabetes. Type I also is called **juvenile diabetes** because it is found mainly in young people. The difference between insulin-dependent diabetes and non-insulin-dependent diabetes is that in the former, the pancreas produces little or no insulin, whereas in the latter, often referred to as adult-onset diabetes, the insulin-producing cells function adequately but the body is unable to use insulin correctly.

Although there is a genetic predisposition to diabetes, adult-onset diabetes is related closely to overeating, obesity, and lack of physical activity. In most cases, this condition can be corrected through a special diet, weight loss, and regular exercise.

A diet high in water-soluble fibers (found in fruits, vegetables, oats, and beans) is helpful in treating diabetes. A simple aerobic exercise program (walking, cycling, or swimming four to five times a week) often is prescribed because it increases the body's sensitivity to insulin. Individuals who have high blood glucose levels should consult a physician to decide on the best treatment.

According to research published in 1991 in the *New England Journal of Medicine*,[11] aerobic exercise helps prevent diabetes in middle-aged men. The protective effect is even greater in those with risk factors such as obesity, high blood pressure, and family propensity.

The preventive effect is attributed to less body fat and better sugar and fat metabolism resulting from the regular exercise program. At 3,500 calories per week, the risk was cut in half, as compared to sedentary men. This preventive effect, according to one of the authors of the study, should hold for women, too.

● Hypertension

Some 60,000 miles of blood vessels run through the human body. As the heart forces the blood through these vessels, the fluid is under pressure.

Blood pressure is measured in milliliters of mercury (mm Hg), usually expressed in two numbers — **systolic blood pressure**, which is the higher number, and the lower **diastolic blood pressure**. Ideal blood pressure is 120/80 or lower (see Table 9.7).

Standards

A few years ago, a systolic pressure of 100 plus your age was the acceptable standard. **Hypertension**, about 160/96, was viewed as the point at which the

Table 9.6	Blood Glucose Guidelines

Amount	Rating
≤120	Desirable
121–159	Borderline high
≥160	High

TERMS

Very low-density lipoproteins (VLDLs) Triglyceride, cholesterol, and phospholipid-transporting molecules in the blood; carry only a small amount of cholesterol.

Diabetes mellitus A disease in which the body doesn't produce or properly utilize insulin.

Insulin Used to convert sugar and starch into energy for the cells.

Juvenile diabetes (Type I) Insulin-dependent diabetes. *See also* Diabetes mellitus.

Blood pressure A measure of the force exerted against the walls of the vessels by the blood flowing through them.

Systolic blood pressure Pressure exerted by the blood against the walls of the arteries during the forceful contraction (systole) of the heart.

Diastolic blood pressure Pressure exerted by the blood against the walls of the arteries during the relaxation phase (diastole) of the heart.

Hypertension Chronically elevated blood pressure.

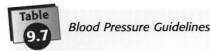

Table 9.7 *Blood Pressure Guidelines*

Rating	Systolic	Diastolic
Ideal	≤120	≤80 mm Hg
Borderline high	121–139	81–89 mm Hg
Hypertension	≥140	≥90 mm Hg

pressure doubled the mortality risk. Readings between 140/90 and 160/96 (either number being in that range) were classified as mild hypertension.

This is no longer the case. Statistical evidence now indicates that blood pressure readings above 140/90 increase the risk for disease and premature death. Consequently, the American Heart Association revised its standards and now considers all blood pressures above 140/90 as hypertension.

Even though the threshold for hypertension has been set at 140/90, many experts believe that the lower the blood pressure, the better. Even if the pressure is around 90/50, as long as that person does not have any symptoms of **hypotension**, he or she need not be concerned. Typical symptoms of hypotension are dizziness, lightheadedness, and fainting.

Hypertensive people who are physically active have a lower relative risk of mortality from all causes than inactive individuals with normal blood pressure.

Blood pressure also may fluctuate during a regular day. Many factors affect blood pressure, and one single reading may not be a true indicator of your real pressure. For example, physical activity and stress increase blood pressure, and rest and relaxation decrease it. Consequently, several measurements should be taken before diagnosing high pressure.

Incidence and Pathology

Based on 1996 estimates by the American Heart Association, nearly 50 million Americans (age 6 and older) are hypertensive. In 1993, 37,520 Americans were killed by high blood pressure. As a disease, hypertension has been referred to as the silent killer. It does not hurt, it does not make you feel sick, and, unless you check it, years may go by before you even

realize you have a problem. High blood pressure is a risk factor not only for CHD, but also for congestive heart failure, strokes, and kidney failure. The relative risk for mortality by systolic blood pressure and various fitness levels is shown in Figure 9.9.

All inner walls of arteries are lined by a layer of smooth endothelial cells. Blood lipids cannot penetrate the lining, and they build up unless damage is done to the cells. High blood pressure is thought to be a leading contributor to destruction of this lining. As blood pressure rises, so does the risk for **atherosclerosis**. The higher the pressure, the greater is the damage to the arterial wall, making the vessels susceptible to fat deposits, especially if serum cholesterol also is high. Blockage of the coronary vessels decreases blood supply to the heart muscle and can lead to heart attacks. When brain arteries are involved, strokes may follow.

A clear example of the connection between high blood pressure and atherosclerosis can be seen by comparing blood vessels in the human body. Even when atherosclerosis is present throughout major arteries, fatty plaques rarely are seen in the pulmonary artery, which goes from the right part of the heart to the lungs. The pressure in this artery normally is below 40 mm Hg, and at such low pressure significant deposits do not occur. This is one of the reasons people with low blood pressure have a lower incidence of cardiovascular disease.

Constantly elevated blood pressure also causes the heart to work much harder. At first the heart does well, but in time this continual strain produces an enlarged heart, followed by congestive heart failure. Furthermore, high blood pressure damages blood vessels to the kidneys and eyes, which may result in kidney failure and loss of vision.

Treatment

Of all hypertension, 90% has no definite cause. This essential hypertension is treatable. Aerobic exercise, weight reduction, a low-sodium/high-potassium diet, stress reduction, no smoking, a diet designed to lower blood lipids, lower caffeine and alcohol intake, and antihypertensive medication all have been used effectively to treat essential hypertension.

The remaining 10% of hypertensive cases is caused by pathological conditions such as narrowing of the kidney arteries, glomerulonephritis (a kidney disease), tumors of the adrenal glands, and narrowing of the aortic artery. With this type of hypertension, the pathological cause has to be treated before the blood pressure problem can be corrected.

Antihypertensive medicines often are the first choice of treatment, but they produce many side effects, such as lethargy, sleepiness, sexual difficulties, higher blood cholesterol and glucose levels, lower potassium levels, and elevated uric acid levels. A physician may end up treating these side effects as much as the hypertension itself. Because of the multiple side effects, about half of the patients stop taking the medication within the first year of treatment.

Another factor contributing to elevated blood pressure is too much sodium in the diet (salt, or sodium chloride, contains approximately 40% sodium). With high sodium intake, the body retains more water, which increases the blood volume and, in turn, drives up the pressure. High intake of potassium seems to regulate water retention and lower the pressure slightly.

Although sodium is essential for normal body functions, the body can function with as little as 200 mg, or a tenth of a teaspoon daily. Even under strenuous conditions of job and sports participation that incite heavy perspiration, the amount of sodium required is seldom more than 3,000 mg per day. Yet, sodium intake in the typical American diet ranges between 6,000 and 20,000 mg per day!

In underdeveloped countries and American Indian tribes where no salt is used in cooking or added at the table, and the only sodium comes from food in its natural form, daily intake rarely is more than 2,000 mg. Blood pressure in these people does not get higher with age, and hypertension is practically unknown. These findings suggest that the human body may be able to handle 2,000 mg per day, but intakes higher than that over the years may cause a gradual rise in blood pressure.

Where does all the sodium come from? The answer is found in Table 9.8. Most people do not realize the amount of sodium in various foods (the list in Table 9.8 does not include salt added at the table).

When treating high blood pressure (unless it is extremely high), before recommending medication, many sports medicine physicians recommend a combination of aerobic exercise, weight loss, and less sodium in the diet. In most instances this treatment brings blood pressure under control.

TERMS

Hypotension   Low blood pressure.

Atherosclerosis   Fatty/cholesterol deposits in the walls of the arteries, leading to plaque formation.

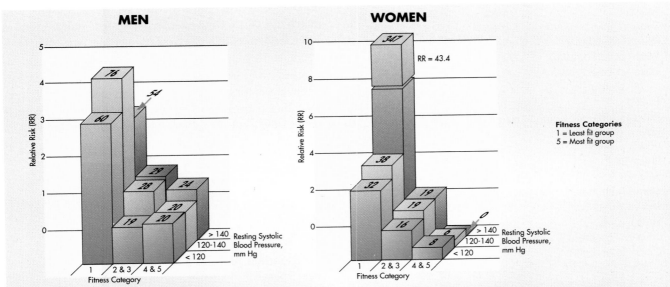

All-cause death rates per 10,000 person-years of follow-up for each cell; 1 person-year indicates one person who was followed up 1 year later. Fitness group 1 is the least fit group; fitness group 5 is the most fit group.

Source: *Physical Fitness and All-Cause Mortality: A Prospective Study of Healthy Men and Women,* by S. N. Blair, H. W. Kohl III, R. S. Paffenbarger, Jr., D. G. Clark, K. H. Cooper, and L. W. Gibbons, in *Journal of the American Medical Association,* 262 (1989) 2395–2401. © American Medical Association. Reproduced by permission.

Figure 9.9 ● *Relative risks of all-cause mortality by physical fitness and systolic blood pressure.*

Table 9.8 *Sodium and Potassium Levels of Selected Foods*

Food	Serving Size	Sodium (mg)	Potassium (mg)
Apple	1 med.	1	182
Asparagus	1 cup	2	330
Avocado	1/2	4	680
Banana	1 med.	1	440
Bologna	3 oz.	1,107	133
Bouillon Cube	1	960	4
Cantaloupe	1/4	17	341
Carrot (raw)	1	34	225
Cheese			
American	2 oz.	614	93
Cheddar	2 oz.	342	56
Muenster	2 oz.	356	77
Parmesan	2 oz.	1,056	53
Swiss	2 oz.	148	64
Chicken (light meat)	6 oz.	108	700
Corn (canned)	1/2 cup	195	80
Corn (natural)	1/2 cup	3	136
Frankfurter	1	627	136
Haddock	6 oz.	300	594
Hamburger (reg)	1	500	321
Lamb (leg)	6 oz.	108	700
Milk (whole)	1 cup	120	351
Milk (skim)	1 cup	126	406
Orange	1 med.	1	263
Orange Juice	1 cup	1	200
Peach	1 med.	2	308
Pear	1 med.	2	130
Peas (canned)	1/2 cup	200	82
Peas (boiled-natural)	1/2 cup	2	178
Pizza (cheese - 14" diam.)	1/8	456	85
Potato	1 med.	6	763
Potato Chips	10	150	226
Potato (french fries)	10	5	427
Pork	6 oz.	96	438
Roast Beef	6 oz.	98	448
Salami	3 oz.	1,047	170
Salmon (canned)	6 oz.	198	756
Salt	1 tsp.	2,132	0
Soups			
Chicken Noodle	1 cup	979	55
Clam Chowder (New England)	1 cup	914	146
Cream of Mushroom	1 cup	955	98
Vegetable Beef	1 cup	1,046	162
Soy Sauce	1 tsp.	1,123	22
Spaghetti (tomato sauce and cheese)	6 oz.	648	276
Strawberries	1 cup	1	244
Tomato (raw)	1 med.	3	444
Tuna (drained)	3 oz.	38	255

The link between hypertension and obesity seems to be quite strong. Not only does blood volume increase with excess body fat, but every additional pound of fat requires an estimated extra mile of blood vessels to feed this tissue. Furthermore, blood capillaries are constricted by the adipose tissues as these vessels run through them. As a result, the heart muscle must work harder to pump the blood through a longer, constricted network of blood vessels.

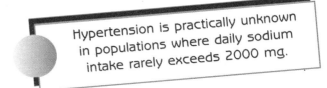

Hypertension is practically unknown in populations where daily sodium intake rarely exceeds 2000 mg.

The role of regular physical activity and aerobic exercise in managing blood pressure is becoming more important each day. On the average, fit individuals have a lower blood pressure than unfit people do. An 18-year follow-up study on exercising and nonexercising subjects showed much lower blood pressures in the active group.[12] The exercise group had an average resting blood pressure of 120/79 as compared to 150/90 for the nonexercise group (see Table 9.9).

Aerobic exercise often is prescribed for hypertensive patients. Several studies have shown that nearly 90% of hypertensive patients who begin a moderate aerobic exercise program can expect a decrease in blood pressure after only a few weeks of training. The research data also show that exercise, not weight loss, is the major contributor to the lowered blood pressure of exercisers. If aerobic exercise is discontinued, these changes are not maintained.

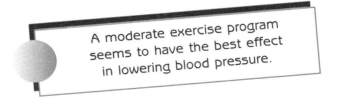

A moderate exercise program seems to have the best effect in lowering blood pressure.

Research presented by Dr. Larry Gibbons (Aerobics Research Institute, Dallas, Texas) at the 1990 American College of Sports Medicine meeting also indicates that exercise programs for hypertensive patients should be of moderate intensity. Training at about 50% of heart rate reserve seems to have the same effect in lowering blood pressure as training at a 70% heart rate reserve. High-intensity training in hypertensive patients actually may cause the blood

Table 9.9   *Effects of a Regular Aerobic Exercise Program on Resting Blood Pressure*

	Initial	Final
Exercise Group		
Age	44.6	68.0
Blood Pressure	120/79	120/78
Nonexercise Group		
Age	51.6	69.7
Blood Pressure	135/85	150/90

Note

The aerobic exercise program consisted of an average four training sessions per week, each 66 minutes long, at about 76 percent of heart rate reserve.

Based on data from "The Effect of Physical Activity on Aerobic Power in Older Men (A Longitudinal Study)," by F. W. Kash, J. L. Boyer, S. P. Van Camp, L. S. Verity, and J. P. Wallace, *The Physician and Sports Medicine*, 18:4 (1990), 73–83.

pressure to rise slightly. Even so, a person may be better off to be highly fit and have high blood pressure than to be unfit and have low blood pressure. As illustrated in Figure 9.9, the death rates for unfit individuals with low systolic blood pressure are much higher than in highly fit people with high systolic blood pressure.

Most important is a preventive approach. Keeping blood pressure under control is easier than trying to bring it down once it is high. Regardless of your past blood pressure history, high or low, you should have it checked routinely. Regular physical exercise, weight control, a low-salt diet, no smoking, and stress management are the keys to controlling blood pressure.

Those who are taking medication for hypertension should not stop unless the prescribing physician gives the go-ahead. If it is not treated properly, high blood pressure can kill. By combining medication with the other treatments, drug therapy eventually may be reduced or completely eliminated.

Excessive Body Fat

Body composition refers to the ratio of lean body weight to fat weight. If the body contains too much fat, the person is considered overweight or obese (see guidelines in Chapter 6, Table 6.8).

Although some experts recognize obesity as an independent risk factor for CHD, the risks attributed to obesity may actually be caused by other risk factors that usually accompany excessive body fat. Risk factors such as high blood lipids, hypertension, and diabetes, usually improve with increased physical activity. As discussed in Chapter 8, overweight people who are physically active do not appear to be at increased risk for premature death.

Attaining recommended body composition helps improve some of the CHD risk factors and also helps to reach a better state of health and wellness. People who have a weight problem and want to get down to recommended weight, must:

1. Increase daily physical activity and participate in aerobic and strength-training programs.
2. Follow a diet low in fat and refined sugars and high in complex carbohydrates and fiber.
3. Reduce total caloric intake moderately while still getting the necessary nutrients to sustain normal body functions.

Additional recommendations for weight reduction and weight control are discussed in Chapter 8.

Smoking

More than 48 million adults and 3.5 million adolescents in the United States smoke. Cigarette smoking is the single largest preventable cause of illness and premature death in the United States. Smoking has been linked to cardiovascular disease, cancer, bronchitis, emphysema, and peptic ulcers. In relation to coronary disease, not only does smoking speed up the process of atherosclerosis, but it also carries a threefold increase in the risk of sudden death following a myocardial infarction.

Smoking prompts the release of nicotine and some other 1,200 toxic compounds into the bloodstream. Similar to hypertension, many of these substances are destructive to the inner membrane that protects the walls of the arteries. As mentioned, once the lining is damaged, cholesterol and triglycerides can be deposited readily in the arterial wall. As the plaque builds up, it obstructs blood flow through the arteries.

Furthermore, smoking encourages the formation of blood clots, which can completely block an artery already narrowed by atherosclerosis. In addition, carbon monoxide, a byproduct of cigarette smoke, decreases the blood's oxygen-carrying capacity. A combination of obstructed arteries, less oxygen, and nicotine in the heart muscle heightens the risk for a serious heart problem.

Smoking also increases heart rate, raises blood pressure, and irritates the heart, which can trigger fatal cardiac **arrhythmias**. Another harmful effect is a decrease in HDL-cholesterol, the "good" type that helps control blood lipids. Smoking actually presents a much greater risk of death from heart disease than from lung disease.

Pipe and cigar smoking and chewing tobacco also increase the risk for heart disease. Even if the smoker inhales no smoke, he or she absorbs toxic substances through the membranes of the mouth, and these end up in the bloodstream. Individuals who use tobacco in any of these three forms also have a much greater risk for cancer of the oral cavity.

The risk for both cardiovascular disease and cancer starts to decrease the moment you quit smoking. The risk approaches that of a lifetime nonsmoker 10 and 15 years, respectively, after quitting. A more thorough discussion of the harmful effects of cigarette smoking, the benefits of quitting, and a complete program for quitting are detailed in Chapter 12.

● Tension and Stress

Tension and stress have become a part of life. Everyone has to deal daily with goals, deadlines, responsibilities, pressures. Almost everything in life (whether positive or negative) is a source of stress. The stressor itself is not what creates the health hazard but, rather, the individual's response to it.

The human body responds to stress by producing more **catecholamines** to prepare the body for "fight or flight." These hormones increase heart rate, blood pressure, and blood glucose levels, enabling the person to take action. If the person fights or flees, the higher levels of catecholamines are metabolized and the body is able to return to a normal state. If, however, a person is under constant stress and unable to take action (as in the death of a close relative or friend, loss of a job, trouble at work, financial insecurity), the catecholamines remain elevated in the bloodstream.

People who are not able to relax will have a constant low-level strain on the cardiovascular system that could manifest itself in heart disease. In addition, when a person is in a stressful situation, the coronary arteries that feed the heart muscle constrict, reducing the oxygen supply to the heart. If the blood vessels are largely blocked by atherosclerosis, abnormal heart rhythms or even a heart attack may follow.

Individuals who are under a lot of stress and do not cope well with it need to take measures to counteract the effects of stress in their lives. One way is to identify the sources of stress and learn how to cope with them. People need to take control of themselves, examine and act upon the things that are most important in their lives, and ignore less meaningful details.

Physical activity is one of the best ways to relieve stress. When a person takes part in physical activity, the body metabolizes excess catecholamines and is able to return to a normal state. Exercise also steps up muscular activity, which contributes to muscular relaxation after completing the physical activity.

Many executives in large cities are choosing the evening hours for their physical activity programs, stopping after work at the health or fitness club. In doing this, they are able to "burn up" the excess tension accumulated during the day and enjoy the evening hours. This has proven to be one of the best stress management techniques. More information on stress management techniques is presented in Chapter 11.

● Personal and Family History

Individuals who have had cardiovascular problems are at higher risk than those who have never had a problem. People with this history should control the other risk factors as much as they can. Most risk factors are reversible, so this will greatly decrease the risk for future problems. The more time that has passed since the cardiovascular problem occurred, the lower is the risk for recurrence.

Genetic predisposition toward heart disease has been demonstrated clearly and seems to be gaining in importance. All other factors being equal, a person with blood relatives who now have or did have heart disease run a greater risk than someone with no such history. Premature CHD is defined as a heart attack before age 55 in a close male relative or before age 65 in a close female relative. The younger the age at which the cardiovascular incident happened to the relative, the greater is the risk for the disease.

In some cases there is no way of knowing whether a person's true genetic predisposition or simply poor lifestyle habits led to a heart problem. A person may have been physically inactive, been overweight, smoked, and had bad dietary habits, leading to heart attack. Regardless, blood relatives fall in the family history category. Because we have no reliable way to differentiate all the factors contributing to cardiovascular disease, a person with a family history should watch all other factors closely and maintain as low a risk level as possible. In addition, the person should have a blood chemistry analysis annually to make sure the body is handling blood lipids properly.

● Age

Age is a risk factor because of the higher incidence of heart disease in older people. This tendency may be induced partly by other factors stemming from changes in lifestyle as we get older — less physical activity, poor nutrition, obesity, and so on.

Young people should not think they are exempt from heart disease. The process begins early in life. Autopsies conducted on soldiers killed at age 22 and younger revealed that approximately 70% had early stages of atherosclerosis. Other studies found elevated blood cholesterol levels in children as young as 10 years old.

Although the aging process cannot be stopped, it certainly can be slowed down. Physiological versus chronological age is important in preventing disease. Some individuals in their 60s or older have the body of a 20-year-old. And 20-year-olds often are in such poor condition and health that they almost seem to have the body of 60-year-olds. Risk factor management and positive lifestyle habits are the best means of slowing down the natural aging process.

● A Final Word on Coronary Risk Reduction

Most of the risk factors for CHD are reversible and preventable. Just because a person has a family history of heart disease and possibly some of the other risk factors because of neglect in lifestyle, this does not mean the person is doomed. A healthier lifestyle — free of cardiovascular problems — is something over which you have much control. You are encouraged to be persistent. Willpower and commitment are required to develop patterns that eventually will turn into healthy habits contributing to total well-being.

TERMS

Arrhythmias Irregular heart rhythms.
Catecholamines Class of hormones including epinephrine and norepinephrine.

Notes

1. S. N. Blair, H. W. Kohl III, R. S. Paffenbarger, Jr, D. G. Clark, K. H. Cooper, and L. W. Gibbons, "Physical Fitness and All-Cause Mortality: A Prospective Study of Healthy Men and Women," *Journal of the American Medical Association,* 262 (1989), 2395–2401.
2. R. S. Paffenbarger, Jr, R. T. Hyde, A. L. Wing, I. Lee, D. L. Jung, and J. B. Kampert, "The Association of Changes in Physical-Activity Level and Other Lifestyle Characteristics with Mortality Among Men," *New England Journal of Medicine,* 328 (1993), 538–545.
3. P. A. Romm, M. K. Hong, and C. E. Rackley, "High-Density-Lipoprotein Cholesterol and Risk of Coronary Heart Disease," *Practical Cardiology,* 16 (1990), 28–40.
4. C. J. Gluek, "Nonpharmacologic and Pharmacologic Alteration of High Density Lipoprotein Cholesterol: Therapeutic Approaches to Prevention of Atherosclerosis," *American Heart Journal,* 110 (1985), 1107–1115.
5. J. M. Gaziano and C. H. Hennekens, "A New Look at What Can Unclog Your Arteries," *Executive Health Report,* 27:8 (1991), 16.
6. Gaziano and Hennekens.
7. Romm et al.
8. American Heart Association, *Heart and Stroke Facts* (Dallas: AHA, 1993).
9. R. J. Barnard, "Effects of Lifestyle Modification on Serum Lipids," *Archives of Internal Medicine* 151 (1991), 1389–1394.
10. R. Superko, "Platelets and Lipid Interaction with a Vessel Wall," presented in symposium at American College of Sports Medicine Annual Meeting, 1991.
11. S. P. Helmrich, D. R. Ragland, R. W. Leung, and R. S. Paffenbarger, "Physical Activity and Reduced Occurrences of Non-Insulin-Dependent Diabetes Mellitus," *New England Journal of Medicine,* 325 (1991), 147–152.
12. F. W. Kash, J. L. Boyer, S. P. Van Camp, L. S. Verity, and J. P. Wallace, "The Effect of Physical Activity on Aerobic Power in Older Men (A Longitudinal Study)," *Physician and Sports Medicine* 18:4 (1990), 73–83.

Suggested Readings

American Heart Association. *Heart and Stroke Statistical Update*: 1997 (Statistical Supplement). Dallas: AHA, 1996.

Blair, S. N., K. H. Cooper, L. W. Gibbons, L. R. Gettman, S. Lewis, and N. N. Goodyear. "Changes in Coronary Heart Disease Risk Factors Associated with Increased Treadmill Time in 753 Men." *American Journal of Epidemiology*, 3 (1983), 352–359.

Blair, S. N., N. N. Goodyear, L. W. Gibbons, and K. H. Cooper. "Physical Fitness and Incidence of Hypertension in Healthy Normotensive Men and Women." *Journal of the American Medical Association*, 252 (1984), 487–490.

Blankenhorn, D. H., et al. "Beneficial Effects of Combined Colestipol-Niacin Therapy on Coronary Atherosclerosis and Coronary Venous Bypass Grafts. *Journal of the American Medical Association*, 257 (1987), 3233–3240.

Blankenhorn, D. H., and H. N. Hodis. "Status Report on Coronary Atherosclerosis Regression: Clinical Implications." *Practical Cardiology*, 16:11 (1990), 41–56.

Dietrich, E. B. *The Arizona Heart Institute's Heart Test*. New York: International Heart Foundation, 1981.

Frick, M. H., et al. "Helsinki Heart Study: Primary-Prevention Trial with Gemfibrozil in Middle-Aged Men with Dyslipidemia." *New England Journal of Medicine*, 317 (1987), 1237–1245.

Gibbons, L. W., S. Blair, K. H. Cooper, and M. Smith. "Association Between Coronary Heart Disease Risk Factors and Physical Fitness in Healthy Adult Women." *Circulation*, 5 (1993), 977–983.

Gordon, D. J., et al. "High-Density Lipoprotein Cholesterol and Coronary Heart Disease in Hypercholesterolemic Men: The Lipid Research Clinics Coronary Primary Prevention Trial." *Circulation*, 74 (1986), 1217–1225.

Guss, S. B. "Heart Attack Risk Score." *Cardiac Alert*, 1983.

Hoeger, W. W. K. "Self-Assessment of Cardiovascular Risk." *Corporate Fitness & Recreation*, 5:6 (1986), 1316.

"How Good is 'Good' Cholesterol?" *Health Letter*, April 9, 1982.

Hubert, H. B., M. Feinleib, P. M. MacNamara, and W. P. Castelli. "Obesity as an Independent Risk Factor for Cardiovascular Disease: A 26-year Follow-up of Participants in the Framingham Heart Study." *Circulation*, 5 (1983), 968–977.

Kannel, W. B., D. McGee, and T. Gordon. "A General Cardiovascular Risk Profile: The Framingham Study." *American Journal of Cardiology*, 7 (1976), 46–51.

Kostas, G. "Three Nutrients May Help Control Blood Pressure." *Aerobics News* 1:7 (1986), 6.

Leon, A., J. Connett, D. R. Jacobs, and R. Rauramaa. "Leisure-time Physical Activity Levels and Risk of Coronary Heart Disease and Death: The Multiple Risk Factor Intervention Trial." *Journal of the American Medical Association*, 258 (1987), 2388–2395.

Manninen, V., et al. "Lipid Alterations and Decline in the Incidence of Coronary Heart Disease in the Helsinki Heart Study." *Journal of the American Medical Association*, 260 (1988), 641–651.

Multiple Risk Factor Intervention Trial Research Group: Risk Factor Changes and Mortality Results. *Journal of the American Medical Association*, 248 (1982), 1465–1477.

Neufeld, H. N., and U. Gouldbourt. "Coronary Heart Disease: Genetic Aspects." *Circulation*, 5 (1983), 943–954.

Ornish, D. S., E. Brown, L. W. Scherwitz, et al., "Can Lifestyle Changes Reverse Coronary Heart Disease? Lifestyle Heart Trial." *Lancet*, 336 129-133.

Page, L. B. "On Making Sense of Salt and Your Blood Pressure." *Executive Health*, August 1982.

Peters, R. K., L. D. Cady, Jr., D. P. Bischoff, L. Bernstein, and M.C. Pike. "Physical Fitness and Subsequent Mycardial Infarction in Healthy Workers." *Journal of the American Medical Association*, 249 (1983), 3052–3056.

Powell, K. E., P. D. Thompson, C. J. Caspersen, and J. S. Kendrick. "Physical Activity and the Evidence of Coronary Heart Disease." *Public Health Reviews*, 8 (1987), 253–287.

Romm, P. A., M. K. Hong, and C. E. Rackley. "High-Density-Lipoprotein Cholesterol and Risk of Coronary Heart Disease." *Practical Cardiology*, 16 (1990), 28–40.

Sobolski, J., et al. "Protection Against Ischemic Heart Disease in the Belgian Physical Fitness Study: Physical Fitness Rather than Physical Activity." *American Journal of Epidemiology*, 125 (1987), 601–610.

Van Camp, S. P. "The Fixx Tragedy: A Cardiologist's Perspective." *Physician and Sportsmedicine*, 12 (1984), 153–155.

Whaley, M. H. and S. N. Blair. "Epidemiology of Physical Activity, Physical Fitness and Coronary Heart Disease." *Certified News*, 5:2 (1995), 1–7.

Wiley, J. A., and T. C. Camacho. "Lifestyle and Future Health: Evidence from the Alameda County Study." *Preventive Medicine*, 9 (1980), 121.

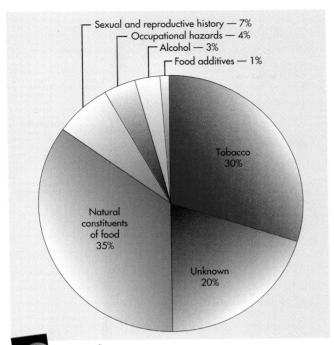

Figure 10.6 ● *Estimate of relative role of major cancer-causing factors.*

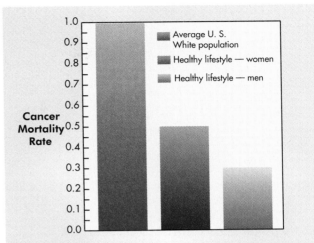

Note: Healthy lifestyle factors include proper nutrition, abstinence from cigarette smoking, regular sleep (7–8 hours per night), and regular physical activity.

Source: "Health Practices and Cancer Mortality Among Active California Mormons," *Journal of the National Cancer Institute*, 81 (1989), 1807–1814.

Figure 10.7 ● *Effects of a healthy lifestyle on cancer mortality rate.*

scientific studies.[3] A group of about 10,000 members of the Church of Jesus Christ of Latter Day Saints (commonly referred to as the Mormon church) in California was reported to have only about one-third (men) to one-half (women) the rate of cancer mortality as the general White population (Figure 10.7). In this study the investigators looked at three general health habits in the participants: lifetime abstinence from smoking, regular physical activity, and sleep. In addition, healthy lifestyle guidelines instituted by the church since 1833 include abstaining from all forms of tobacco, alcohol, caffeine, and drugs, and adhering to a well-balanced diet based on grains, fruits, and vegetables, and moderate amounts of poultry and red meat.

Equally important is that more than 8 million Americans with a history of cancer were alive in 1996, nearly 5 million of whom were considered cured. For most patients, "cured" means 5 years without symptoms after treatments stop. Life expectancy for these individuals is the same as for those who never have had cancer.[4]

● Guidelines for Cancer Prevention

The biggest factor in fighting cancer today is health education. People need to be informed about the risk factors for cancer and the guidelines for early detection. The most effective way to protect against cancer is to change negative lifestyle habits and behaviors. Following are guidelines for preventing cancer.

Dietary Changes

The diet should be low in fat and high in fiber, and contain vitamins A and C from natural sources. Protein intake should be within the RDA guidelines. **Cruciferous vegetables** are encouraged. Alcohol should be consumed in moderation, and obesity should be avoided.

High fat intake has been linked primarily to breast, colon, and prostate cancers. Total fat intake should be limited to less than 20% of total daily calories.[5] Low intake of fiber seems to increase the

TERMS

Nonmelanoma skin cancer Spreads or grows directly from the original site but does not metastasize to other regions of the body.

Cruciferous vegetables Plants that produce cross-shaped leaves (cauliflower, broccoli, cabbage, Brussels sprouts, and kohlrabi); these vegetables seem to have a protective effect against cancer.

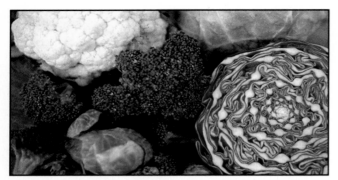

Cruciferous vegetables are recommended in a cancer-prevention diet.

risk for colon cancer. Also recommended is the consumption of at least 25 grams of fiber daily.[6] Foods high in vitamins A and C may deter larynx, esophagus, and lung cancers. Salt-cured, smoked, and nitrite-cured foods have been associated with cancer of the esophagus and stomach. Vitamin C seems to discourage the formation of **nitrosamines**. These potentially cancer-causing compounds are formed when nitrites and nitrates, which are used to prevent the growth of harmful bacteria in processed meats, combine with other chemicals in the stomach.

Carrots, squash, sweet potatoes, and cruciferous vegetables (cauliflower, broccoli, cabbage, Brussels sprouts, and kohlrabi) seem to protect against cancer. These vegetables contain a lot of beta-carotene (a precursor to vitamin A) and vitamin C. Researchers believe the antioxidant effect of these vitamins protects the body from oxygen-free radicals.

As discussed in Chapter 7, during normal metabolism most of the oxygen in the human body is converted into stable forms of carbon dioxide and water. A small amount, however, ends up in an unstable form known as oxygen-free radicals, which are thought to attack and damage the cell membrane and DNA, leading to the formation of cancers. Antioxidants absorb free radicals before they can cause damage, and they also interrupt the sequence of reactions once damage has begun.

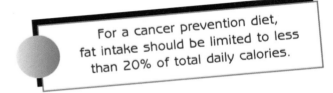

For a cancer prevention diet, fat intake should be limited to less than 20% of total daily calories.

A promising new horizon in cancer prevention is the recent discovery of **phytochemicals**. These compounds, found in abundance in fruits and vegetables, seem to exert a powerful effect in cancer prevention. Phytochemicals exert their protective action by:[7, 8]

- Removing **carcinogens** from cells before they cause damage.
- Activating enzymes that detoxify cancer-causing agents.
- Keeping carcinogens from locking onto cells.
- Preventing carcinogens from binding to DNA.
- Breaking up cancer-causing precursors to benign forms.
- Disrupting the chemical combination of cell molecules that can produce carcinogens.
- Keeping small tumors from accessing capillaries (small blood vessels) to get oxygen and nutrients.

Examples of phytochemicals and their effects are found in Table 10.1.

Table 10.1   *Selected Phytochemicals, Their Effects, and Sources*

Phytochemical	Effects	Good Sources
Sulforaphane	Removes carcinogens from cells	Broccoli
PEITC	Keeps carcinogens from binding to DNA	Broccoli
Genistein	Prevents small tumors from accessing capillaries to get oxygen and nutrients	Soybeans
flavenoids	Helps keep cancer-causing hormones from locking onto cells	Most fruits and vegetables
p-coumaric and chlorogenic acids	Disrupts the chemical combination of cell molecules that can produce carcinogens	Strawberries, green peppers, tomatoes, pineapples
Capsaicin	Keeps carcinogens from binding to DNA	Hot chili peppers

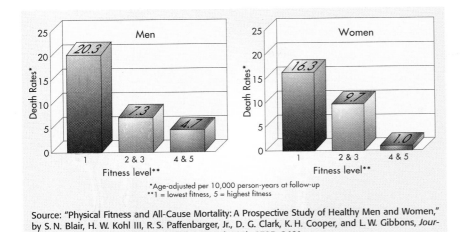

Source: "Physical Fitness and All-Cause Mortality: A Prospective Study of Healthy Men and Women," by S. N. Blair, H. W. Kohl III, R. S. Paffenbarger, Jr., D. G. Clark, K. H. Cooper, and L. W. Gibbons, *Journal of the American Medical Association*, 262 (1989), 2395–2401.

Figure 10.8 • *Association between physical activity and cancer.*

Early Detection

Fortunately, many cancers can be controlled or cured through early detection. The real problem comes when cancerous cells spread, because they are difficult to wipe out then. Therefore, effective prevention, or at least early detection, is crucial. Herein lies the importance of periodic screening.

Other Factors

The contribution of many of the other much-publicized factors is not as significant as those just pointed out. Intentional food additives, saccharin, processing agents, pesticides, and packaging materials currently used in the United States and other developed countries seem to have minimal consequences. High levels of tension and stress and poor coping may affect the autoimmune system negatively and render the body less effective in dealing with the various cancers.

Genetics plays a role in susceptibility in about 10% of all cancers. Most of the effect is seen in the early childhood years. Some cancers are a combination of genetic and environmental liability. Genetics may add to the environmental risk of certain types of cancers. The biggest carcinogenic exposure in the workplace is cigarette smoke. Environment, however, means more than pollution and smoke. It incorporates diet, lifestyle-related events, viruses, and physical agents such as x-rays and exposure to the sun.

Warning Signals

Everyone should become familiar with the following seven warning signals for cancer and bring them to a physician's attention if any are present:

1. Change in bowel or bladder habits.
2. Sore that does not heal.
3. Unusual bleeding or discharge.
4. Thickening or lump in breast or elsewhere.
5. Indigestion or difficulty in swallowing.
6. Obvious change in wart or mole.
7. Nagging cough or hoarseness.

Furthermore, the American Medical Association has developed a questionnaire to alert people to symptoms that may indicate a serious health problem. The questionnaire is given in Figure 10.13 at the end of this chapter. Although in most cases nothing serious will be found, any of the symptoms calls for a physician's attention as soon as possible. Finally, the Recommendations for Early Detection of Cancer by the American Cancer Society, outlined in Table 10.2, should be heeded in regular physical examinations as part of a cancer-prevention program.

Scientific evidence and testing procedures for prevention and early detection of cancer do change. Studies continue to provide new information. The intent of cancer prevention programs is to educate and guide individuals toward a lifestyle that will help prevent cancer and enable early detection of malignancy.

Treatment of cancer always should be left to specialized physicians and cancer clinics. Current treatment modalities include surgery, radiation, radioactive substances, chemotherapy, hormones, and immunotherapy.

TERMS

Melanoma The most virulent, rapidly spreading form of skin cancer.

Ultraviolet B rays (UVB) Sunrays that cause sunburn and encourage skin cancers.

Sun protection factor (SPF) Degree of protection offered by ingredients in sunscreen lotion; at least SPF 15 is recommended.

Table 10.2   *Recommendations for the Early Detection of Cancer*

Test or Procedure	Sex	Age	Frequency
Sigmoidoscopy, preferably flexible	Male & female	50 and over	Every 3–5 years, based on advice of physician
Fecal occult blood test	Male & female	50 and over	Every year
Digital rectal examination	Male & female	40 and over	Every year
Prostate examination*	Male	50 and over	Every year
Pap test	Female		All women who are, or have been, sexually active, or have reached age 18, should have an annual Pap test and pelvic examination. After a woman has had >3 consecutive satisfactory normal annual examinations, the Pap test may be performed less frequently at the discretion of her physician
Pelvic examination	Female	18–40	Every 1–3 years with Pap test
		Over 40	Every year
Endometrial tissue sample	Female	At menopause, women at high risk+	At menopause and thereafter at the discretion of the physician
Breast self-examination	Female	20 and over	Every month
Breast clinical examination	Female	20–40	Every 3 years
		Over 40	Every year
Mammography++	Female	40–49	Every 1–2 years
		50 and over	Every year
Health counseling and cancer checkup§	Male & female	Over 20	Every 3 years
	Male & female	Over 40	Every year

* Annual digital rectal examination and prostate-specific antigen should be performed in men 50 years and older. If either is abnormal, further evaluation should be considered.

+ History of infertility, obesity, failure to ovulate, abnormal uterine bleeding, or unopposed estrogen therapy or tamoxifen therapy.

++ Screening mammography should begin by age 40

§ To include examination for cancers of the thyroid, testicles, ovaries, lymph nodes, oral region, and skin

Source: American Cancer Society, *Textbook of Clinical Oncology* (Atlanta: ACS, 1995).

● Cancer Questionnaire: Assessing Your Risks*

The Texas Division of the American Cancer Society designed a simple self-testing questionnaire to help people assess their risk for cancer (Figure 10.9). Some people have a greater than average risk for developing certain cancers. These people are identified by risk factors for certain common types of cancer. These are the major risk factors and by no means represent the only ones that might be involved. The

---

* Cancer Questionnaire: Assessing Your Risks obtained from the Texas Division of the American Cancer Society and reproduced with permission. (NOTE: This questionnaire is not available nationwide; distribution is limited to Texas residents only.)

instructions given to people who take this questionnaire are:

Men should complete the questions for lung, colon-rectum, and skin cancer. In addition, three major cancer sites for women are included with space to enter the score totals.

Check your own risks against the answers contained on this questionnaire. Individual numbers for specific questions are not to be interpreted as a precise measure of relative risk, but the totals for a given site should give you a general indication of your risk. An explanation of the risk factors for each type of cancer follows the questionnaire. If you are at higher risk, you are advised to discuss the results with your physician.

ASSESSING YOUR RISKS

Read each question concerning each site and its specific risk factors. Be honest in your responses. Place the number in parentheses (risk points) in the correct space provided to the left of each question. For example, Question #2 on lung cancer: If you are 53 years old (age 50 to 59), then enter 5 (risk points) as your score on the left. At the end of each site, total your number of points for that site. Record the final number of points in your cancer profile (Figure 10.12) and in the fitness and wellness profile in Appendix A. Figure A.1

Lung Cancer

1. Sex
   a. Male (2)
   b. Female (1)

2. Age
   a. 39 or less (1)
   b. 40-49 (2)
   c. 50-59 (5)
   d. 60+ (7)

3. Smoking status
   a. Smoker (8)
   b. Nonsmoker (1)

4. Type of smoking
   a. Current cigarettes or little cigars (10)
   b. Pipe and/or cigar, but not cigarettes (3)
   c. Ex-cigarette smoker (2)

5. Amount of cigarettes smoked per day
   a. 0 cigarettes (1)
   b. Less than 1 pack per day (5)
   c. 1 pack (9)
   d. 1-2 packs (15)
   e. 2+ packs (20)

6. Type of cigarette
   a. High tar/nicotine (10)*
   b. Medium T/N (9)
   c. Low T/N (7)
   d. Nonsmoker (1)

7. Duration of smoking
   a. Never smoked (1)
   b. Ex-smoker (3)
   c. Up to 15 years (5)
   d. 15-25 years (10)
   e. 25+ years (20)

8. Type of industrial work
   a. Mining (3)
   b. Asbestos (7)
   c. Uranium and radioactive products (5)

Total

Colon-Rectum Cancer

1. Age
   a. 39 or less (10)
   b. 40-59 (20)
   c. 60+ (50)

2. Has anyone in your immediate family ever had:
   a. Colon cancer (20)
   b. One or more polyps of the colon (10)
   c. Neither (1)

3. Have you ever had:
   a. Colon cancer (100)
   b. One or more polyps of the colon (40)
   c. Ulcerative colitis (20)
   d. Cancer of the breast or uterus (10)
   e. None (1)

4. Bleeding from the rectum (other than obvious hemorrhoids or piles)
   a. Yes (75)
   b. No (1)

Total

Skin Cancer

1. Frequent work or play in the sun:
   a. Yes (10)
   b. No (1)

2. Work in mines, around coal tars, or around radioactivity:
   a. Yes (10)
   b. No (1)

3. Complexion — fair and/or light skin:
   a. Yes (10)
   b. No (1)

Total

Source: Texas Division of the American Cancer Society. Reproduced with permission. (NOTE: This questionnaire is not available nationwide; distribution is limited to Texas residents only.)

Figure 10.9 ● *Cancer questionnaire: Assessing Your Risks.*

Breast Cancer

1. Age group
   a. 20-34 (10)
   b. 35-49 (40)
   c. 50+ (90)

2. Race group
   a. Oriental (5)
   b. Black (20)
   c. White (25)
   d. Mexican American (10)

3. Family history
   a. Mother, sister, aunt, or grandmother with breast cancer (30)
   b. None (10)

4. Your History
   a. Previous lumps or cysts (25)
   b. No breast disease (10)
   c. Previous breast cancer (100)

5. Maternity
   a. 1st pregnancy before 25 (10)
   b. 1st pregnancy after 25 (15)
   c. No pregnancies (20)

   Total

Cervical Cancer

(Lower portion of uterus. These questions would not apply to a woman who has had a total hysterectomy.)

1. Age group
   a. Less than 25 (10)
   b. 25-39 (20)
   c. 40-54 (30)
   d. 55+ (30)

2. Race
   a. Oriental (10)
   b. Puerto Rican (20)
   c. Black (20)
   d. White (10)
   e. Mexican American (20)

3. Number of pregnancies
   a. 0 (10)
   b. 1-3 (20)
   c. 4 and over (30)

4. Viral infections
   a. Herpes and other viral infections or ulcer formations on the vagina (10)
   b. Never (1)

5. Age at first intercourse
   a. Before 15 (40)
   b. 15-19 (30)
   c. 20-24 (20)
   d. 25 and over (10)
   e. Never (5)

6. Bleeding between periods or after intercourse
   a. Yes (40)
   b. No (1)

   Total

Endometrial Cancer

(Body of uterus. These questions do not apply to a woman who has had a total hysterectomy.)

1. Age group
   a. 39 or less (5)
   b. 40-49 (20)
   c. 50+ (60)

2. Race
   a. Oriental (10)
   b. Black (10)
   c. White (20)
   d. Mexican American (10)

3. Births
   a. None (15)
   b. 1 to 4 (7)
   c. 5 or more (5)

4. Weight
   a. 50 or more pounds overweight (50)
   b. 20-49 pounds overweight (15)
   c. Underweight for height (10)
   d. Normal (10)

5. Diabetes (elevated blood sugar)
   a. Yes (3)
   b. No (1)

6. Estrogen hormone intake
   a. Yes, regularly (15)
   b. Yes, occasionally (12)
   c. None (10)

7. Abnormal uterine bleeding
   a. Yes (40)
   b. No (1)

8. Hypertension (high blood pressure)
   a. Yes (3)
   b. No (1)

   Total

Figure 10.9 ● *Cancer questionnaire: Assessing Your Risks (continued).*

● Cancer Questionnaire Interpretation

The following interpretation of the cancer questionnaire is to summarize, explain new evidence, and provide valuable information on the individual risk that a person may have for each type of cancer. Potential cancer risk is based on individual lifestyle and medical history.

Lung Cancer

1. **Sex.** Men have a higher risk of lung cancer than women, equating them for type, amount and duration of smoking. Since more women are smoking cigarettes for a longer duration than previously, their incidence of lung and upper respiratory tract (mouth, tongue, and larynx) cancer is increasing.

2. **Age.** The occurrence of lung and upper respiratory tract cancer increases with age.

3. **Smoking status.** Cigarette smokers have up to twenty times or even greater risk than nonsmokers. However, the rates of ex-smokers who have not smoked for ten years approach those of non-smokers.

4. **Type of smoking.** Pipe and cigar smokers are at a higher risk for lung cancer than nonsmokers. Cigarette smokers are at a much higher risk than nonsmokers or pipe and cigar smokers. All forms of tobacco, including chewing, markedly increase the user's risk of developing cancer of the mouth.

5. **Amount of cigarettes smoked per day.** Male smokers of less than one-half pack per day have five times higher lung cancer rates than non-smokers. Male smokers of one to two packs per day have fifteen times higher lung cancer rates than nonsmokers. Smokers of more than two packs per day are twenty times more likely to develop lung cancer than nonsmokers.

6. **Type of cigarette.** Smokers of low-tar/nicotine cigarettes have slightly lower lung cancer rates.

7. **Duration of smoking.** The frequency of lung and upper respiratory tract cancer increases with the duration of smoking.

8. **Type of industrial work.** Exposures to materials used in the industries mentioned in the questionnaire have been demonstrated to be associated with lung cancer. Smokers who work in these industries may have greatly increased risks. Exposures to materials in other industries may also carry a higher risk.

Total Risk:

24 or less . . . . You have a low risk for lung cancer (low risk category).

25-49 . . . . You may be a light smoker and would have a good chance of kicking the habit (light risk).

50-74 . . . . As a moderate smoker, your risks of lung and upper respiratory tract cancer are increased. If you stop smoking now, these risks will decrease (moderate risk).

75 or over . . . . As a heavy cigarette smoker, your chances of getting lung and upper respiratory tract cancer are greatly increased. Your best bet is to stop smoking now — for the health of it. See your doctor if you have a nagging cough, hoarseness, persistent pain, or a sore in the mouth or throat (high risk).

Colon-Rectum Cancer

1. **Age.** Colon cancer occurs more frequently after the age of 50.

2. **Family predisposition.** Colon cancer is more common in families with a previous history of this disease.

3. **Personal history.** Polyps and bowel diseases are associated with colon cancer.

4. **Rectal bleeding.** Rectal bleeding may be a sign of colorectal cancer.

Total Risk:

29 or less . . . . You are at a low risk for colon-rectal cancer.

30-69 . . . . This is a moderate risk category. Testing by your physician may be indicated.

70 or over . . . . This is a high-risk category. You should see your physician for the following tests: digital rectal exam, guaiac slide test, and protoscopic exam.

In addition to the risk factors mentioned in the questionnaire, a diet high in fat and low in fiber as well as a history of breast or endometrial cancer also increase the risk for colon-rectum cancer.

Skin Cancer

1. **Sun exposure.** Excessive ultraviolet light causes cancer of the skin. Protect yourself with a sun screen medication.

2. **Work environment.** Working in mines, around coal tar, or around radioactive materials can cause cancer of the skin.

3. **Complexion.** Persons with light complexions need more protection than others.

Total Risk:

Numerical risks for skin cancer are difficult to state. For instance, a person with a dark complexion can work longer in the sun and be less likely to develop cancer than a light-complected person. Furthermore, a person wearing a long sleeved shirt and wide-brimmed hat may work in the sun and be less at risk than a person who wears a bathing suit for only a short period. The risk greatly increases with age.

If you answer "yes" to any question, you need to protect your skin from the sun or any other toxic material. Changes in moles, warts, or skin sores are very important and should be seen by your doctor.

Breast Cancer

1. **Age.** The risk for breast cancer significantly increases after age 50.

2. **Race.** Breast cancer occurs more frequently in white women than any other group.

3. **Family history.** The risk for breast cancer is higher in women with a family history of this type of cancer. The risk is even higher if more than one family member has developed breast cancer, and is also enhanced by the closeness in terms of immediacy, e.g., mother, sister, aunt, or grandmother.

4. **Personal history.** A previous history of breast or ovarian cancer would indicate a greater risk.

5. **Maternity.** The risk is greater in women who have never had children and in women who bear children after age 30.

Total Risk:

Under 100 . . . . Low-risk women should practice monthly breast self-examination (BSE — see Figure 10.10) and have their breasts examined by a doctor

HOW TO EXAMINE YOUR BREASTS

1
In the shower: Check for any lump or thickening.

2
Before a mirror: Look for any changes in contour of your breasts, a swelling or dimple in the skin.

3
Lying down: Put pillow under right shoulder. With fingers flat, examine right breast, press gently in small circular motions; then squeeze nipple to check for discharge. Now do left breast.

Reproduced by permission from American Cancer Society, Atlanta, GA.

Figure 10.10 • *Breast self-examination.*

as a part of a cancer-related check-up.

100-199 . . . . . Moderate-risk women should practice monthly BSE and have their breasts examined by a doctor as part of a cancer-related checkup. Periodic breast x-rays should be included as your doctor may advise.

200 or over . . . High-risk women should practice monthly BSE and have the above examinations more often. See your doctor for the recommended (frequency of breast physical examinations and x-ray) examinations related to you.

Other possible risk factors for breast cancer not listed in the questionnaire are a diet high in fat, onset of menstruation prior to age 13, chronic cystic disease, and ionizing radiation.

Cervical Cancer

1. **Age.** The highest occurrence is in the 40 and over age group. The numbers represent the relative rates of cancer for different age groups. A 45-year-old woman has a risk three times higher than a 20-year-old.
2. **Race.** Puerto Ricans, Blacks, and Mexican Americans have higher rates of cervical cancer.
3. **Number of pregnancies.** Women who have delivered more children have a higher occurrence.
4. **Viral infections.** Viral infections of the cervix and vagina are associated with cervical cancer.
5. **Age at first intercourse.** Women with earlier intercourse and with more sexual partners are at a higher risk.
6. **Bleeding.** Irregular bleeding may be a sign of uterine cancer.

Total Risk:

40-69 . . . . This is a low-risk group. Ask your doctor for a pap test. You will be advised how often you should be tested after your first test.

70-99 . . . . In this moderate-risk group, more frequent pap tests may be required.

100 or over . . . You are in a high-risk group and should have a pap test (and pelvic exam) as advised by your doctor.

Endometrial Cancer

1. **Age.** Endometrial cancer is seen in older age groups. The numbers by the age groups represent relative rates of endometrial cancer at different ages. A 50-year-old woman has a risk twelve times higher than a 35-year-old woman.
2. **Race.** Caucasians have a higher occurrence.
3. **Births.** The fewer children one has delivered, the greater the risk of endometrial cancer.
4. **Weight.** Women who are overweight are at greater risk.
5. **Diabetes.** Cancer of the endometrium is associated with diabetes.
6. **Estrogen use.** Cancer of the endometrium may be associated with prolonged continuous estrogen hormone intake. This occurs in only a small number of women. You should consult your physician before starting or stopping any estrogen medication.
7. **Abnormal bleeding.** Women who do not have cyclic regular menstrual periods are at greater risk.
8. **Hypertension.** Cancer of the endometrium is associated with high blood pressure.

Total Risk:

49-59 . . . . You are at low risk for developing endometrial cancer.

60-99 . . . . Your risks are slightly higher (moderate risk). Report any abnormal bleeding immediately to your doctor. Tissue sampling at menopause is recommended.

100 or over . . . Your risks are much greater (high risk). See your doctor for tests as appropriate.

Additional risk factors that may be associated with endometrial cancer, not included in the questionnaire, are infertility, a prolonged history of failure to ovulate, and menopause after age 55.

● Other Cancer Sites

Risk factors and prevention techniques for other types of cancer not contained in the cancer questionnaire have been outlined in *The Causes of Cancer*[13] book published by the American Cancer Society, as well as in a series of pamphlets on "Facts on Cancer" (one each for selected cancer sites). These types of cancer are discussed next, along with the risk factors associated with each type and preventive techniques to decrease risk. Unlike the previous questionnaire, no numeric weights for the different risk factors have been assigned. However, as you read the information, rate yourself on a scale from 1 to 3 (1 = low risk, 2 = moderate risk, 3 = high risk) for each cancer site, and record your results in Figure 10.12.

Prostate Cancer

The prostate gland is actually a cluster of smaller glands that encircles the top section of the urethra (urinary channel) at the point where it leaves the bladder. The function of the prostate is not quite clear, but the muscles of these small glands help squeeze prostatic secretions into the urethra.

Risk Factors

1. **Advancing age.** The highest incidence of prostate cancer is found in men over 55. The incidence is also higher among Blacks than Whites, and more married than single men develop this type of cancer.

2. **A history of venereal disease.** Herpes Simplex Virus Type 2 and Cytomegalovirus (herpes virus) have been linked to prostate cancer.

3. **A history of prostate infections** (more than two).

4. **A diet high in fat.**

Prevention and Warning Signals

Prostate cancer is difficult to control because the causes are not known. Death rates can be lowered through early detection and awareness of the warning signals. Detection is made by a rectal exam of the gland and should be conducted once a year after the age of 40. Possible warning signals include: difficulties in urination (especially at night), painful urination, blood in the urine, and constant pain in the lower back or hip area.

Testicular Cancer

Testicular cancer accounts for only 1% of all male cancers. However, it is the most common type of cancer seen in men between ages 25 and 35. The incidence is slightly higher in Whites than Blacks, and it is rarely seen in middle-aged and older men. The malignancy rate of testicular tumors is 96%, but this type of cancer is highly curable if it is diagnosed early.

Risk Factors

1. Undescended testicle not corrected before age 6.
2. Atrophy of the testicle following mumps or virus infection.
3. Family history of testicular cancer.
4. Recurrent injury to the testicle.
5. Abnormalities of the endocrine system (e.g., high hormone levels of pituitary gonadotropin or androgens).
6. Incomplete testicular development.

Prevention and Warning Signals

The incidence of testicular cancer is quite high in males born with an undescended testicle. Therefore, this condition should be corrected early in life. Parents of infant males need to make sure that the child is checked by a physician to ensure that the testes have descended into the scrotum. Testicular self-examination (TSE) once a month following a warm bath or shower (when the scrotal skin is relaxed) is recommended (see Figure 10.11). Each testicle is gently examined by rolling it between the thumb and fingers. The individual should feel for a firm lump about the size of a pea. Although most lumps are noncancerous, if detected, a physician should be promptly consulted.

Some of the warning signs associated with testicular cancer are: a small lump found on the testicle, slight enlargement (usually painless) and change in consistency of the testis, sudden build-up of blood or fluid in the scrotum, groin and lower abdominal pain or discomfort accompanied by a sensation of dragging and heaviness, breast enlargement or tenderness, and enlarged lymph glands.

Early diagnosis of testicular cancer is essential, as this type of cancer spreads rapidly to other parts of the body. Because in most cases no early symptoms or pain are associated with testicular cancer, most people do not see a physician for months following the discovery of a lump or a slightly enlarged testis. Unfortunately, this delay allows almost 90% of testicular cancer to metastasize (spread) before a diagnosis is made.

Pancreatic Cancer

The pancreas is a thin gland that lies behind the stomach. This gland releases insulin and pancreatic juice. Insulin regulates blood sugar, and pancreatic juice contains enzymes that aid in food digestion.

TESTICULAR SELF-EXAM

How do I do this examination?

Here's how to go about it: Roll each testicle between your thumb and first three fingers until you have felt the entire surface (see illustration below). The testicles should feel round and smooth, like hard-boiled eggs.

These are the things you have to be on the lookout for:

- Lumps

- Irregularities

- A change in the size of the testicle

- Pain in the testicle

- A dragging or heavy sensation.

How often do I have to do this exam?

Do it at least once a month. It helps to pick a regular day of the month — the day of your birthday, the first of the month, the first Sunday, or some other day that's easy for you to remember. You can do the exam more often if you like.

 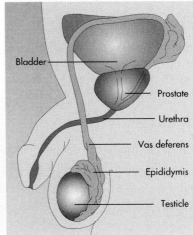

Bladder — Prostate — Urethra — Vas deferens — Epididymis — Testicle

Figure 10.11 • *Testicular self-examination.*

Possible Risk Factors

1. Increased incidence between ages 35 and 70, but significantly higher around age 55.
2. Cigarette smoking.
3. High cholesterol diet.
4. Exposure to unspecified environmental agents.

Prevention and Warning Signals

Detection of pancreatic cancer is difficult because (a) no symptoms are evoked in the early disease process, and (b) advanced disease symptoms are similar to those of other diseases. Warning signals that may be related to pancreatic cancer include pain in the abdomen or lower back, jaundice, loss of weight and appetite, nausea, weakness, agitated depression, loss of energy and feeling weary, dizziness, chills, muscles spasms, double vision, and coma.

Kidney and Bladder Cancer

The kidneys are the organs that filter the urine, and the bladder stores and empties the urine. Most of these two types of cancer are caused by environmental factors. Bladder cancer occurs most frequently between the ages of 50 and 70. Eighty percent of bladder cancers are seen in men, and the incidence is twice as high in White males than in Black males.

Risk Factors

1. Congenital (inborn) abnormalities of either organ (these conditions are detected by a physician).
2. Exposure to certain chemical compounds such as aniline dyes, naphthalenes, or benzidines.
3. Heavy cigarette smoking.

4. History of schistosomiasis (a parasitic bladder infection).

5. Frequent urinary tract infections, particularly after age 50.

Prevention and Warning Signals

Avoiding cigarette smoking and occupational exposure to cancer-causing chemicals is important to decrease risk. Bloody urine, especially repeated occurrences, is always a warning sign and requires immediate evaluation.

Oral Cancer

Oral cancer includes the mouth, lips, tongue, salivary glands, pharynx, larynx, and floor of the mouth. Most of these cancers seem to be related to cigarette smoking and excessive alcohol consumption.

Risk Factors

1. Heavy smoking and/or drinking.
2. Broken or ill-fitting dentures.
3. Broken tooth that irritates the inside of the mouth.
4. Chewing and dipping tobacco.
5. Excessive sun exposure (lip cancer).

Prevention and Warning Signals

Regular examinations and good dental hygiene help in the prevention and early detection of oral cancer. Warning signals may include: a nonhealing sore or white patch in the mouth, a lump, problems with chewing and swallowing, a constant feeling of having "something" in the throat. A person with any of those conditions should be evaluated by a physician or dentist. A tissue biopsy is normally conducted to diagnose the presence of cancer.

Esophageal and Stomach Cancer

The incidence of gastric cancer in the United States has dropped about 40% in the last 30 years. Cancer experts attribute this drastic decrease to changes in dietary habits and more refrigeration. This type of cancer is more common in men, and the incidence is also higher in Black males than in White males.

Risk Factors

1. A diet high in starch and low in fresh fruits and vegetables.

2. High consumption of salt-cured, smoked, and nitrate-cured foods.
3. Stomach acid imbalance.
4. History of pernicious anemia.
5. Chronic gastritis or gastric polyps.
6. Family history of these types of cancer.

Prevention and Warning Signals

Prevention is accomplished primarily by increasing dietary intake of complex carbohydrates and fiber and decreasing the intake of salt-cured, smoked, and nitrate-cured foods. In addition, regular guaiac testing for occult blood (hemoccult test) is recommended. Warning signals for this type of cancer include: indigestion for two weeks or longer, blood in the stools, vomiting, rapid weight loss.

Ovarian Cancer

The ovaries are part of the female reproductive system that produces and releases the egg and the hormone estrogen. Ovarian cancer develops more frequently after menopause, and the highest incidence is seen between ages 55 and 64.

Risk Factors

1. Women over 50 years old.
2. History of ovarian problems.
3. Extensive history of menstrual irregularities.
4. Family history of ovarian cancer.
5. Personal history of breast, bowel, or endometrial cancer.
6. Nulliparity (not having given birth to a child).

Prevention and Warning Signals

In most cases, there are no signs or symptoms related to ovarian cancer. Therefore, regular pelvic examinations to detect signs of enlargement or other abnormalities are highly recommended. Some warning signals may be: an enlarged abdomen, abnormal vaginal bleeding, unexplained digestive disturbances in women over 40, normal-sized ovaries (premenopause size) after menopause.

Thyroid Cancer

The thyroid gland, located in the lower portion of the front of the neck, helps regulate growth and metabolism. Thyroid cancer occurs almost twice as often in women as in men, and the incidence is also higher in Whites than Blacks.

Risk Factors

1. Increased age.
2. Radiation therapy of the head and neck region received in childhood or adolescence.
3. Family history of thyroid cancer.

Prevention and Warning Signals

Regular inspection for thyroid tumors is done by palpation of the gland and surrounding areas during a physical examination. Thyroid cancer is slow-growing; therefore, it is highly treatable. However, any unusual lumps in front of the neck should be promptly reported to a physician. Although thyroid cancer does not have many warning signals (besides a lump), these may include: difficulty in swallowing, choking, labored breathing, persistent hoarseness.

Liver Cancer

The incidence of liver cancer in the United States is very low. Men are more prone to liver cancer, and the disease is more common after age 60.

Risk Factors

1. History of cirrhosis of the liver.
2. History of hepatitis B virus.
3. Exposure to vinyl chloride (industrial gas used in plastics manufacturing) and aflatoxin (natural food contaminant).

Prevention and Warning Signals

Prevention consists primarily of avoiding the risk factors and being aware of warning signals. Possible signs and symptoms are a lump or pain in the upper right abdomen (which may radiate into the back and the shoulder), fever, nausea, rapidly deteriorating health, jaundice, and liver tenderness.

Leukemia

Leukemia is a type of cancer that interferes with blood-forming tissues (bone marrow, lymph nodes, and spleen), by producing too many immature white blood cells. People who have leukemia cannot fight infection very well. The causes of leukemia are mostly

unknown, although suspected risk factors have been identified.

Risk Factors

1. Inherited susceptibility, but not directly transmitted from parent to child.
2. Greater incidence in children with Down syndrome (mongolism) and a few other genetic abnormalities.
3. Excessive exposure to ionizing radiation.
4. Environmental exposure to chemicals such as benzene.

Prevention and Warning Signals

Detection is not easy because early symptoms may be associated with serious ailments. Early warning signals include: fatigue, pallor, weight loss, easy bruising, nose bleeds, paleness, loss of appetite, repeated infections, hemorrhages, night sweats, bone and joint pain, fever. At a more advanced stage, fatigue increases, hemorrhages become more severe, pain and high fever continue, the gums swell, and various skin disorders occur.

Lymphomas

Lymphomas are cancer of the lymphatic system. The lymphatic system consists of lymph nodes found throughout the body and a network of vessels that link these nodes. The lymphatic system participates in the body's immune reaction to foreign cells, substances, and infectious agents.

Risk Factors

As with leukemia, the causes of lymphomas are unknown at this time. Some researchers suspect that a form of herpes virus, referred to as Epstein-Barr, is active in the initial stages of lymphosarcomas. Other researchers suggest that certain external factors may alter the immune system, making it more susceptible to the development and multiplication of cancer cells.

Prevention and Warning Signals

Prevention of lymphomas is limited because little is known about its causes. Enlargement of a lymph node or cluster of lymph nodes is the first sign of lymphoma. Other signs and symptoms may be: enlarged spleen or liver, weakness, fever, back or abdominal pain, nausea/vomiting, unexplained weight loss, unexplained itching and sweating, fever at night that lasts for a long time.

● What Can You Do?

If you are at high risk for any of the cancer sites, you are advised to discuss this with your physician. An ounce of prevention is worth a pound of cure. Although cardiovascular disease is the number-one killer in the country, cancer is the number-one fear.

Of all cancers, 60% to 80% are preventable, and about 50% are curable. Most cancers are lifestyle-related, so being aware of the risk factors and following the screening guidelines (Table 10.2) and basic recommendations for cancer prevention will greatly decrease the risk for developing cancer.

Notes

1. G. Cowley, "The Secrets of a Cancer Cell's Success," *Newsweek*, April 25, 1994, pp. 48–49.
2. American Cancer Society, *Cancer Facts & Figures – 1997* (New York: ACS, 1997).
3. J. E. Enstrom, "Health Practices and Cancer Mortality Among Active California Mormons," *Journal of the National Cancer Institute*, 81 (1989), 1807–1814.
4. American Cancer Society.
5. J. H. Weisburger and G. M. Williams, "Causes of Cancer," *American Cancer Society Textbook of Clinical Oncology* (Atlanta: ACS, 1995), 10–39.
6. Weisburger and Williams.
7. S. Begley, "Beyond Vitamins" *Newsweek*, April 25, 1994, pp. 45–49.
8. "Antioxidant Vitamins: Are They the Only Cancer-Phyters?" *Cancer Smart*, 1:3(1995),4–5.
9. "Your Barbecue Grill: A Smoking Gun?" *Cancer Smart*, 1:2(1995), 4–5.
10. Weisburger and Williams.
11. S. N. Blair, H. W. Kohl III, R. S. Paffenbarger, Jr., D. G. Clark, K. H. Cooper, and L. W. Gibbons, "Physical Fitness and All-Cause Mortality: A Prospective Study of Healthy Men and Women," *Journal of the American Medical Association*, 262 (1989), 2395–2401.
12. I-Min Lee, "Exercise and Physical Health: Cancer and Immune Function," *Research Quarterly for Exercise and Sport*, 66 (1995), 286–291.
13. Weisburger and Williams.

Suggested Readings

American Cancer Society. Facts [on selected cancer sites]. New York: ACS, 1978 and 1983.

American Cancer Society. *Textbook of Clinical Oncology*. Atlanta: ACS, 1995.

American Cancer Society. *Cancer Book*. New York: ACS, 1986.

American Cancer Society, Texas Division. *Cancer: Assessing Your Risk*. Dallas: ACS, 1982.

Feng, J. et al. "The RNA Component of Human Telomerase." *Science*, 269 (1995), 1236–1241.

Greenwald, P. "Assessment of Risk Factors for Cancer." *Preventive Medicine*, 9 (1980), 260–263.

Hammond, E. C., and H. Seidman. "Smoking and Cancer in the United States." *Preventive Medicine*, 9 (1980), 169–173.

Higginson, J. "Proportion of Cancers Due to Occupation." *Preventive Medicine*, 9 (1980), 180–188.

Paffenbarger, R. S., R. T. Hyde, A. L. Wing, and C. H. Steinmetz. "A Natural History of Athleticism and Cardiovascular Health." *Journal of the American Medical Association*, 252 (1984), 491–495.

"Physical Activity and Cancer." *Physical Activity and Fitness Research Digest*. Washington, DC: President's Council on Physical Fitness and Sport, June 1995.

Rothman, K. J. "The Proportion of Cancer Attributable to Alcohol Consumption." *Preventive Medicine*, 9 (1980), 174–179.

Weisburger, J. H., D. M. Hegsted, G. B. Gori, and B. Lewis. "Extending the Prudent Diet to Cancer Prevention." *Preventive Medicine*, 9 (1980), 297–304.

Williams, C. L. "Primary Prevention of Cancer Beginning in Childhood." *Preventive Medicine*, 9 (1980), 275–280.

Williams, P. A. "A Productive History and Physical Examination in the Prevention and Early Detection of Cancer." *Cancer*, 47 (1981), 1146–1150.

Stress Assessment and Management Techniques

11

*L*earning to live and get ahead today is nearly impossible without stress. To succeed in an unpredictable world that changes with every new day, working under pressure has become the rule rather than the exception for most people. As a result, stress has become one of the most common problems we face. Current estimates indicate that the annual cost of stress and stress-related diseases in the United States exceeds $100 billion, a direct result of health-care costs, lost productivity, and absenteeism.

The good news is that stress can be self-controlled. Most people have accepted stress as a normal part of daily life, and even though everyone has to deal with it, few seem to understand it and know how to cope effectively. Stress should not be avoided entirely, as a certain amount is necessary for optimum health, performance, and well-being. It is difficult to succeed and have fun in life without "hits, runs, and errors."

Just what is **stress**? Dr. Hans Selye, one of the foremost authorities on stress, defined it as "the nonspecific response of the human organism to any demand that is placed upon it."[1] "Nonspecific" indicates that the body reacts in a similar fashion regardless of the nature of the event that leads to the stress response.

Objectives

- Define stress, eustress, and distress.
- Explain the role of stress in maintaining health and optimal performance.
- Identify the major sources of stress in life.
- Define the two major types of behavior patterns.
- Learn to lower your vulnerability to stress.
- Develop time-management skills.
- Define the role of physical exercise in reducing stress.
- Learn to use various stress-management techniques.

In simpler terms, stress is the body's mental, emotional, and physiological response to any situation that is new, threatening, frightening, or exciting.

The body's response to stress has been the same ever since humans were first put on the earth. Stress prepares the organism to react to the stress-causing event, also called the **stressor**. The problem, though, is the way in which we react to stress. Many people thrive under stress; others under similar circumstances are unable to handle it. An individual's reaction to a stress-causing agent determines whether stress is positive or negative.

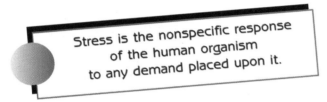

Stress is the nonspecific response of the human organism to any demand placed upon it.

Dr. Selye defined the ways in which we react to stress as either eustress or distress. In both cases, the nonspecific response is almost the same. In the case of **eustress**, *health and performance continue to improve even as stress increases.* On the other hand, **distress** refers to *the unpleasant or harmful stress under which health and performance begin to deteriorate.* The relationship between stress and performance is illustrated in Figure 11.1.

Stress is a fact of modern life, and every person does need an optimal level of stress that is most conducive to adequate health and performance. When stress levels reach mental, emotional, and physiological limits, however, stress becomes distress and the person no longer functions effectively.

Chronic distress raises the risk for many health disorders, including coronary heart disease, hypertension, eating disorders, ulcers, diabetes, asthma, depression, migraine headaches, sleep disorders, and chronic fatigue and may even play a role in the development of certain types of cancers. Recognizing this turning point and overcoming the problem quickly and efficiently are crucial in maintaining emotional and physiological stability.

● Sources of Stress

During recent years several instruments have been developed to assess sources of stress in life. One of the instruments used most often is the **Life Experiences Survey**, presented in Figure 11.2. This survey identifies a person's life changes within the last 12 months that may have an impact on that person's physical and psychological well-being.

TERMS

Stress The mental, emotional, and physiological response of the body to any situation that is new, threatening, frightening, or exciting.

Stressor Stress-causing event.

Eustress Positive stress: health and performance continue to improve, even as stress increases.

Distress Negative stress. Refers to unpleasant or harmful stress under which health and performance begin to deteriorate.

Life Experiences Survey Questionnaire used to assess sources of stress in life.

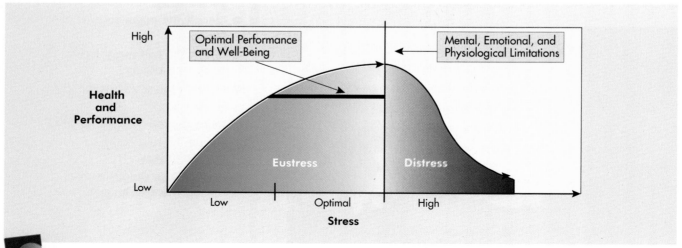

Figure 11.1 ● *Relationship between stress and health and performance.*

THE LIFE EXPERIENCES SURVEY

Section I

1. Marriage	−3	−2	−1	0	+1	+2	+3
2. Detention in jail or comparable institution	−3	−2	−1	0	+1	+2	+3
3. Death of spouse	−3	−2	−1	0	+1	+2	+3
4. Major change in sleeping habits (much more or much less sleep)	−3	−2	−1	0	+1	+2	+3
5. Death of close family member:							
a. mother	−3	−2	−1	0	+1	+2	+3
b. father	−3	−2	−1	0	+1	+2	+3
c. brother	−3	−2	−1	0	+1	+2	+3
d. sister	−3	−2	−1	0	+1	+2	+3
e. grandmother	−3	−2	−1	0	+1	+2	+3
f. grandfather	−3	−2	−1	0	+1	+2	+3
g. other (specify)	−3	−2	−1	0	+1	+2	+3
6. Major change in eating habits (much more or much less food intake)	−3	−2	−1	0	+1	+2	+3
7. Foreclosure on mortgage or loan	−3	−2	−1	0	+1	+2	+3
8. Death of close friend	−3	−2	−1	0	+1	+2	+3
9. Outstanding personal achievement	−3	−2	−1	0	+1	+2	+3
10. Minor law violations (traffic tickets, disturbing the peace, etc.)	−3	−2	−1	0	+1	+2	+3
11. Male: Wife/girlfriend's pregnancy	−3	−2	−1	0	+1	+2	+3
12. Female: Pregnancy	−3	−2	−1	0	+1	+2	+3
13. Changed work situation (different work responsibility, major change in working conditions, working hours, etc.)	−3	−2	−1	0	+1	+2	+3
14. New job	−3	−2	−1	0	+1	+2	+3
15. Serious illness or injury of close family member:							
a. father	−3	−2	−1	0	+1	+2	+3
b. mother	−3	−2	−1	0	+1	+2	+3
c. sister	−3	−2	−1	0	+1	+2	+3
d. brother	−3	−2	−1	0	+1	+2	+3
e. grandfather	−3	−2	−1	0	+1	+2	+3
f. grandmother	−3	−2	−1	0	+1	+2	+3
g. spouse	−3	−2	−1	0	+1	+2	+3
h. other (specify)	−3	−2	−1	0	+1	+2	+3
16. Sexual difficulties	−3	−2	−1	0	+1	+2	+3
17. Trouble with employer (in danger of losing job, being suspended, demoted, etc.)	−3	−2	−1	0	+1	+2	+3
18. Trouble with in-laws	−3	−2	−1	0	+1	+2	+3
19. Major change in financial status (a lot better off or a lot worse off)	−3	−2	−1	0	+1	+2	+3
20. Major change in closeness of family members (increased or decreased closeness)	−3	−2	−1	0	+1	+2	+3
21. Gaining a new family member (through birth, adoption, family member moving in, etc.)	−3	−2	−1	0	+1	+2	+3
22. Change of residence	−3	−2	−1	0	+1	+2	+3
23. Marital separation from mate (due to conflict)	−3	−2	−1	0	+1	+2	+3
24. Major change in church activities (increased or decreased attendance)	−3	−2	−1	0	+1	+2	+3
25. Marital reconciliation with mate	−3	−2	−1	0	+1	+2	+3
26. Major change in number of arguments with spouse (a lot more or a lot less arguments)	−3	−2	−1	0	+1	+2	+3
27. Married Male: Change in wife's work outside the home (beginning work, ceasing work, changing to a new job, etc.)	−3	−2	−1	0	+1	+2	+3

(Continued)

From "Assessing the Impact of Life Changes: Development of the Life Experiences Survey," by I. G. Sarason, *Journal of Consulting and Clinical Psychology* 46 (1978), 932–946. Copyright © 1978 by American Psychological Association. Reprinted by permission of the publisher and the author.

 Figure 11.2 •

THE LIFE EXPERIENCES SURVEY

28.	Married Female: Change in husband's work (loss of job, beginning new job, retirement, etc.)	−3	−2	−1	0	+1	+2	+3
29.	Major change in usual type and/or amount of recreation	−3	−2	−1	0	+1	+2	+3
30.	Borrowing more than $10,000 (buying home, business etc.)	−3	−2	−1	0	+1	+2	+3
31.	Borrowing less than $10,000 (buying car, TV, getting school loan, etc.)	−3	−2	−1	0	+1	+2	+3
32.	Being fired from job	−3	−2	−1	0	+1	+2	+3
33.	Male: Wife/girlfriend having abortion	−3	−2	−1	0	+1	+2	+3
34.	Female: Having abortion	−3	−2	−1	0	+1	+2	+3
35.	Major personal illness or injury	−3	−2	−1	0	+1	+2	+3
36.	Major change in social activities, e.g., parties, movies, visiting (increased or decreased participation)	−3	−2	−1	0	+1	+2	+3
37.	Major change in living conditions of family (building new home, remodeling, deterioration of home, neighborhood, etc.)	−3	−2	−1	0	+1	+2	+3
38.	Divorce	−3	−2	−1	0	+1	+2	+3
39.	Serious injury or illness of close friend	−3	−2	−1	0	+1	+2	+3
40.	Retirement from work	−3	−2	−1	0	+1	+2	+3
41.	Son or daughter leaving home (due to marriage, college, etc.)	−3	−2	−1	0	+1	+2	+3
42.	Ending of formal schooling	−3	−2	−1	0	+1	+2	+3
43.	Separation from spouse (due to work, travel, etc.)	−3	−2	−1	0	+1	+2	+3
44.	Engagement	−3	−2	−1	0	+1	+2	+3
45.	Breaking up with boyfriend/girlfriend	−3	−2	−1	0	+1	+2	+3
46.	Leaving home for the first time	−3	−2	−1	0	+1	+2	+3
47.	Reconciliation with boyfriend/girlfriend	−3	−2	−1	0	+1	+2	+3
48.	Others	−3	−2	−1	0	+1	+2	+3
49		−3	−2	−1	0	+1	+2	+3
50.		−3	−2	−1	0	+1	+2	+3

Section 2

51.	Beginning a new school experience at a higher academic level (college, graduate school, professional school, etc.)	−3	−2	−1	0	+1	+2	+3
52.	Changing to a new school at the same academic level undergraduate, graduate, etc.)	−3	−2	−1	0	+1	+2	+3
53.	Academic probation	−3	−2	−1	0	+1	+2	+3
54.	Being dismissed from dormitory or other residence	−3	−2	−1	0	+1	+2	+3
55.	Failing an important exam	−3	−2	−1	0	+1	+2	+3
56.	Changing a major	−3	−2	−1	0	+1	+2	+3
57.	Failing a course	−3	−2	−1	0	+1	+2	+3
58.	Dropping a course	−3	−2	−1	0	+1	+2	+3
59.	Joining a fraternity/sorority	−3	−2	−1	0	+1	+2	+3
60.	Financial problems concerning school (in danger of not having sufficient money to continue)	−3	−2	−1	0	+1	+2	+3

Total Negative Points: ☐

Total Positive Points: ☐

Category	Negative Score		Total Score	
	Men	Women	Men	Women
Poor	≥13	≥15	≥27	≥27
Fair	7–12	8–14	17–26	18–26
Average	6	7	16	17
Good	1–5	1–6	5–15	6–16
Excellent	0	0	1–4	1–5

Figure 11.2 ● *Continued.*

The Life Experiences Survey is divided into two sections. Section 1, to be completed by all respondents, contains a list of 47 life events plus three blank spaces for other events experienced but not listed in the survey. Section 2 contains an additional 10 questions designed for students only (students should fill out both sections).

The survey requires the person to rate the extent to which the life events he or she experienced had a positive or negative impact on his or her life at the time these events occurred. The ratings are on a 7-point scale. A rating of –3 indicates an extremely undesirable impact. A rating of zero (0) suggests neither a positive nor a negative impact. A rating of +3 indicates an extremely desirable impact.

After determining the life events that have taken place, the negative and the positive points are added together separately. Both scores are expressed as positive numbers (for example — positive ratings: 2, 1, 3, 3 = 9 points positive score; negative ratings: –3, –2, –2, –1, –2 = 10 points negative score). A final "total life change" score can be obtained by adding the positive score and the negative score together as positive numbers (total life change score: 9 + 10 = 19 points).

Because negative and positive changes alike can produce nonspecific responses, the total life change score is a good indicator of total life stress. Most research in this area, however, suggests that the negative change score is a better predictor of potential physical and psychological illness than the total change score.

More research is necessary to establish the role of total change and the role of the ratio of positive to negative stress. Therefore, only the negative score is used as part of the stress profile. To obtain a stress rating, the end of Figure 11.2 presents the various stress categories based on the survey's results.

● Behavior Patterns

Common life events are not the only source of stress in life. All too often individuals bring on stress as a result of their behavior patterns. The two main types of behavior patterns are Type A and Type B. Each type is based on several characteristics that are used to classify people into one of these behavioral patterns.

Several attempts have been made to develop an objective scale to identify Type A individuals properly, but these questionnaires are not as valid and reliable as researchers would like them to be. Consequently, the main assessment tool to determine behavioral type is still the **Structured Interview**. During the Structured Interview a person is asked to reply to several questions that describe Type A and Type B behavior patterns. The interviewer notes not only the responses to the questions but also mental, emotional, and physical behaviors the individual exhibits as he or she replies to each question.

Based on the answers and the associated behaviors, the interviewer rates the person along a continuum, ranging from Type A to Type B. Along this continuum behavioral patterns are classified into five categories: A-1, A-2, X (a mix of Type A and Type B), B-3, and B-4. The Type A-1 exhibits all of the Type A characteristics, and the B-4 shows a relative absence of Type A behaviors. The Type A-2 does not exhibit a complete Type A pattern, and the Type B-3 exhibits only a few Type A characteristics.

Type A *behavior characterizes a primarily hard-driving, overambitious, aggressive, at times hostile and overly competitive person.* Type A individuals often set their own goals, are self-motivated, try to accomplish many tasks at the same time, are excessively achievement-oriented, and have a high degree of time urgency.

A Type A person is usually hard-driving, overambitious, aggressive, and, at times, hostile and overly competitive.

In contrast, **Type B** *behavior is characteristic of calm, casual, relaxed, easy-going individuals.* Type B people take one thing at a time, do not feel pressured or hurried, and seldom set their own deadlines.

Over the years, experts have indicated that individuals classified as Type A are under too much stress and have a significantly higher incidence of

TERMS

Structured interview   Assessment tool used in determining behavioral patterns (Type A and B personality).

Type A   Behavior pattern characteristic of a hard-driving, overambitious, aggressive, at times hostile, and overly competitive person.

Type B   Behavior pattern characteristic of a calmed, casual, relaxed, and easy-going individual.

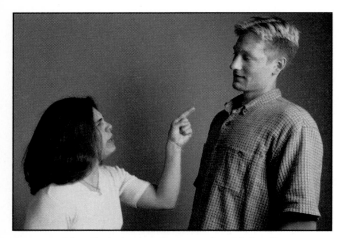

Angry and hostile behaviors increase the risk for disease.

coronary heart disease. Based on these findings, Type A individuals have been counseled to lower their stress level by modifying many of their Type A behaviors.

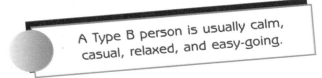

A Type B person is usually calm, casual, relaxed, and easy-going.

Many of the Type A characteristics are learned behaviors. Consequently, if people can learn to identify the sources of stress and make changes in their behavioral responses, they can move along the continuum and respond more like Type B's. The debate, however, has centered on which Type A behaviors should be changed, because not all of them are undesirable.

Scientific evidence further indicates that not all typical Type A people are at higher risk for disease. Type A individuals who commonly express anger and hostility are the ones at higher risk. Therefore, many behavioral modification counselors now work on changing the latter behaviors to prevent disease.

We also know that many individuals perform well under pressure. They typically are classified as Type A but do not demonstrate any of the detrimental effects of stress. Drs. Robert and Marilyn Kriegel came up with the term Type C to characterize people with these behaviors.[2]

Type C individuals are just as highly stressed as Type A's but do not seem to be at higher risk for disease than Type B's. *The keys to successful Type C performance seem to be commitment, confidence, and control.* Type C people are highly committed to

what they are doing, have a great deal of confidence in their ability to do their work, and are in constant control of their actions. In addition, they enjoy their work and maintain themselves in top physical condition to be able to meet the mental and physical demands of their work.

Type C people usually are highly committed to what they are doing, have a great deal of confidence in their ability, and are in control.

Because of the results of recent studies, Type A behavior by itself is no longer viewed as a major risk factor for coronary heart disease. Many experts now believe that emotional stress is far more likely than physical stress to trigger a heart attack. People who are impatient and readily annoyed when they have to wait for someone or something — an employee, a traffic light, in a restaurant line — are especially vulnerable.

Research also is focusing on individuals who have anxiety, depression, and feelings of helplessness when they encounter setbacks and failures in life. People who lose control of their lives, those who give up on their dreams in life, knowing that they could and should be doing better, probably are more likely to have heart attacks than hard-driving people who enjoy their work.

● Vulnerability to Stress

Researchers have identified a number of factors that can affect the way in which people handle stress. How people deal with these factors actually can increase or decrease vulnerability to stress. The questionnaire provided in Figure 11.3 lists these factors so you can determine your vulnerability rating. Many of the items on this questionnaire are related to health, social support, self-worth, and nurturance (sense of being needed). All of the factors are crucial for a person's physical, social, mental, and emotional well-being. The questionnaire will help you

TERMS

Type C Behavior pattern of individuals who are just as highly stressed as the Type A but do not seem to be at higher risk for disease than the Type B.

STRESS VULNERABILITY QUESTIONNAIRE

Item	Strongly Agree	Mildly Agree	Mildly Disagree	Strongly Disagree
1. I try to incorporate as much physical activity* as possible in my daily schedule.	1	2	3	4
2. I exercise aerobically 20 minutes or more at least three times per week.	1	2	3	4
3. I regularly sleep 7 to 8 hours per night.	1	2	3	4
4. I take my time eating at least one hot, balanced meal a day.	1	2	3	4
5. I drink fewer than two cups of coffee (or equivalent) per day.	1	2	3	4
6. I am at recommended body weight.	1	2	3	4
7. I enjoy good health.	1	2	3	4
8 I do not use tobacco in any form.	1	2	3	4
9. I limit my alcohol intake to no more than one drink per day.	1	2	3	4
10. I do not use hard drugs (chemical dependency).	1	2	3	4
11. I have someone I love, trust, and can rely on for help if I have a problem or need to make an essential decision.	1	2	3	4
12. There is love in my family.	1	2	3	4
13. I routinely give and receive affection.	1	2	3	4
14. I have close personal relationships with other people who provide me with a sense of emotional security.	1	2	3	4
15. There are people close by whom I can turn to for guidance in time of stress.	1	2	3	4
16. I can speak openly about feelings, emotions, and problems with people I trust.	1	2	3	4
17. Other people rely on me for help.	1	2	3	4
18. I am able to keep my feelings of anger and hostility under control.	1	2	3	4
19. I have a network of friends who enjoy the same social activities I do.	1	2	3	4
20. I take time to do something fun at least once a week.	1	2	3	4
21. My religious beliefs provide guidance and strength to my life.	1	2	3	4
22. I often provide service to others.	1	2	3	4
23. I enjoy my job (major or school).	1	2	3	4
24. I am a competent worker.	1	2	3	4
25. I get along well with co-workers (or students).	1	2	3	4
26. My income is sufficient for my needs.	1	2	3	4
27. I manage time adequately.	1	2	3	4
28. I have learned to say "no" to additional commitments when I am already pressed for time.	1	2	3	4
29. I take daily quiet time for myself.	1	2	3	4
30. I practice stress management as needed.	1	2	3	4

Total Points: ☐

Scoring:

0–30 points . . . . Excellent (great resistance to stress)
31–40 points . . . . Good (little vulnerability to stress)
41–50 points . . . . Average (somewhat vulnerable to stress)
51–60 points . . . . Fair (vulnerable to stress)
≥61 points . . . . Poor (highly vulnerable to stress)

*Walk instead of driving, avoid escalators and elevators, or walk to neighboring offices, homes, and stores.

Figure 11.3 ●

identify specific areas in which you can make improvements to help you cope more efficiently.

The benefits of physical fitness are discussed extensively in this book. Further, social support, self-worth, and nurturance are essential to cope effectively with stressful life events. These factors render a supportive and protective role in people's lives. The more integrated people are in society, the less vulnerable they are to stress and illness.

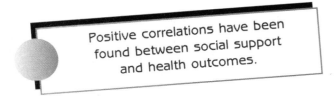

Positive correlations have been found between social support and health outcomes. People can draw upon social support to weather crises. Knowing that someone else cares, that people are there to lean on, that support is out there, is valuable for survival (or growth) in times of need.

As you take the test, you will notice that many of the items describe situations and behaviors that are within your own control. To make yourself less vulnerable to stress, you will want to improve the behaviors that make you more vulnerable to stress. You should start by modifying the behaviors that are easiest to change before undertaking some of the most difficult ones. After completing the questionnaire,

record the results in Figure 11.4 and in your fitness and wellness profile in Appendix A.

● Time Management

According to Benjamin Franklin, "Time is the stuff life is made of." The present "hurry-up" style of life of the American people is not conducive to wellness. The hassles involved in getting through a routine day often lead to stress-related illnesses. People who do not manage their time properly will quickly experience chronic stress, fatigue, despair, discouragement, and illness.

Based on a 1990 Gallup Poll, almost 80% of Americans reported that time moves too fast for them, and 54% felt they had to get everything done. The younger the respondents, the more they struggled with lack of time. Almost half wished they had more time for exercise and recreation, hobbies, and family.

Healthy and successful people are good time managers, able to maintain a pace of life within their comfort zone. In a survey of 1954 Harvard graduates from the school of business, only 27% had reached the goals they established in college. Every one had rated himself as a superior time manager, and only 8% of the remaining graduates perceived themselves as superior time managers. The successful graduates attributed their success to "smart work," not necessarily "hard work."

Name: _____

	Date		
Life Experiences Survey			
Score (negative)	☐	☐	☐
Stress Rating	☐	☐	☐
Stress Vulnerability Questionnaire			
Score	☐	☐	☐
Rating	☐	☐	☐
Stress Management Technique(s) to be used	☐	☐	☐

Figure 11.4 ● *Stress profile.*

Five Steps to Time Management

Trying to achieve one or more goals in a limited time can create a tremendous amount of stress. Many people just don't seem to have enough hours in the day to accomplish their tasks. The greatest demands on our time, nonetheless, frequently are self-imposed: trying to do too much, too fast, too soon.

Some time killers, such as eating, sleeping, and recreation, are necessary for health and wellness, but, in excess, they'll lead to stress in life. You can follow five basic steps to make better use of your time:

1. **Find the time killers.** Many people do not know how they spend each part of the day. Keep a 4- to 7-day log, and record your activities at half-hour intervals. A form is provided in Figure 11.5 to do this (make as many copies as the number of days you wish to evaluate). As you go through your typical day, record the activities so you will remember all of them. At the end of each day, decide when you wasted time. You may be shocked by the amount of time you spent on the phone, sleeping (more than 8 hours per night), or watching television.

2. **Set long-range and short-range goals.** Setting goals requires some in-depth thinking and helps put your life and daily tasks in perspective. What do I want out of life? Where do I want to be 10 years from now? Next year? Next week? Tomorrow? You can use the form provided in Figure 11.6 to list these goals.

3. **Identify your immediate goals,** and prioritize them for today and this week (use Figure 11.7 — make as many copies as necessary). Each day sit down and determine what you need to accomplish that day and that week. Rank your "today" and "this week" tasks in four categories: (a) top-priority, (b) medium-priority, (c) low-priority, and (d) "trash."

    Top-priority tasks are the most important ones. If you were to reap most of your productivity from 30% of your activities, which would they be? Medium-priority activities are those that must be done but can wait a day or two. Low-priority activities are those to be done only upon completing all top- and middle-priority activities. Trash are activities that are not worth your time (for example, cruising the hallways).

4. **Use a daily planner to help you organize and simplify your day.** In this way you can access your priority list, appointments, notes, references, names, places, phone numbers, and addresses conveniently from your coat pocket or purse. Many individuals think that planning daily and weekly activities is a waste of time. A few minutes to schedule your time each day, however, may pay off in hours saved.

    As you plan your day, be realistic and find your comfort zone. Determine what is the best way to organize your day. Which is the most productive time for work, study, errands? Are you a morning person, or are you getting most of your work done when people are quitting for the day? Pick your best hours for top-priority activities. Be sure to schedule enough time for exercise and relaxation. Recreation is not necessarily wasted time. You need to take care of your physical and emotional well-being. Otherwise your life will be seriously imbalanced.

5. **Nightly audits.** Take 10 minutes each night to figure out how well you accomplished your goals that day. Successful time managers evaluate themselves daily. This simple task will help you see the entire picture. Cross off the goals you accomplished, and carry over to the next day those you did not get done. You also may realize that some goals can be moved down to low-priority or be trashed.

COMMON TIME KILLERS

- watching television
- listening to radio/music
- sleeping
- eating
- daydreaming
- shopping
- socializing/parties
- recreation
- talking on the telephone
- worrying
- procrastination
- drop-in visitors
- confusion (unclear goals)
- indecision (what to do next)
- interruptions
- perfectionism (every detail must be done)

Time-Management Skills

In addition to the five major steps, the following can help you make better use of your time:

- **Delegate.** If possible, delegate activities that someone else can do for you. Having another person type your paper while you prepare for an exam might be well worth the expense and your time.

- **Say "no."** Learn to say *no* to activities that keep you from getting your top priorities done. You can do only so much in a single day. Nobody has enough time to do everything he or she would like to get done. Don't overload either. Many people are afraid to say no because they feel guilty if they do. Think ahead, and think of the consequences. Are you doing it to please others? What will it do to your well-being? Can you handle one more task? At some point you have to balance your activities and look at life and time realistically.

> Learn to say no to activities that keep you from getting your priorities done.

- **Protect against boredom.** Doing nothing can be a source of stress. People need to feel that they are contributing and that they are productive members of society. It also is good for self-

Planning and prioritizing your daily activities simplifies your days.

esteem and self-worth. Set realistic goals, and work toward them each day.

- **Plan ahead for disruptions.** Even a careful plan of action can be disrupted. An unexpected phone call or visitor can ruin your schedule. Planning your response ahead will help you deal with these saboteurs.

- **Get it done.** Select only one task at a time, concentrate on it, and see it through. Many people do a little here, do a little there, then do something else. In the end, nothing gets done. An exception to working on just one task at a time is when you are doing a difficult task. Rather than "killing yourself," interchange with another activity that is not as hard.

- **Eliminate distractions.** If you have trouble adhering to a set plan, remove distractions and trash activities from your eyesight. Television, radio, magazines, open doors, or studying in a park might distract you and become time killers.

- **Set aside "overtimes."** Regularly schedule time you did not think you would need as overtime to complete unfinished projects. Most people under-schedule rather than overschedule time. The result is usually late-night burnout! If you schedule overtimes and get your tasks done, enjoy some leisure time, get ahead on another project, or work on some of your trash priorities.

- **Plan time for you.** Set aside special time for yourself daily. Life is not meant to be all work. Use your time to walk, read, or listen to your favorite music.

- **Reward yourself.** As with any other healthy behavior, positive change or a job well done deserves a reward. We often overlook the value of rewards, even if they are self-given. People practice behaviors that are rewarded and discontinue those that are not.

One more activity that you should perform weekly is to go through the list of strategies in Figure 11.8 to determine if you are becoming a good time manager. Provide a yes or no answer to each statement. If you are able to answer yes to most questions, congratulations. You are becoming a good time manager.

Keep a 4- to 7-day log, and record at half-hour intervals the activities you do (make additional copies of this form as needed). Record the activities as you go through your typical day, so you will remember them all. At the end of each day, decide when you wasted time. Using a highlighter, identify the time killers on this form and plan necessary changes for the next day.

Name: _____   Date:_____

Time	
6:00	
6:30	
7:00	
7:30	
8:00	
8:30	
9:00	
9:30	
10:00	
10:30	
11:00	
11:30	
12:00	
12:30	
1:00	
1:30	
2:00	
2:30	
3:00	
3:30	
4:00	
4:30	
5:00	
5:30	
6:00	
6:30	
7:00	
7:30	
8:00	
8:30	
9:00	
9:30	
10:00	
10:30	
11:00	
11:30	
12:00	

Figure 11.5 • *Finding your time killers.*

On a weekly basis, go through the list of strategies given below and write a "Yes" or "No" in response to each statement. If you are able to answer "Yes" to most questions, congratulations. You are becoming a good time manager.

Strategy Date:																
1. I evaluate my time killers periodically																
2. I have written down my long-range goals																
3. I have written down my short-range goals																
4. I use a daily planner																
5. I conduct nightly audits																
6. I conduct weekly audits																
7. I delegate activities that others can do																
8. I have learned to say no to additional tasks when I'm already in "overload"																
9. I plan activities to avoid boredom																
10. I plan ahead for distractions																
11. I work on one task at a time until it's done																
12. I have removed distractions from my work																
13. I set aside "overtimes"																
14. I set aside special time for myself daily																
15. I reward myself for a job well done																

Figure 11.8 • *Evaluation of time-management skills.*

● Coping with Stress

The ways in which people perceive and cope with stress seems to be more important in the development of disease than the amount and type of stress itself. If individuals perceive stress as a definite problem in their lives, when it interferes with optimal level of health and performance, several excellent stress management techniques can help them cope more effectively.

First, of course, the person must recognize that a problem exists. Many people either do not want to believe they are under too much stress or they fail to recognize some of the typical symptoms of distress.

Noting some of the stress-related symptoms (see below) will help a person respond more objectively and initiate an adequate coping response.

> The ways in which people perceive and cope with stress seem to be more important in the development of disease than the amount and type of stress itself.

When people have stress-related symptoms, they first should try to identify and remove the stressor or stress-causing agent. This is not as simple as it may seem, because in some situations eliminating the stressor is not possible, or a person may not even know the exact causing agent. If the cause is unknown, keeping a log of the time and days when the symptoms occur, as well as the events preceding and following the onset of symptoms, may be helpful.

For instance, a couple noted that every afternoon around 6 o'clock, the wife became nauseated and had abdominal pain. After seeking professional help, both were instructed to keep a log of daily events. It soon became clear that the symptoms did not occur on weekends but always started just before the husband came home from work during the week. Following some personal interviews with the couple, it was determined that the wife felt a lack of attention from her husband and responded subconsciously by becoming ill to the point at which she required personal care and affection from her husband. Once the stressor was identified, appropriate behavior changes were initiated to correct the situation.

In many instances, however, the stressor cannot be removed. Examples of situations in which little or nothing can be done to eliminate the stress-causing agent are the death of a close family member, first year on the job, an intolerable boss, a change in work responsibility. Nevertheless, stress can be managed through relaxation techniques.

The body responds to stress by activating the **fight-or-flight** mechanism, which prepares a person

COMMON SYMPTOMS OF STRESS

- headaches
- muscular aches (mainly in neck, shoulders, and back)
- grinding teeth
- nervous tick, finger tapping, toe tapping
- increased sweating
- increase in or loss of appetite
- insomnia
- nightmares
- fatigue
- dry mouth
- stuttering
- high blood pressure
- tightness or pain in the chest
- impotence
- hives
- dizziness
- depression
- irritation
- anger
- hostility
- fear, panic, anxiety
- stomach pain, flutters
- nausea
- cold, clammy hands
- poor concentration
- pacing
- restlessness
- rapid heart rate
- low-grade infection
- loss of sex drive
- rash or acne

TERMS

Fight or flight Physiological response of the body to stress which prepares the individual to take action by stimulating the vital defense systems.

to take action by stimulating the vital defense systems. This stimulation originates in the hypothalamus and the pituitary gland in the brain. The hypothalamus activates the sympathetic nervous system, and the pituitary activates the release of catecholamines (hormones) from the adrenal glands.

These hormonal changes increase heart rate, blood pressure, blood flow to active muscles and the brain, glucose levels, oxygen consumption, and strength — all necessary for the body to fight or flee. For the body to relax, one of these actions must take place. If the person fights or flees, the body relaxes and stress dissipates but if the person is unable to take action, the muscles tense up and tighten (see Figure 11.9). This increased tension and tightening can be dissipated effectively through some coping techniques.

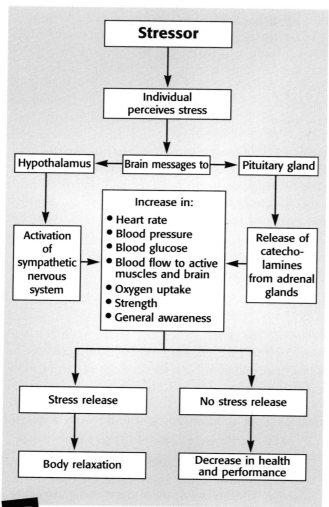

Figure 11.9 • *Physiological response to stress: fight or flight mechanism.*

● Relaxation Techniques

Although benefits are reaped immediately after engaging in any of the several relaxation techniques, several months of regular practice may be necessary for total mastery. The relaxation exercises that follow should not be considered cure-alls or panaceas. If these exercises do not prove to be effective, more specialized textbooks and professional help are called for. In some instances a person's symptoms may not be caused by stress but, rather, may be related to a different medical disorder.

Biofeedback

Clinical application of biofeedback in treating various medical disorders has become popular in the last few years. Besides its successful application in managing stress, it is used commonly in treating medical disorders such as essential hypertension, asthma, heart rhythm and rate disturbances, cardiac neurosis, eczematous dermatitis, fecal incontinence, insomnia, and stuttering. **Biofeedback** as a treatment modality has been defined as:[3]

> A process in which a person learns to reliably influence physiological responses of two kinds: either responses which are not ordinarily under voluntary control or responses which ordinarily are easily regulated but for which regulation has broken down due to trauma or disease.

In simpler terms biofeedback is the interaction with the interior self. This interaction allows a person to learn the relationship between the mind and the biological response. The person actually can "feel" how thought processes influence biological responses (such as heart rate, blood pressure, body temperature, and muscle tension) and how biological responses influence the thought process.

As an illustration of this process, consider the association between a strange noise in the middle of a dark, quiet night and the heart rate response. At first the heart rate shoots up because of the stress the unknown noise induces. The individual may even feel the heart palpitating in the chest and, while still uncertain about the noise, attempts not to panic to prevent an even faster heart rate. Upon realizing that all is well, the person can take control and influence the heart rate to come down. The mind now is able to exert almost complete control over the biological response.

Complex electronic instruments are required to conduct biofeedback. The process itself entails a three-stage, closed-loop feedback system:

1. A biological response to a stressor is detected and amplified.
2. The response is processed.
3. Results of the response are fed back to the individual immediately.

The person uses this new input and attempts to change the physiological response voluntarily, which, in turn, is detected, amplified, and processed. The results then are fed back to the person. The process continues with the intent of teaching the person to reliably influence for the better the physiological response (see Figure 11.10). The most common methods used to measure physiological responses are heart rate, finger temperature, blood pressure equipment, electromyograms, and electroencephalograms.

Physical Activity

Although biofeedback has significant applications in treating various medical disorders, including stress, it requires adequately trained personnel and, in many cases, costly equipment. Therefore, several alternative methods that yield similar results frequently are substituted for biofeedback. For example, research has shown that physical exercise and progressive muscle relaxation, used successfully in stress management, seem to be just as effective as biofeedback in treating essential hypertension.

Physical activity is one of the simplest tools to control stress. The value of exercise in reducing stress is related to several factors, the main one being a decrease in muscular tension.

> You cannot hit your boss or the car in front of you, but you can certainly "hit" the swimming pool, the tennis ball, the weights, or the jogging trail.

For example, a person can be distressed because he or she has had a miserable 8 hours of work in a smoke-filled room with an intolerable boss. To make matters worse, it is late and on the way home the car in front is going much slower than the speed limit. The fight-or-flight mechanism is activated, catecholamines rise, heart rate and blood pressure shoot up, breathing quickens and deepens, muscles tense up, and all systems say "go." No action can be initiated or stress dissipated, though, because the person just cannot hit the boss or the car in front.

A real remedy would be to take action by "hitting" the swimming pool, the tennis ball, the weights, or the jogging trail. By engaging in physical activity, a person is able to reduce the muscular tension and metabolize the increased catecholamines that brought about the physiological changes triggering the fight-or-flight mechanism. Although exercise does not solve problems at work or take care of slow drivers on the road, it certainly can help a person cope with stress, preventing it from becoming a chronic problem.

The early evening hours are becoming the most popular time to exercise for a lot of highly stressed executives. On the way home from work, they stop at the health club or the fitness center. Exercising at this time helps them to dissipate the stress accumulated during the day.

Figure 11.10 ● *Biofeedback mechanism.*

TERMS

Biofeedback Stress management technique. A process in which a person learns to reliably influence physiological responses of two kinds: either responses which are not ordinarily under voluntary control or responses that ordinarily are easily regulated but for which regulation has broken down as a result of trauma or disease.

Physical activity is an excellent tool to control stress.

Most people can relate to exercise as a means of managing stress by remembering how good they felt the last time they concluded a strenuous exercise session after a long, difficult day at the office. A fatigued muscle is a relaxed muscle. For this reason, many people have said that the best part of exercise is the shower afterward.

Not only does evening exercise help to get rid of the stress, but it also provides an opportunity to enjoy the evening more. At home, the family will appreciate Dad or Mom coming home more relaxed, leaving work problems behind, and being able to dedicate all energy to family activities.

Research also has shown that physical exercise requiring continuous and rhythmic muscular activity, such as aerobic exercise, stimulates alpha-wave activity in the brain. These are the same wave patterns seen commonly during meditation and relaxation.

Further, during vigorous aerobic exercise lasting 30 minutes or longer, morphine-like substances referred to as **endorphines** are thought to be released from the pituitary gland in the brain. These substances not only act as painkillers but also seem to induce the soothing, calming effect often associated with aerobic exercise.

Another way that exercise helps to lower stress is by deliberately diverting stress to various body systems. Dr. Hans Selye explains in his book, *Stress Without Distress,*[4] that when accomplishing one specific task becomes difficult, a change in activity can be as good or better than rest itself. For example, if a person is having trouble with a task and does not seem to be getting anywhere, jogging or swimming for a while is better than sitting around and getting frustrated. In this way the mental strain is diverted to the working muscles, and one system helps the other to relax.

Other psychologists indicate that when muscular tension is removed from the emotional strain, the emotional strain disappears. In many cases the change of activity suddenly clears the mind and helps put the pieces together.

Researchers have found that physical exercise gives people a psychological boost because exercise:

- Lessens feelings of anxiety, depression, frustration, aggression, anger, and hostility.
- Alleviates insomnia.
- Provides an opportunity to meet social needs and develop new friendships.
- Allows the person to share common interests and problems.
- Develops discipline.
- Provides the opportunity to do something enjoyable and constructive that will lead to better health and total well-being.

Beyond the short-term benefits of exercise in lessening stress, another benefit of a regular aerobic exercise program is in actually strengthening the cardiovascular system itself. Because the cardiovascular system seems to be affected seriously by stress, a stronger system should be able to cope more effectively. For instance, good cardiovascular endurance has been shown to lower resting heart rate and blood pressure. Because both heart rate and blood pressure rise in stressful situations, initiating the stress response at a lower baseline will counteract the negative effects of stress. Cardiovascularly fit individuals can cope more effectively and are less affected by the stresses of daily living.

Progressive Muscle Relaxation

Progressive muscle relaxation was developed by Dr. Edmund Jacobsen in the 1930s. This technique enables individuals to relearn the sensation of deep relaxation. The technique involves *progressively contracting and relaxing muscle groups throughout the body.* As chronic stress leads to high levels of muscular tension, acute awareness of how progressively tightening and relaxing the muscles feels releases the tension on the muscles and teaches the body to relax at will.

Feeling the tension during the exercises also helps the person to be more alert to signs of distress because this tension is similar to that experienced in stressful situations. In everyday life these feelings then can cue the person to do relaxation exercises.

Relaxation exercises should be done in a quiet, warm, well-ventilated room. The recommended exercises and the duration of the routine vary from one person to the next. Most important is that the individual pay attention to the sensation he or she feels each time the muscles are tensed and relaxed.

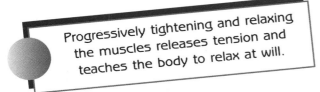

Progressively tightening and relaxing the muscles releases tension and teaches the body to relax at will.

The exercises should encompass all muscle groups of the body. An example of a sequence of progressive muscle relaxation exercises is given next. The instructions for these exercises can be read to the person or memorized or tape-recorded. At least 20 minutes should be set aside to complete the entire sequence. Doing the exercises any faster will defeat their purpose. Ideally, the sequence should be done twice a day.

The individual performing the exercises stretches out comfortably on the floor, face up, with a pillow under the knees, and assumes a passive attitude, allowing the body to relax as much as possible. Each muscle group is to be contracted in sequence, taking care to avoid any strain. Muscles should be tightened to only about 70% of the total possible tension to avoid cramping or some type of injury to the muscle itself.

To produce the relaxation effects, the person must pay attention to the sensation of tensing up and relaxing. The person holds each contraction about 5 seconds and then allows the muscles to go totally limp. The person should take enough time to contract and relax each muscle group before going on to the next. An example of a complete progressive muscle relaxation sequence is:

1. Point your feet, curling the toes downward. Study the tension in the arches and the top of the feet. Hold, and continue to note the tension, then relax. Repeat once again.

2. Flex the feet upward toward the face, and note the tension in your feet and calves. Hold, and relax. Repeat once more.

3. Push your heels down against the floor as if burying them in the sand. Hold, and note the tension at the back of the thigh. Relax. Repeat once more.

4. Contract the right thigh by straightening the leg, gently raising the leg off the floor. Hold, and study the tension. Relax. Repeat with the left leg. Hold and relax. Repeat each leg again.

5. Tense the buttocks by raising your hips ever so slightly off the floor. Hold, and note the tension. Relax. Repeat once again.

6. Contract the abdominal muscles. Hold them tight and note the tension. Relax. Repeat one more time.

7. Suck in your stomach. Try to make it reach your spine. Flatten your lower back to the floor. Hold, and feel the tension in the stomach and lower back. Relax. Repeat once more.

8. Take a deep breath and hold it, then exhale. Repeat. Note your breathing becoming slower and more relaxed.

9. Place your arms at the side of your body and clench both fists. Hold, study the tension, and relax. Repeat a second time.

10. Flex the elbow by bringing both hands to the shoulders. Hold tight and study the tension in the biceps. Relax. Repeat one more time.

11. Place your arms flat on the floor, palms up, and push the forearms hard against the floor. Note the tension on the triceps. Hold, and relax. Repeat once more.

12. Shrug your shoulders, raising them as high as possible. Hold, and note the tension. Relax. Repeat once again.

Practicing regular progressive muscle relaxation helps reduce stress.

TERMS

Endorphines Morphine-like substances released from the pituitary gland in the brain during prolonged aerobic exercise. They are thought to induce feelings of euphoria and natural well-being.

Progressive muscle relaxation Stress management technique involving progressive contraction and relaxation of muscle groups throughout the body.

13. Gently push your head backward. Note the tension in the back of the neck. Hold, relax. Repeat one more time.

14. Gently bring the head against the chest, push forward, hold, and note the tension in the neck. Relax. Repeat a second time.

15. Press your tongue toward the roof of your mouth. Hold, study the tension, and relax. Repeat once more.

16. Press your teeth together. Hold, and study the tension. Relax. Repeat one more time.

17. Close your eyes tightly. Hold them closed and note the tension. Relax, leaving your eyes closed. Do this one more time.

18. Wrinkle your forehead and note the tension. Hold, and relax. Repeat one more time.

Each muscle contraction should be performed at 70% of maximal capacity for about five seconds.

When time is a factor during the daily routine and an individual is not able to go through the entire sequence, he or she may do only the exercises specific to the area that feels most tense. Performing a partial sequence is better than not doing the exercises at all. Completing the entire sequence, of course, yields the best results.

Breathing Techniques For Relaxation

Breathing exercises also can be an antidote to stress. These exercises have been used for centuries in the Orient and India to improve mental, physical, and emotional stamina. In breathing exercises the person concentrates on "breathing away" the tension and inhaling fresh air to the entire body. Breathing exercises can be learned in only a few minutes and require considerably less time than the progressive muscle relaxation exercises.

As with any other relaxation technique, these exercises should be done in a quiet, pleasant, well-ventilated room. Any of the three examples of breathing exercises presented here will help relieve tension induced by stress.

1. **Deep breathing.** Lie with your back flat against the floor, and place a pillow under your knees, feet slightly separated, with toes pointing outward.

(The exercise also may be done while sitting up in a chair or standing straight up). Place one hand on your abdomen and the other hand on your chest.

In breathing exercises, concentrate on "breathing away" the tension and inhaling fresh air to the entire body.

Slowly breathe in and out so the hand on your abdomen rises when you inhale and falls as you exhale. The hand on the chest should not move much at all. Repeat the exercise about 10 times. Next, scan your body for tension, and compare your present tension with the tension you felt at the beginning of the exercise. Repeat the entire process once or twice more.

2. **Sighing.** Using the abdominal breathing technique, breathe in through your nose to a specific count (e.g., 4, 5, or 6). Now exhale through pursed lips to double the intake count (e.g., 8, 10, or 12). Repeat the exercise eight to 10 times whenever you feel tense.

3. **Complete natural breathing.** Sit in an upright position or stand straight up. Breathing through your nose, gradually fill your lungs from the bottom up. Hold your breath for several seconds. Now exhale slowly by allowing your chest and abdomen to relax completely. Repeat the exercise eight to 10 times.

Breathing exercises help dissipate stress.

Autogenic Training

Autogenic training is basically *a form of self-suggestion, in which people are able to place themselves in an autohypnotic state* by repeating and concentrating on feelings of heaviness and warmth in the extremities. This technique was developed by Johannes Schultz, a German psychiatrist, who noted that hypnotized individuals developed sensations of warmth and heaviness in the limbs and torso. The sensation of warmth is caused by dilation of blood vessels, which increases blood flow to the limbs. Muscular relaxation produces the feeling of heaviness.

In this technique the person lies down or sits in a comfortable position, eyes closed, and concentrates progressively on six fundamental stages:

1. **Heaviness**

    My right (left) arm is heavy.
    Both arms are heavy.
    My right (left) leg is heavy.
    Both legs are heavy.
    My arms and legs are heavy.

2. **Warmth**

    My right (left) arm is warm.
    Both arms are warm.
    My right (left) leg is warm.
    Both legs are warm.
    My arms and legs are warm.

3. **Heart**

    My heartbeat is calm and regular (repeat four or five times).

4. **Respiration**

    My body breathes itself (repeat four or five times).

5. **Abdomen**

    My abdomen is warm (repeat four or five times).

6. **Forehead**

    My forehead is cool (repeat four or five times).

The autogenic training technique is more difficult to master than any of those mentioned previously. The person should not move too fast through the entire exercise, as this actually may interfere with learning and relaxation. Each stage must be mastered before proceeding to the next.

Meditation

Meditation is *a mental exercise that can bring about psychological and physical benefits.* The objective of meditation is to gain control over one's attention, clearing the mind and blocking out the stressor(s) responsible for the higher tension. This technique can be learned rather quickly and can be used frequently during times of increased tension and stress.

Initially the person who is learning to meditate should choose a room that is comfortable, quiet, and free of all disturbances (including telephones). After learning the technique, the person will be able to meditate just about anywhere. A time block of approximately 15 minutes, twice a day, is needed to meditate.

1. Sit in a chair in an upright position with the hands resting either in your lap or on the arms of the chair. Close your eyes and focus on your breathing. Allow your body to relax as much as possible. Do not try to consciously relax, because trying means work. Rather, assume a passive attitude and concentrate on your breathing.

2. Allow the body to breathe regularly, at its own rhythm, and repeat in your mind the word "one" every time you inhale, and the word "two" every time you exhale. Paying attention to these two words keeps distressing thoughts from entering into your mind.

3. Continue to breathe in this way about 15 minutes. Because the objective of meditation is to bring about a hypometabolic state leading to body relaxation, do not use an alarm clock to remind you that the 15 minutes have expired. The alarm will only trigger your stress response again, defeating the purpose of the exercise. Opening your eyes once in a while to keep track

TERMS **Breathing exercise** Stress management technique in which the individual concentrates on "breathing away" the tension and inhaling fresh air to the entire body.

Autogenic training Stress management technique; form of self-suggestion where an individual is able to place himself/herself in an autohypnotic state by repeating and concentrating on feelings of heaviness and warmth in the extremities.

Meditation Stress management technique used to gain control over one's attention, clearing the mind and blocking out the stressor(s) responsible for the increased tension.

of the time is fine, but do not rush or anticipate the end of the 15 minutes. This time has been set aside for meditation, and you need to relax, take your time, and enjoy the exercise.

> Stress is not what makes people ill but, rather, the way they react to the stress-causing agent.

Which Technique Is Best?

Each person reacts to stress differently. Therefore, the best coping strategy depends mostly on the individual. Which technique is used does not really matter as long as it works. An individual may want to experiment with all of them to find out which works best. A combination of two or more works best for many people.

All of the coping strategies discussed here help to block out stressors and promote mental and physical relaxation by diverting the attention to a different, nonthreatening action. Some of the techniques are easier to learn and may take less time per session. Regardless of which technique you select, the time spent doing stress management exercises (several times a day, as needed) is well worth the effort when stress becomes a significant problem in life.

People need to learn to relax and take time out for themselves. Stress is not what makes people ill but, rather, the way they react to the stress-causing agent. Individuals who learn to be diligent and start taking control of themselves find that they can enjoy a better, happier, and healthier life.

Notes

1. H. Selye, *Stress Without Distress* (New York: Signet, 1974).

2. R. J. Kriegel and M. H. Kriegel, *The C Zone: Peak Performance Under Stress* (Garden City, NY: Anchor Press/Doubleday, 1984).

3. E. B. Blanchard and L. H. Epstein, *A Biofeedback Primer* (Reading, MA: Addison-Wesley, 1978).

4. Selye.

Suggested Readings

Andrasik, F., D. Coleman, and L. H. Epstein. "Biofeedback: Clinical and Research Considerations." In *Behavioral Medicine: Assessment and Treatment Strategies*, edited by D. M. Doleys, R. L. Meredith, and A. R. Ciminero. New York: Plenum Press, 1982.

Blue Cross Association. *Stress.* Chicago: BCA, 1974.

Brown, B. *New Mind, New Body.* New York: Harper & Row, 1974.

Chesney, M. A., J. R. Eagleston, and R. H. Roseman. "Type A Assessment and Intervention." In *Medical Psychology: Contributions to Behavioral Medicine*, edited by C. K. Prokop and L. A. Bradley. New York: Academic Press, 1981.

Gauron, E. F. *Mental Training for Peak Performance.* Lansing, NY: Sport Science Associates, 1984.

Girdano, D., and G. Everly. *Controlling Stress and Tension: A Holistic Approach.* Englewood Cliffs, NJ: Prentice Hall, 1992.

Greenberg, J. S. *Comprehensive Stress Management.* Dubuque, IA: Wm. C. Brown Co., 1993.

Luthe, W. "Autogenic Training: Method, Research and Applications in Medicine." *American Journal of Psychotherapy,* 17 (1963), 174-195.

McKay, M., M. Davis, and P. Fanning. *Thoughts and Feelings: The Act of Cognitive Stress Intervention.* Richmond, CA: New Harbinger Publications, 1981.

Miller, L. H., and A. D. Smith. "Vulnerability Scale." *Stress Audit,* 1983.

Sarason, I. G., J. H. Johnson, and J. M. Siegel. "Assessing the Impact of Life Changes: Development of the Life Experiences Survey." *Journal of Consulting and Clinical Psychology,* 46 (1978), 932-946.

Schafer, W. *Stress Management for Wellness.* Fort Worth, TX: HBJ College Publishers, 1995.

Selye, H. *The Stress of Life.* New York: McGraw-Hill Book Co., 1978.

Smith, J. S. *Creative Stress Management: The 1-2-3 Cope System.* Englewood Cliffs, NJ: Prentice Hall, 1993.

Staff. "How Running Relieves Stress." *Runner* 8:11 (1986), 38-43, 82.

Turk, D. C., and R. D. Kerns. "Assessment in Health Psychology: A Cognitive-Behavioral Perspective." In *Measurement Strategies in Health Psychology*, edited by P. Karoly. New York: John Wiley & Sons, 1985.

Smoking Cessation

12

*P*eople throughout the world have used tobacco for hundreds of years. Before the 18th century they smoked tobacco primarily in the form of pipes or cigars. Cigarette smoking per se did not become popular until the mid-1800s, and its use started to increase dramatically at the turn of the century.

In 1900, 2.5 billion cigarettes were consumed in the United States, as compared to 640 billion in 1981. This figure dropped to 487 billion in 1995. Nonetheless, more than 48 million Americans over age 18 still smoked in 1994.

The harmful effects of cigarette smoking and tobacco use in general were not exactly known until the early 1960s, when researchers began to show a link between tobacco usage and disease. In 1964, the U. S. Surgeon General issued the first major report presenting scientific evidence that cigarettes were indeed a major health hazard in our society.

Objectives

- Understand the detrimental health effects of tobacco use in general.
- Recognize cigarette smoking as the largest preventable cause of premature illness and death in the United States.
- Learn the fundamental reasons for which people smoke.
- Understand the benefits and the significance of a smoking cessation program.
- Learn how to implement a smoking cessation program, either for yourself (if you smoke), or to help others go through the quitting process.

Tobacco use in all its forms now is considered a significant threat to life. Estimates indicate that 10% of the 5 billion people presently living on the earth will die as a result of smoking-related illnesses, killing approximately 3 million people each year.[1]

● Morbidity and Mortality

Illegal drug overdoses kill about 17,500 people per year in the United States. Drug felonies and drug-related murders kill another 1,600 people each year. This brings drug-related deaths to a grand total of 19,100. Citizens and the government have mounted a tremendous campaign to eradicate illegal drug use in America.

At the same time, cigarettes, a legal drug, kill about 26 times as many people as all illegal drugs combined. Cigarette smoking is the largest preventable cause of illness and premature death in the United States. When considering all related deaths, smoking is responsible for more than 400,000 unnecessary deaths each year — enough deaths to wipe out the entire population of Miami and Miami Beach in a single year.

Death rates from heart disease, cancer, stroke, aortic aneurysm, chronic bronchitis, emphysema, and peptic ulcers have increased. Figure 12.1 illustrates normal and diseased **alveoli** seen with emphysema. Cigarette smoking by pregnant women has been linked to retarded fetal growth, higher risk for spontaneous abortion, and prenatal death. Smoking also is the most prevalent cause of injury and death from

fire. The average life expectancy for a chronic smoker is as much as 18 years shorter than for a nonsmoker, and the death rate among chronic smokers during the most productive years of life, between ages 25 and 65, is twice that of the national average.

Based on a 1993 report by U.S. government physicians, each cigarette shortens life by 7 minutes. This figure represents 5 million years of potential life that Americans lose to smoking each year.

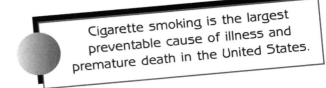

Cigarette smoking is the largest preventable cause of illness and premature death in the United States.

According to estimates by the American Heart Association, more than 30%, or 120,000 fatal heart attacks in the United States annually, result from smoking. The risk for heart attack is 50% to 100% higher for smokers than for nonsmokers. The mortality rate following heart attacks also is higher for smokers, as the attacks usually are more severe and the risk for deadly arrhythmias is much greater.

Cigarette smoking affects the cardiovascular system by increasing heart rate, blood pressure, and susceptibility to atherosclerosis, blood clots, coronary artery spasm, cardiac arrhythmia, and arteriosclerotic peripheral vascular disease. Evidence also indicates that smoking decreases high-density lipoprotein (HDL) cholesterol, the "good" cholesterol that lowers the risk for heart disease. Smoking further increases the amount of fatty acids, glucose, and various hormones in the blood. The carbon monoxide in smoke hinders the capacity of the blood to carry oxygen to body tissues. Finally, both carbon monoxide and nicotine may damage the inner walls of the arteries and thus encourage the buildup of fat on these walls.

Smoking also causes increased adhesiveness and clustering of platelets in the blood, decreases platelet survival and clotting time, and increases blood thickness. All of these effects can precipitate a heart attack.

The American Cancer Society reports that 83% of lung cancer and 30% of all cancers are attributable to smoking. Cancer kills about 142,000 people in the United States each year. Lung cancer is the leading killer by cancer, responsible for 30% of all cancer deaths. Cigarette smoking also leads to chronic obstructive pulmonary disease, the third leading cause of death in the United States (also see Chapter 1).

Mucus and pus secretion

Overinflated (obstructed) alveoli

Bronchus

Normal alveoli

Figure 12.1 ● *Normal and diseased alveoli in lungs.*

Reproduced by permission from "If You Smoke" slide show by Gordon Hewlett.

Normal lung (left) is contrasted with diseased lung (right). The white growth near the top of the diseased lung is cancer; the dark appearance on the bottom half is emphysema.

The largest carcinogenic exposure in the workplace is cigarette smoke. In a 1990 report, the Environmental Protection Agency (EPA) estimated that secondhand smoke is responsible for 3,000 or more lung cancer deaths in the United States each year.

Research presented at the 1990 World Conference on Lung Health also reveals that nonsmokers who live with smokers have a 20% to 30% greater risk of dying from heart disease than do other nonsmokers. Results of this research suggest further that the number of deaths from heart disease attributed to passive smoking is 10 times that of cancer.

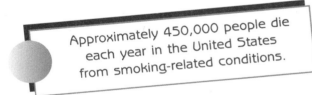

Approximately 450,000 people die each year in the United States from smoking-related conditions.

Although half of all cancers are now curable, the 5-year survival rate for lung cancer is less than 13%. Tobacco use also increases the risk for cancer of the oral cavity, larynx, esophagus, bladder, pancreas, and kidneys.

Even though many tobacco users are aware of the health consequences of cigarette smoking, they may fail to realize the risk of pipe smoking, cigar smoking, and tobacco chewing. As a group in general, the risk for heart disease and lung cancer is lower than for cigarette smokers. Nevertheless, blood nicotine levels in pipe and cigar smokers have been shown to approach those of cigarette smokers, as nicotine still is absorbed through the membranes of the mouth. Therefore, these tobacco users still have a higher risk for heart disease than nonsmokers do.

Cigarette smokers who substitute pipe or cigar smoking for cigarettes usually continue to inhale the smoke, which actually results in more **nicotine** and **tar** brought into the lungs. Consequently, the risk for disease is even higher if pipe or cigar smoke is inhaled. The risk and mortality rates for lip, mouth, and larynx cancer for pipe smoking, cigar smoking, and tobacco chewing are actually higher than for cigarette smoking.

● Economic Impact

The economic impact of cigarette smoking on the health-care system is staggering. In 1992, the Surgeon General calculated the lifetime excess medical care costs for smokers at $501 billion above that of nonsmokers. Other estimates indicate that the American people pay over $68 billion annually for tobacco-related health-care costs and lost productivity. Each pack of cigarettes sold represents about $2.59 in treatment of smoking-related illness and lost productivity.[2]

Heavy smokers use the health-care system, especially hospitals, twice as much as nonsmokers do. The yearly cost to a given company has been estimated to be between $624 and $4,611 per smoking employee. These costs include employee health care, absenteeism, additional health insurance, morbidity/disability and early mortality, on-the-job lost time, property damage/maintenance and depreciation, workers compensation, and the impact of secondhand smoke.

In the summer of 1985, more than 1,500 people worldwide died in major airplane accidents. These accidents generated a tremendous amount of media attention, and planes were grounded for safety reasons. Imagine what the coverage and concern would be if 400,000 people each year were to die in the

TERMS

Alveoli   Air sacs in the lungs where gas exchange (oxygen and carbon dioxide) takes place.

Nicotine   Poisonous compound found in tobacco leaves.

United States alone because of airplane accidents! People would not even consider flying any more. Most individuals would think of it as a form of suicide. Or think of the public outrage if close to 400,000 Americans were to die annually in a meaningless war, or if a single nonprescription drug would cause more than 138,000 cancer deaths and 120,000 fatal heart attacks. The American public would never tolerate these situations. We probably would mount an intense fight to prevent these deaths.

Yet, are we not committing a form of slow suicide by smoking cigarettes? Isn't tobacco a nonprescription drug available to almost anyone who wishes to smoke, killing more than 400,000 people each year? If cigarettes were invented today, the tobacco industry would be put on trial for mass murder.

● Trends

The fight against all forms of tobacco use has been gaining momentum in the last few years. This was not always the case. It has been difficult to fight an industry that has as great a financial and political influence as the tobacco industry has in the United States. Tobacco is the sixth largest cash crop in the United States, producing 2.5% of the gross national product. It has influenced elections cleverly by emphasizing the individual's right to smoke, avoiding the fact that so many people die because of its use.

In 1990, Philip Morris, one of the largest tobacco-producing companies in the world, ranked seventh among Fortune 500 companies. Nearly 70% of the profits came from the sale of cigarettes. In 1992, Philip Morris donated about $17 million to "bribing" leading organizations until they no longer question the detrimental effects of tobacco use. Among the organizations receiving donations from Philip Morris in 1992 were: United Way, YMCA, Salvation Army, Pediatric AIDS Foundation, Red Cross, Cystic Fibrosis Foundation, March of Dimes, Easter Seals, Muscular Dystrophy Association, Multiple Sclerosis Society, Hemophilia Foundation, United Cerebral Palsy, American Civil Liberties Union, American Bar Association, Task Force for Battered Women, Boy Scouts, Boys and Girls Club, and Big Brothers and Big Sisters.

> We call Colombian drug runners uncivilized scums (for about 19,100 illegal drug-related deaths per year), but we welcome Philip Morris with glee and we call it civic pride.[3]

Tobacco was socially accepted for many years. In the 1980s, however, cigarette smoking no longer was acceptable in many social circles. Nonsmokers and ex-smokers alike are fighting for their right to clean air and health. If every smoker were to give up cigarettes, in one year alone sick time would drop by approximately 90 million days, heart conditions would decrease by 280,000, chronic bronchitis and emphysema would number 1 million fewer cases, and total death rates from cardiovascular disease, cancer, and peptic ulcers would fall off drastically.[4]

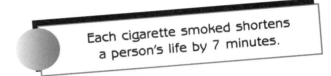

Each cigarette smoked shortens a person's life by 7 minutes.

Many smokers are unaware of or simply do not care to realize how much cigarette smoke bothers nonsmokers. Smokers sometimes think that blowing the smoke off to the side is enough to get it out of the way. As a matter of fact, it is not enough. Smokers do not comprehend this until they quit and later find themselves in that situation. At times, ex-smokers are bothered even by someone smoking several yards away and all of a sudden come to realize why cigarette smoke is so unpleasant and undesirable to most people.

In recent years, the Food and Drug Administration (FDA) Drug Abuse Advisory Committee has taken a strong stance against the use of all forms of tobacco products in the United States. The American Heart Association (AHA) commends the work initiated by the FDA, but the AHA has further stated that the FDA and the federal government have an obligation to take regulatory action against the national problem of nicotine addiction and abuse from cigarettes and tobacco products in general. In a 1992 statement before the FDA Drug Abuse Advisory Committee, the AHA indicated:

> It is a national health travesty that a product (tobacco) which accounts for over 430,000 deaths in the U.S. each year has escaped regulation under every major health and safety law enacted by congress to protect the public health.[4]

● Smokeless Tobacco

Smokeless tobacco often is promoted as a safe alternative to cigarette smoking. According to the

Advisory Committee to the U.S. Surgeon General, smokeless tobacco represents a significant health risk and is just as addictive as cigarette smoking.

Unlike smoking, the use of smokeless tobacco has increased during the last 15 years. Currently, some 15 million Americans use tobacco in this form. The greatest concern is the increase in use of "spit" tobacco, especially by young people.

More than 2 million people under age 25 use spit tobacco, including nearly 20% of all males in grades 9 through 12. One-third of those who use spit tobacco started at age 5, and the average starting age was 9. Spit tobacco contains 2.5 times as much nicotine as a similarly priced pack of cigarettes.

Using smokeless tobacco can lead to gingivitis and periodontitis. It carries a fourfold increase in oral cancer, and in some cases even premature death. People who chew or dip also have a higher rate of cavities, sore gums, bad breath, and stained teeth. They can't smell or taste as well. Consequently, they tend to add more sugar and salt to food. These practices alone increase the risk for being overweight and having high blood pressure.

Nicotine addiction and its related health risks hold true for smokeless tobacco users. Nicotine blood levels approach those of cigarette smokers, increasing the risk for diseases of the cardiovascular system. Further, research has revealed changes in heart rate and blood pressure similar to those of cigarette smokers.

Using tobacco in any form can be addictive and poses a serious threat to health and well-being. Completely eliminating its use in any form is the single most important lifestyle change a tobacco user can make to improve health, quality of life, and longevity.

● Why Do People Smoke?

People typically begin to smoke without realizing its detrimental effects on their health and life in general. Although people start to smoke for many different reasons, the three fundamental instigators are peer pressure, the desire to appear "grown up," and rebellion against authority. Unfortunately, smoking only three packs of cigarettes can lead to physiological addiction, turning smoking into a nasty habit that has become the most widespread example of drug dependency in the United States.

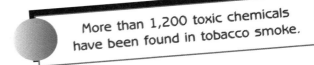

More than 1,200 toxic chemicals have been found in tobacco smoke.

When tobacco leaves are burned, hot air and gases containing tar (chemical compounds) and nicotine are released in the smoke. More than 1,200 toxic chemicals have been found in tobacco smoke. **Tar** contains about 30 chemical compounds that are proven **carcinogens**.

The drug nicotine has strong addictive properties. Within seconds of inhalation, nicotine affects the central nervous system and can act simultaneously as a tranquilizer and a stimulant. The stimulating effect produces strong physiological and psychological dependency. The physical addiction to nicotine is six to eight times more powerful than the addiction to alcohol, and most likely greater than for some of the hard drugs currently used.

The psychological dependency develops over a longer time. People smoke to help themselves relax, and they also gain a certain amount of pleasure from the ritual of smoking. Smokers automatically associate many activities of daily life with cigarettes. Typical associated activities are: coffee drinking, alcohol drinking, social gatherings, after a meal, talking on

Smokeless tobacco can lead to gum and teeth damage as well as oral cancer (pictured).

TERMS

Tar Chemical compound that forms during the burning of tobacco leaves.

Carcinogens Substances that contribute to the formation of cancers.

the telephone, driving, reading, watching television. In many cases the social rituals of smoking are the most difficult to eliminate. The dependency is so strong that even years after people have stopped smoking, they still may crave cigarettes when they engage in some social activities.

"Why-Do-You Smoke?" Test

Most people smoke for a variety of reasons. To find out why people smoke, the National Clearinghouse for Smoking and Health developed a simple "Why-Do-You-Smoke Test."

This test contained in Figure 12.2 lists some statements by people describing what they get out of smoking cigarettes. Smokers are to indicate how often they have the feelings described in each statement when smoking.*

The scores obtained on this test give an indication for each of six factors that describe people's feelings when they smoke. The first three highlight the positive feelings people derive from smoking. The fourth factor relates to reducing tension and relaxing. The fifth reveals the extent of dependence on cigarettes. The sixth factor differentiates habit smoking and purely automatic smoking. Each of the remaining factors fits one of the six reasons for smoking discussed next. A score of 11 or above on any factor indicates that smoking is an important source of satisfaction for you. The higher you score (15 is the highest), the more important a given factor is in your smoking, and the more useful the discussion of that factor can be in your attempt to quit.

If you do not score high on any of the six factors, chances are that you do not smoke much or have not been smoking for very many years. If so, giving up smoking, and staying off, should be fairly easy.

1. **Stimulation.** If you score high or fairly high on this factor, you are one of those smokers who is stimulated by the cigarette; you think it helps wake you up, organize your energies, and keep you going. If you try to give up smoking, you may want a safe substitute — a brisk walk or moderate exercise, for example — whenever you feel the urge to smoke.

2. **Handling.** Handling things can be satisfying, but you can keep your hands busy in many ways without lighting up or playing with a cigarette. Why not toy with a pen or pencil? Try doodling. Play with a coin, a piece of jewelry, or some other harmless object.

3. **Accentuation of pleasure/pleasurable relaxation.** Finding out whether you use the cigarette to feel good — get real, honest pleasure from smoking (Factor 3) — or to keep from feeling bad (Factor 4) is not always easy. About two-thirds of smokers score high or fairly high on accentuation of pleasure, and about half of those also score as high or higher on reduction of negative feelings. Those who do get real pleasure from smoking often find that honest consideration of the harmful effects of their habit is enough to help them quit. They substitute social and physical activities and find they do not seriously miss their cigarettes.

4. **Reduction of negative feelings, or "crutch."** Many smokers use cigarettes as a kind of crutch during moments of stress or discomfort. Ironically, the heavy smoker — the person who tries to handle severe personal problems by smoking many times a day — is apt to discover that cigarettes do not help in dealing with problems effectively. This kind of smoker may stop smoking readily when everything is going well but may be tempted to start again in a time of crisis. Again, physical exertion or social activity may be a useful substitute for cigarettes, even in times of tension.

5. **Craving or dependence.** Quitting smoking is difficult for people who score high on this factor. The craving for a cigarette begins to build up the moment the cigarette is put out, so tapering off is not likely to work. This smoker must go **cold turkey.** If you are dependent on cigarettes, you may try smoking more than usual for a day or two to spoil the taste for cigarettes, then isolating yourself completely from cigarettes until the craving is gone.

6. **Habit.** If you are smoking from habit, you no longer get much satisfaction from the cigarettes.

---

* This test, as well as much of the remaining information in this chapter, is written directly to smokers, though nonsmokers will gain an understanding of smokers by reading it.

 TERMS

Cold turkey Elimination of a negative behavior all at once.

WHY-DO-YOU-SMOKE?

		Always	Fre-quently	Occa-sionally	Seldom	Never
A.	I smoke cigarettes to keep myself from slowing down.	5	4	3	2	1
B	Handling a cigarette is part of the enjoyment of smoking it.	5	4	3	2	1
C.	Smoking cigarettes is pleasant and relaxing.	5	4	3	2	1
D.	I light up a cigarette when I feel angry about something.	5	4	3	2	1
E.	When I have run out of cigarettes, I find it almost unbearable until I can get them.	5	4	3	2	1
F.	I smoke cigarettes automatically without even being aware of it.	5	4	3	2	1
G.	I smoke cigarettes to stimulate me, to perk myself up.	5	4	3	2	1
H.	Part of the enjoyment of smoking a cigarette comes from the steps I take to light up.	5	4	3	2	1
I.	I find cigarettes pleasurable.	5	4	3	2	1
J.	When I feel uncomfortable or upset about something, I light up a cigarette.	5	4	3	2	1
K.	I am very much aware of the fact when I am not smoking a cigarette.	5	4	3	2	1
L	I light up a cigarette without realizing I still have one burning in the ashtray.	5	4	3	2	1
M.	I smoke cigarettes to give me a "lift."	5	4	3	2	1
N.	When I smoke a cigarette, part of the enjoyment is watching the smoke as I exhale it.	5	4	3	2	1
O.	I want a cigarette most when I am comfortable and relaxed.	5	4	3	2	1
P.	When I feel "blue" or want to take my mind off cares and worries, I smoke cigarettes.	5	4	3	2	1
Q.	I get a real gnawing hunger for a cigarette when I haven't smoked for a while.	5	4	3	2	1
R.	I've found a cigarette in my mouth and didn't remember putting it there.	5	4	3	2	1

Scoring Your Test:

Enter the numbers you have circled on the test questions in the spaces provided below, putting the number you circled for question A on line A, for question B on line B, etc. Add the three scores on each line to get a total for each factor. For example, the sum of your scores for lines A, G, and M gives you your score on "Stimulation," lines B, H, and N give the score on "Handling," etc. Scores can vary from 3 to 15. Any score 11 and above is high; any score 7 and below is low.

```
A _____  + G _____  + M _____  = _____   Stimulation
B _____  + H _____  + N _____  = _____   Handling
C _____  + I _____  + O _____  = _____   Pleasure/Relaxation
D _____  + J _____  + P _____  = _____   Crutch: Tension Reduction
E _____  + K _____  + Q _____  = _____   Craving: Psychological Addiction
F _____  + L _____  + R _____  = _____   Habit
```

From *A Self-Test for Smokers.* Washington, DC: (U.S. Department of Health and Human Services, 1983).

Figure 12.2 ● *Test: "Why do you smoke?"*

You light them frequently without even realizing you are doing it. You may have an easy time quitting and staying off if you can break the habitual patterns you have built up. Cutting down gradually may be effective if you change the way you smoke cigarettes and the conditions under which you smoke them. The key to success is to become aware of each cigarette you smoke. You can do this by asking yourself, "Do I really want this cigarette?" You may be surprised at how many you do not want.

● Smoking Cessation

Quitting cigarette smoking is not easy. Only about 20% of smokers who try to quit the first time each year succeed. The addictive properties of nicotine and smoke make quitting difficult.

The American Psychiatric Association and the National Institute on Drug Abuse have indicated that nicotine is perhaps the most addictive drug known to humans. The 1988 Surgeon General's Report on Nicotine Addiction concluded that:[5]

- Cigarettes and other forms of tobacco are addicting.
- Nicotine is the drug responsible for the addictive behavior.
- Pharmacologic and behavioral traits that determine addiction to tobacco are similar to those that determine addiction to drugs such as heroin and cocaine.

Smokers develop a tolerance to nicotine and smoke. They become dependent on both and get physical and psychological withdrawal symptoms when they stop smoking. Even though giving up smoking can be extremely difficult, it by no means is impossible, as attested by those who have quit.

During the last three decades, cigarette smoking in the United States has been declining gradually among smokers of all ages with the exception of young women. Surveys have shown that between 75% and 90% of all smokers would like to quit. Forty percent of the adult population — 53% of men and 32% of women — smoked in 1964 when the U.S. Surgeon General first reported the link between smoking and increased risk for disease and mortality. By 1994, only 25.5%, or 48 million adults, smoked. Among men, 25.3 million (28.2%) were smokers, and 22.7 million (23.1%) women

smoked. More than 38 million Americans have given up cigarettes. Over 40% of all adults who have ever smoked have quit since 1964.

More than 95% of successful ex-smokers have been able to do it on their own, either by quitting

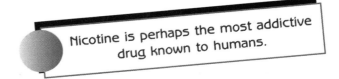
Nicotine is perhaps the most addictive drug known to humans.

cold turkey or by using self-help kits available from organizations such as the American Cancer Society, the American Heart Association, and the American Lung Association. Only 3% of ex-smokers have done so as a result of formal cessation programs. Smokers' information and treatment centers commonly are listed in the yellow pages of the telephone book.

"Do You Want To Quit?" Test

The most important factor in quitting cigarette smoking is the person's sincere desire to do so. Although some smokers can simply quit, this is not the case in most instances. Those who can quit easily are primarily light or casual smokers. They realize that the pleasure of an occasional cigarette is not worth the added risk for disease and premature death. For heavy smokers, quitting most likely will be a difficult battle. Even though many do not succeed the first time around, the odds of quitting are much better for those who try to stop repeatedly.

To find out a smoker's preparedness to quit, the "Do You Want To Quit?" test contained in Figure 12.3, developed by the National Clearinghouse for Smoking and Health, will measure the smoker's attitude toward the four primary reasons he or she wants to quit smoking. The results give an indication of whether you are ready to start the program. On this test, the higher you score in any category, say "Health," the more important that reason is to you. A score of 9 or above in one of these categories indicates that this is one of the most important reasons you may want to quit.

1. **Health.** Knowing the harmful consequences of cigarettes, many people have stopped smoking and many others are considering doing so. If your score on the health factor is 9 or above, the health hazards of smoking may be enough to make you want to quit now. If your score on this

DO YOU WANT TO QUIT?

	Strongly Agree	Mildly Agree	Mildly Disagree	Strongly Disagree
A. Cigarette smoking might give me a serious illness.	4	3	2	1
B. My cigarette smoking sets a bad example for others.	4	3	2	1
C. I find cigarette smoking to be a messy kind of habit.	4	3	2	1
D. Controlling my cigarette smoking is a challenge to me.	4	3	2	1
E. Smoking causes shortness of breath.	4	3	2	1
F. If I quit smoking cigarettes, it might influence others to stop.	4	3	2	1
G. Cigarettes damage clothing and other personal property.	4	3	2	1
H. Quitting smoking would show that I have willpower.	4	3	2	1
I. My cigarette smoking will have a harmful effect on my health.	4	3	2	1
J. My cigarette smoking influences others close to me to take up or continue smoking.	4	3	2	1
K. If I quit smoking, my sense of taste or smell would improve.	4	3	2	1
L. I do not like the idea of feeling dependent on smoking.	4	3	2	1

Scoring Your Test:

Write the number you have circled after each statement on the test in the corresponding space to the right. Add the scores on each line to get your totals. For example, the sum of your scores A, E, I gives you your score for the Health factor. Scores can vary from 3 to 12. Any score of 9 or over is high, and a score of 6 or under is low.

A _____ + G _____ + M _____ = _____ Health

B _____ + H _____ + N _____ = _____ Example

C _____ + I _____ + O _____ = _____ Aesthetics

D _____ + J _____ + P _____ = _____ Mastery

From *A Self-Test for Smokers* by National Clearinghouse for Smoking and Health, Washington, DC: (U.S. Department of Health and Human Services, 1983).

Figure 12.3 • *Test: "Do you want to quit?"*

factor is low (6 or below), consider the hazards of smoking. You may be lacking important information or may even have incorrect information. If so, health considerations are not playing the role they should be in your decision to keep smoking or to quit.

2. **Example.** Some people stop smoking because they want to set a good example for others. Parents quit to make it easier for their children to resist starting to smoke. Doctors quit to be role models for their patients. Teachers quit to discourage their students from smoking. Sports stars want to set an example for their young fans. Husbands quit to influence their wives to quit, and vice versa. Examples have a significant influence on our behavior. Research shows that almost twice as many high school students smoke if both parents are smokers, compared to those whose parents are nonsmokers or former smokers.

   If your score is low (6 or lower), you might not be interested in giving up smoking to set an example for others. Perhaps you do not realize how important your example could be.

3. **Aesthetics.** People who score high (9 or above) in this category recognize and are disturbed by some of the unpleasant aspects of smoking. The smell of stale smoke on their clothing, bad breath, and stains on their fingers and teeth might be reason enough to consider quitting.

4. **Mastery.** If you score 9 or above on this factor, you are bothered by knowing that you cannot control your desire to smoke. You are not your own master. Awareness of this challenge to your self-control may make you want to quit.

Breaking the Habit

The following seven-step plan has been developed as a guide to help you quit smoking. The total program should be completed in 4 weeks or less. Steps one through four combined should take no longer than 2 weeks. A maximum of two additional weeks is allowed for the rest of the program.

Step One

Decide positively that you want to quit. Avoid negative thoughts of how difficult this can be. Think positive. You can do it.

Now prepare a list of the reasons you smoke and why you want to quit (see Figure 12.4). Make several copies of the list and keep them in places where you commonly smoke. Review the reasons for quitting frequently, as this will motivate and prepare you psychologically for cessation.

When the reasons for quitting outweigh the reasons for smoking, you will have an easier time quitting. Try to read as much information as possible on the detrimental effects of tobacco and the benefits of quitting.

Step Two

Initiate a personal diet and exercise program. About one-third of the people who quit smoking gain weight. This could be caused by one or a combination of several reasons: (a) Food becomes a substitute for cigarettes; (b) appetite increases; and (c) basal metabolism may slow down.

Giving up one pack of cigarettes a day is the equivalent of losing between 50 and 75 pounds of excess body fat!

If you start an exercise and weight-control program prior to quitting smoking, weight gain should not be a problem. If anything, exercise and lower body weight create more awareness of healthy living and strengthen the motivation for giving up cigarettes.

Even if you gain some weight, the harmful effects of cigarette smoking are much more detrimental to human health than a few extra pounds of body weight. Experts have indicated that, as far as the extra load on the heart is concerned, giving up one pack of cigarettes a day is the equivalent of losing between 50 and 75 pounds of excess body fat!

Step Three

Decide on the approach you will use to stop smoking. You may quit cold turkey or gradually cut down the number of cigarettes you smoke daily. Base your decision on your scores obtained on the "Why Do You Smoke?" test. If you scored 11 points or higher in either the "Crutch: Tension Reduction" or the "Craving: Psychological Addiction" categories, your best chance for success is quitting cold turkey. For any of the other four categories, you may choose either approach.

REASONS FOR SMOKING VERSUS QUITTING

Name: _____ Date:_____

Reasons for Smoking Cigarettes

1. _____

2. _____

3. _____

4. _____

5. _____

6. _____

7. _____

8. _____

9. _____

10. _____

Reasons for Quitting Cigarette Smoking

1. _____

2. _____

3. _____

4. _____

5. _____

6. _____

7. _____

8. _____

9. _____

10. _____

Figure 12.4 ● *Form: Reasons for smoking versus quitting.*

People still argue about which approach is more effective. Quitting cold turkey may cause fewer withdrawal symptoms than tapering off gradually. When cutting down, the fewer the cigarettes you smoke, the more important each one becomes. Therefore, you have a greater chance for relapse and returning to the original number of cigarettes smoked. When the cutting-down approach is accompanied by a definite target date for quitting, the technique has been shown to be quite effective. Smokers who taper off without a target date for quitting are the most likely to relapse.

Step Four

Keep a daily log of your smoking habit for a few days. This will help you understand the situations in which you smoke. To assist you in doing this, make copies of Figure 12.5 or develop your own form. Keep this form with you, and every time you smoke, record the required information. Keep track of the number of cigarettes you smoke, times of day you smoke them, events associated with smoking, amount of each cigarette smoked, and a rating of how badly you needed that cigarette. Rate each cigarette from 1 to 3. A 1 means desperately needed, a 2 means moderately needed, and a 3 means no real need. This daily log will assist you in three ways:

1. You will get to know your habit.
2. It will help you eliminate cigarettes you really do not need.
3. It will aid you in finding positive substitutes for situations that trigger your desire to smoke.

Step Five

Set the target date for quitting. If you are going to taper off gradually, read the instructions under the "Cutting Down Gradually" discussion before you proceed to step six. In setting the target date, a special date may add a little extra incentive. An upcoming birthday, anniversary, vacation, graduation, family reunion — all are examples of good dates to free yourself from smoking. Dates when you are going to be away from events that trigger your desire to smoke may be especially helpful. Once you have set the date, do not change it. Do not let anyone or anything interfere with this date.

Let your friends and relatives know of your intentions, and ask for their support. Consider asking someone else to quit with you. This way, you can support each other in your efforts to stop. Avoid anyone who will not support you in your effort to quit. Unfortunately, other people can be a prime obstacle when you are attempting to quit. Many smokers are intolerable when they first stop smoking, so some friends and relatives prefer that the person continue to smoke.

Step Six

Stock up on low-calorie foods — carrots, broccoli, cauliflower, celery, popcorn (butter- and salt-free), fruits, sunflower seeds (in the shell), sugarless gum — and drink plenty of water. Keep the food handy on the day you stop and the first few days following cessation. Substitute this food for a cigarette when you want one.

Step Seven

On your quit day and the first few days thereafter, do not keep cigarettes handy. Stay away from friends and events that trigger your desire to smoke, and drink large amounts of water and fruit juices. To replace the old behavior with new behavior, replace smoking time with new, positive substitutes that will make smoking difficult or impossible.

When you want a cigarette, take a few deep breaths and then occupy yourself by doing any of a number of things such as talking to someone else, washing your hands, brushing your teeth, eating a healthy snack, chewing on a straw, doing dishes, playing sports, going for a walk or a bike ride, going swimming, and so on. Engage in activities that require the use of your hands. Try gardening, sewing, writing letters, drawing, doing household chores, or washing the car. Visit nonsmoking places such as libraries, museums, stores, and theaters. Plan an outing or a trip away from home. Any of these activities can keep your mind away from cigarettes. Record your choice of activity or substitute under the Remarks/Substitutes column in Figure 12.5.

Quitting Cold Turkey

Many people have found that quitting all at once is the easiest way to do it. Most smokers have tried this approach at least once. Even though it may not work the first time, they do not allow themselves to get discouraged, and they succeed eventually. Many times after several attempts, all of a sudden they are able to overcome smoking without too much difficulty.

On the average, as few as three smokeless days are sufficient to break the physiological addiction to nicotine. The psychological addiction may linger for years but will get weaker as time goes by.

Cutting Down Gradually

Tapering off cigarettes can be done in several ways.

1. Eliminate cigarettes you do not necessarily need (those ranked numbers 3 and 2 on your daily log).
2. Switch to a brand lower in nicotine/tar every couple of days.
3. Smoke less of each cigarette.
4. Smoke fewer cigarettes each day.

Most people prefer a combination of these four suggestions.

Before you start cutting down, set a target date for quitting. Once the date is set, don't change it. The total time until your quit date should be no longer than 2 weeks. Reduce the total number of cigarettes smoked each day by 10% to 25%. As you smoke less, be careful not to take more puffs or inhale more deeply as you smoke, as this would offset the principle of cutting down.

As an aid in tapering off, make several copies of Figure 12.5. (By now you already should have completed the initial daily log of your smoking habit — see Step Four under Breaking the Habit.) Start a new daily log, and every night review your data and set goals for the following day.

Decide which cigarettes will be easiest to give up, what brand you will smoke, the total number of cigarettes to be smoked, and how much of each you will smoke. Write down any comments or situations you may want to avoid, as well as any substitutes you could use to help you in the program. For example, if you always smoke with coffee, substitute juice for coffee. If you smoke while driving, arrange for a ride or take a bus to work. If you smoke with a certain friend at lunch, avoid having lunch with that friend for a week or so. Continue using this log until you have stopped smoking completely.

● Nicotine Substitution Products

Nicotine substitution drug products such as nicotine transdermal patches and nicotine gum have been developed to help people kick the tobacco habit. These products are most effective when used in a physician-supervised cessation program. As with tapering, the amount of nicotine used in these products is decreased gradually until the person no longer craves the drug.

In particular, nicotine patches are used to supply a steady dose of nicotine through the skin. These patches are available in various dosage amounts, delivering anywhere from about 5 to 21 mg of nicotine in a 24-hour period. A typical program lasts between 3 and 10 weeks with an average weekly cost to the consumer of about $35.00. Sales of nicotine patches approximate $1 billion per year.

About three smokeless days are sufficient to break the physiological addiction to nicotine.

Public safety concerns regarding the use of nicotine patches, including indications, precautions, warnings, contraindications, potential abuse, and marketing and labeling issues are monitored and regulated by the FDA. People contemplating their use should pay careful attention to contraindications and potential side effects. Pregnant and lactating women, people with heart disease, high blood pressure, or a recent heart attack should check with their physician prior to using nicotine substitution products. Skin redness, swelling, or rashes sometimes are associated with the use of nicotine patches. Other undesirable side effects are listed on the label and should be monitored closely.

● Life After Cigarettes

When you first quit smoking, you can expect a series of withdrawal symptoms. Among the typical physiological and psychological reactions during the first few days are lower heart rate and blood pressure, headaches, gastrointestinal discomfort, mood changes, irritability, aggressiveness, and difficulty sleeping.

The physiological addiction to nicotine is broken only 3 days following your last cigarette. Therefore, you should not crave cigarettes as much. For the habitual smoker, the psychological dependency could be the most difficult to break. The first few days may not be as difficult as the first few months. Any of the activities in daily life that have been associated with smoking — either stress or relaxation, joy or unhappiness — may trigger a relapse even months, or at times years, after quitting.

DAILY CIGARETTE SMOKING LOG

Today's Date: _____   Quit Date:_____   Decision Date: _____

Cigarettes to be Smoked Today:_____   Brand: _____

No.	Time	Activity	Amount Smoked[a]	Rating[b]	Remarks/Substitutes
1.					
2.					
3.					
4.					
5.					
6.					
7.					
8.					
9.					
10.					
11.					
12.					
13.					
14.					
15.					
16.					
17.					
18.					
19.					
20.					

Additional comments, list of friends, and/or activities to avoid

_____

_____

_____

_____

_____

_____

[a] Amount smoked: entire cigarette, two-thirds, half, etc.
[b] Rating: 1 = desperately needed, 2 = moderately needed, 3 - no real need

Figure 12.5 ●

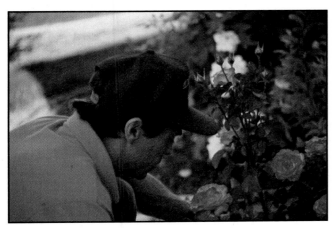

Simple pleasures of life, such as smell and taste, improve with smoking cessation.

Ex-smokers should realize that even though some harm may have been done already, it is never too late to quit. The greatest early benefit is a lower risk for sudden death. Furthermore, the risk for illness starts to decrease the moment you stop smoking. You will have fewer sore throats and sores in the mouth, less hoarseness, no more cigarette cough, and lower risk for peptic ulcers.

Circulation to the hands and feet will improve, as will gastrointestinal and kidney and bladder functions. Everything will taste and smell better. You will have more energy, and you will gain a sense of freedom, pride, and well-being. You no longer will have to worry whether you have enough cigarettes to last through a day, a party, a meeting, a weekend, a trip.

When you first quit and you think how tough it is and how miserable you feel because you cannot have a cigarette, try the opposite: Think of the benefits and how great it is not to smoke! The ex-smoker's risk for heart disease approaches that of a lifetime nonsmoker 10 years following cessation, and cancer 15 years after cessation.

If you have been successful and stopped smoking, a lot of events can still trigger your urge to smoke. When confronted with these events, people rationalize and think, "One cigarette won't hurt. I've been off for months (years in some cases)" or, "I can handle it. I'll smoke just today." It won't work! Before you know it, you will be back to the regular nasty habit. Be prepared to take action in those situations. Find substitutes. In addition to the many things that have been discussed in this chapter, the tips given in Figure 12.6 should help you in retraining yourself to live without cigarettes.

Start thinking of yourself as a nonsmoker — no "buts" about it. Remind yourself of how difficult it has been and how long it has taken you to get to this point. If you have come this far, you certainly can resist brief moments of temptation. It will get easier rather than harder as time goes on.

Notes

1. American Cancer Society, *World Smoking & Health* (Atlanta: ACS, 1993).
2. "Got a Watch?" *University of California at Berkeley Wellness Letter* (February, 1996).
3. American Cancer Society.
4. American Heart Association, *AHA Public Affairs/Coalition on Smoking OR Health Position* (Dallas: AHA, 1996).
5. U.S. Department of Health and Human Services, "Nicotine Addiction, A Report of the Surgeon General" (Atlanta: U.S. Department of Health and Human Services, Centers for Disease Control and Prevention, National Center for Chronic Disease Prevention and Health Promotion, 1988).

Suggested Readings

American Cancer Society. *Quitter's Guide: Seven-Day Plan to Help You Stop Smoking Cigarettes.* New York: ACS, 1978.

American Cancer Society. *Fifty Most Often Asked Questions About Smoking and Health and the Answers.* New York: ACS, 1982.

American Cancer Society. *Cancer Facts & Figures – 1997.* New York: ACS, 1997.

American Heart Association. *Smoking and Heart Disease.* Dallas: AHA, 1981.

American Heart Association. *The Good Life: A Guide to Becoming a Nonsmoker.* Dallas: AHA, 1984.

American Heart Association. *Heart at Work: Smoking Reduction Program — Coordinator's Guide.* Dallas: AHA, 1984.

American Heart Association. *How to Quit.* Dallas: AHA, 1984.

Carroll, C. R. *Drugs in Modern Society.* Dubuque, IA: Wm. C. Brown, 1995.

Channing L. Bete Co. *Smoking and Your Heart.* South Deerfield, MA: Author, 1982.

Girdano, D. A., D. Dusek, and G. S. Everly. *Experiencing Health.* Englewood Cliffs, NJ: Prentice Hall, 1985.

Halper, M. S. *How to Stop Smoking: A Preventive Medicine Institute/Strang Clinic Health Action Plan.* New York: Holt, Rinehart and Winston, 1980.

Hodgson, R. J., and P. Miller. *Self-Watching: Addictions, Habits, Compulsions — What to Do.* New York: Facts on File, 1982.

National Cancer Institute. *Clearing the Air: A Guide to Quitting Smoking.* Bethesda, MD: NCI, 1979.

Public Health Service. *Smoking Tobacco and Health: A Fact Book.* Rockville, MD: U.S. Department of Health and Human Services, 1981.

Public Health Service. *Why People Smoke Cigarettes.* Rockville, MD: U.S. Department of Health and Human Services, 1982.

Public Health Service. *A Self-Test for Smokers.* Rockville, MD: U.S. Department of Health and Human Services, 1983.

Public Health Service. *Chronic Obstructive Lung Disease: A Report of the Surgeon General.* Rockville, MD: U.S. Department of Health and Human Services, 1984.

U.S. Office on Smoking and Health. *Smoking and Health: A Report of the Surgeon General.* Washington, DC: U.S. Department of Health, Education and Welfare, 1979.

TIPS TO HELP STOP SMOKING

The following are different ways smokers retrained themselves to live without cigarettes. Any one or several of these methods in combination might be helpful to you. Check the ones you like and from these develop your own retraining program.

☐ Before you quit smoking, try wrapping your cigarettes with a sheet of paper like a Christmas present. Every time you want a cigarette, unwrap the pack and write down what you are doing, how you feel, and how important this cigarette is to you. Do this for 2 weeks and you'll have cut down as well as developed new insights into your smoking.

☐ If cigarettes give you an energy boost, try gum, modest exercise, a brisk walk, or a new hobby. Avoid eating new foods that are high in calories.

☐ If cigarettes help you relax, try eating, drinking new beverages, or social activities within reasonable bounds.

☐ Try smoking an excess of cigarettes for a day or two before you quit so the taste of cigarettes is spoiled. Another opportune time to quit is when you are ill with a cold or flu and have lost your taste for cigarettes.

☐ On a 3" X 5" card, list what you like and dislike about smoking. Add to it and read it daily.

☐ Make up a short list of luxuries you have wanted or items you would like to purchase for a loved one. Next to each item, write down the cost. Now convert the cost to "packs of cigarettes." If you save the money each day from packs of cigarettes, you will be able to purchase these items. Use a special "piggy bank" for saving your money, or start a "Christmas Club" account at your bank.

☐ Don't smoke after you get a craving for a cigarette until 3 minutes have passed since you got the urge. During those 3 minutes, change your thinking or activity.

☐ Telephone an ex-smoker or somebody you can talk to until the craving subsides.

☐ Plan a memorable day for stopping. You might choose your vacation, New Year's Day, your birthday, a holiday, the birthday of your child, your anniversary. But don't make the date so distant that you lose momentum.

☐ If you smoke under stress at work, pick a date for stopping when you will be away from your work.

☐ Decide whether you are going to stop suddenly or gradually. If it is to be gradual, work out a tapering system so you have intermediate goals.

☐ Don't store cigarettes. Never buy a carton. Wait until one pack is finished before you buy another.

☐ Never carry cigarettes with you at home or at work. Keep your cigarettes as far from you as possible. Leave them with someone or lock them up.

☐ Until you quit, make yourself a "smoking corner" that is far from anything interesting. If you like to smoke with others, always smoke alone. If you like to smoke alone, always smoke with others, preferably if they are nonsmokers. Never smoke while watching television.

☐ Never carry matches or a lighter with you.

☐ Put away your ashtrays or fill them with objects so they cannot be used for ashes. Plant flowers in them or fill them with walnuts. The latter will give you something to do with your hands.

☐ Change your brand of cigarettes weekly so you always are smoking a brand of lower tar and nicotine content than the week before.

☐ Never say, "I quit smoking," because your resolution is broken if you have a cigarette. Better to say, "I don't want to smoke." This way you maintain your resolution even if you accidentally have a cigarette.

☐ Try to help someone else quit smoking, particularly your mate.

☐ Always ask yourself, "Do I need this cigarette or is this just a reflex?"

☐ Each day try to put off lighting your first cigarette.

☐ Decide arbitrarily that you will smoke only on even- or odd-numbered hours of the clock.

☐ Try going to bed early and rising a half hour earlier than usual to avoid hurrying through breakfast and rushing to work.

☐ Keep your hands occupied. Try playing a musical instrument, knitting, or fiddling with hand puzzles.

☐ Take a shower. You cannot smoke in the shower.

☐ Brush your teeth frequently to get rid of the tobacco taste and stains.

☐ If you have a sudden craving for a cigarette, take 10 deep breaths, holding the last breath while you strike a match. Exhale slowly, blowing out the match. Pretend the match was a cigarette by crushing it out in an ashtray. Now immediately get busy on some work or activity.

Figure 12.6 •

TIPS TO HELP STOP SMOKING

☐ Smoke only half a cigarette.

☐ After you quit, start using your lungs. Increase your activities and indulge in moderate exercise, such as short walks before or after a meal.

☐ Bet with someone that you can quit. Put the cigarette money in a jar each morning and forfeit it if you smoke. Keep the money if you don't smoke by the end of the week. Try to extend this period for a month.

☐ If you gain weight because you are not smoking, wait until you get over the craving before you diet. Dieting is easier then.

☐ If you are depressed or have physical symptoms that might be related to your smoking, relieve your mind by discussing this with your physician. It is easier to quit when you know your health status.

☐ After you quit, visit your dentist and have your teeth cleaned to get rid of the tobacco stains.

☐ If the cost of cigarettes is your motivation for quitting, purchase a money order equivalent to a year's supply of cigarettes. Give it to a friend. If you smoke in the next year, he or she cashes the money order and keeps the money. If you don't smoke, he or she gives back the money order at the end of the year.

☐ After you quit, redirect the temptation to smoke by calling or visiting someone.

☐ When you feel irritable or tense, shut your eyes and count backward from 10 to zero as you imagine yourself descending a flight of stairs, or imagine that you are looking at the horizon as the sun sets in the west.

☐ Get out of your old habits. Seek new activities or perform old activities in a new way. Don't rely on the old ways of solving problems. Do things differently.

☐ If you are a "kitchen smoker" in the morning, volunteer your services to a school or nonprofit organization to get you out of the house.

☐ Stock up on light reading materials, crossword puzzles, and vacation brochures that you can read during your coffee breaks.

☐ Frequent places where you can't smoke, such as libraries, buses, theatres, swimming pools, department stores.

☐ Give yourself time to think and get fit by walking one-half hour each day. If you have a dog, take it for a walk with you.

Excerpted from *TIPS*, American Cancer Society, Texas Division. Used by permission.

Figure 12.6 • *(Continued.)*

In small doses, marijuana has a sedative effect. Larger doses produce physical and psychic changes. Studies in the 1960s indicated that the potential effects of marijuana were exaggerated and that the drug was relatively harmless. The drug as it is used today, however, is as much as 10 times stronger than when the initial studies were conducted. Today, 90% of the research shows marijuana to be a dangerous and harmful drug.

The main, and most active, psychoactive and mind-altering ingredient in marijuana is thought to be delta-9-tetrahydrocannabinol (THC). In the 1960s, THC content in marijuana ranged from .02% to 2%. Users called the latter "real good grass." Today's THC content averages 4% to 6%, although it has been reported as high as 20%. The THC content in sinsemilla, a seedless variety of high-potency marijuana grown from the seedless female cannabis plant, is approximately 8% THC.

THC reaches the brain within 30 seconds of inhalation of marijuana smoke, and the psychic and physical changes reach their peak in about 2 or 3 minutes. THC then is metabolized in the liver to waste metabolites, but 30% of it remains in the body a week after marijuana was first smoked. Studies indicate that THC is not completely eliminated until 30 days or longer after an initial dose of the drug. The drug always remains in the system of regular users.

Some of the short-term effects of marijuana are tachycardia, dryness of the mouth, reddening of the eyes, stronger appetite, decrease in coordination and tracking (following a moving stimulus), difficulty in concentration, intermittent confusion, impairment of short-term memory and continuity of speech, and interference with the physical and mental learning process during periods of intoxication. Another common effect is the **amotivational syndrome**. This syndrome persists after periods of intoxication but usually disappears a few weeks after the individual stops using the drug. Long-term harmful effects include atrophy of the brain (leading to irreversible brain damage), less resistance to infectious diseases, chronic bronchitis, lung cancer (marijuana smoke may contain as much as 50% more cancer-producing hydrocarbons than cigarette smoke), and possible sterility and impotence.

One of the most common myths about marijuana use is that it does not lead to addiction. Ample scientific evidence clearly shows that regular users of marijuana do develop physical and psychological

dependence. Similar to cigarette smoking, when regular users go without the drug, they crave the substance, go through mood changes, are irritable and nervous, and develop an obsession to get more.

Cocaine

Similar to marijuana, **cocaine** was thought for many years to be a relatively harmless drug. This misconception came to an abrupt halt in 1986 when two well-known athletes, Len Bias (basketball) and Don Rogers (football), died suddenly following a cocaine overdose. Estimates indicate that between 4 and 8 million Americans use cocaine, 96% of whom had used marijuana previously. Over the years it has been given several different names, including coke, C, snow, blow, toot, flake, Peruvian lady, white girl, and happy dust. The drug usually is sniffed or snorted, but it can be smoked or injected.

An expensive drug, some users pay more than $2,000 per ounce for cocaine. Cocaine used in medical therapy sells for about $100 per ounce. Because of the high cost, cocaine is viewed as a luxury drug. Many users are well-educated, affluent, upwardly mobile professionals who are otherwise law-abiding citizens.

Cocaine has become the fastest growing drug problem in the United States. Each day about 5,000 people try cocaine for the first time. The addiction begins with a desire to get high, often at social gatherings, with the assurance that occasional use is harmless. About one in five of these first-time users will continue to use the drug now and then, and for some it is the beginning of a lifetime nightmare.

The popularity of cocaine is based on the almost universal guarantee that users will find themselves in an immediate state of euphoria and well-being. When

TERMS

Addiction Compulsive and uncontrollable behavior(s) or use of substance(s).

Marijuana A psychoactive drug, prepared from a mixture of crushed leaves, flowers, small branches, stems, and seeds from the hemp plant *cannabis sativa*.

Amotivational syndrome A condition characterized by loss of motivation, dullness, apathy, and no interest in the future.

Cocaine 2-beta-carbomethoxy-3-betabenozoxytropane, the primary psychoactive ingredient derived from coca plant leaves.

cocaine is snorted, it is absorbed quickly through the mucous membranes of the nose into the bloodstream. The drug is usually arranged in fine powder lines one to two inches long. Each line stimulates the autonomic nervous system for about 30 minutes.

Cocaine seems to alleviate fatigue and raise energy levels, as well as lessen the need for food and sleep. Following this stimulation comes a "crash," a state of physiological and psychological depression, often leaving the user with the desire to get more. This can lead to a constant craving for the drug.

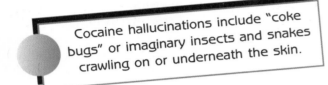

Cocaine hallucinations include "coke bugs" or imaginary insects and snakes crawling on or underneath the skin.

Addiction becomes a lifetime illness and, similar to alcoholism, the individual recovers only by abstaining from the drug completely. A single "backslide" can result in renewed addiction.

Light to moderate cocaine use commonly is associated with feelings of pleasure and well-being. Sustained cocaine snorting can lead to a constant runny nose, nasal congestion and inflammation, and perforation of the nasal septum. Long-term consequences of cocaine use in general include loss of appetite, digestive disorders, weight loss, malnutrition, insomnia, confusion, anxiety, and cocaine psychosis. Cocaine psychosis is characterized by paranoia and hallucinations. In one type of hallucination, referred to as formication or "coke bugs," the chronic user perceives imaginary insects or snakes crawling on or underneath the skin.

High doses of cocaine can cause nervousness, dizziness, blurred vision, vomiting, tremors, seizures, high blood pressure, strokes, angina, and cardiac arrhythmias. Those who use freebase (a purer, more potent, smokable form of cocaine) have an increased risk for lung disease. Intravenous users are at risk for hepatitis, HIV, and other infectious diseases.

Large overdoses of cocaine can precipitate sudden death from respiratory paralysis, cardiac arrhythmias, and severe convulsions. For individuals who lack an enzyme used in metabolizing cocaine, as few as two to three lines of cocaine may be fatal.

Chronic users who constantly crave the drug often turn to crime, including murder, to sustain their habit. Some users view suicide as the only solution to this sad syndrome.

Alcohol

Drinking **alcohol** has been a socially acceptable behavior for centuries. Alcohol is an accepted accompaniment at parties, ceremonies, dinners, sport contests, the establishment of kingdoms or governments, and the signing of treaties between nations. Alcohol also has been used for medical reasons as a mild sedative or as a pain killer for surgery.

For a short period of 14 years, from 1920 to 1933, by constitutional amendment, the sale and use of alcohol were declared illegal in the United States. This amendment was repealed because drinkers and nondrinkers alike questioned the right of government to pass judgment on individual moral standards. In addition, organized crime to smuggle and sell alcohol illegally expanded enormously.

Alcohol is the cause of one of the most significant health-related drug problems in the United States today. An estimated 6 in 10 adults, or more than 100 million Americans 18 years and older, are drinkers. Approximately 10 million of them will develop a drinking problem, including **alcoholism**, in their lifetime. Another 3 million teenagers are thought to have a drinking problem.

The addiction to alcohol develops slowly. Most people think they are in control of their drinking habits and do not realize they have a problem until they become alcoholics, when they find themselves physically and emotionally dependent on the drug. This addiction is characterized by excessive use and constant preoccupation with drinking. Alcohol abuse, in turn, leads to mental, emotional, physical, and social problems.

Alcohol intake impedes peripheral vision, lowers visual and hearing acuity, decreases reaction time,

The sale of alcohol was illegal in the United States between 1920 and 1933.

and impairs concentration and motor performance (including increased swaying and impaired judgment of distance and speed of moving objects). Further, it alleviates fear, increases risk-taking, stimulates urination, and induces sleep.

A single large dose of alcohol also may decrease sexual function. One of the most unpleasant, dangerous, and life-threatening effects of drinking is the **synergistic action** of alcohol when combined with other drugs, particularly central nervous system depressants. Each person reacts to a combination of alcohol and other drugs in a different way. The effects range from loss of consciousness to death.

Long-term effects of alcohol abuse are serious and often life-threatening. Some of these detrimental effects are cirrhosis of the liver; higher risk for oral, esophageal, and liver cancer; cardiomyopathy; elevated blood pressure; greater risk for strokes; inflammation of the esophagus, stomach, small intestine, and pancreas; stomach ulcers; sexual impotence; malnutrition; brain cell damage leading to loss of memory; psychosis; depression; and hallucinations.

Alcohol on Campuses

Alcohol is the number-one drug problem among college students. According to a 1992 national survey, 86.9% of college students reported using alcohol, and 41% of them had engaged in binge drinking (five or more drinks in a row) at least once in the 2 weeks preceding the survey. Alcohol is a factor in about 28% of all college dropouts, costing the federal government more than $3 billion in taxes. Today's student spends more on alcohol than on books.

A second 1992 survey, involving 56,000 college students, showed that gradepoint average (GPA) is related to the average number of drinks per week (see Figure 13.1). Students with a "D" or "F" GPA reported a weekly consumption of almost 11 drinks. Students with "A" GPAs consumed about 3.5 drinks per week. Of greater concern is that 36% indicated driving while intoxicated. This figure translates to about 20,000 college student deaths related to automobile accidents each year. Of the current 12 million college students in the United States, between 2% and 3% will die from alcohol-related causes. This represents approximately the same number as those who will receive advanced degrees (master's and doctorate degrees combined).

Another major concern is that over 50% of college students participate in games that involve heavy drinking (6 to 10 drinks) in a short time. Often students participate because of fear of rejection and peer pressure. Further, up to 48% report getting drunk at least once a month. Excessive drinking can lead to unplanned and unprotected sex (risking HIV

TERMS

Alcohol (ethyl alcohol)   A depressant drug that affects the brain and slows down central nervous system activity; has strong addictive properties.

Alcoholism   Disease in which an individual loses control over drinking alcoholic beverages.

Synergistic action   The effect of mixing two or more drugs which can be much greater than the sum of two or more drugs acting by themselves.

Figure 13.1 • *Average number of drinks by college students per week by gradepoint average.*

infection) or even date rape. Practice common sense when your date drinks.

How to Cut Down Your Drinking*

To find out if drinking is a problem in your life, refer to the questionnaire Alcohol Abuse: Are You Drinking Too Much?, given in Figure 13.2, developed by the American Medical Association.[1] If you respond "yes" twice or more on this questionnaire, you may be jeopardizing your health.

If a person is determined to control the problem, it is not that hard to do. The first and most important step is to want to cut down. If you want to do this but find you cannot, you had better accept the probability that alcohol is becoming a serious problem for you, and you should seek guidance from your physician or from an organization such as Alcoholics Anonymous. The next few suggestions also may help you cut down alcohol intake.

1. **Set reasonable limits for yourself.** Decide not to exceed a certain number of drinks on a given

---

* Reproduced by permission from *Family Medical Guide* by American Medical Association (New York: Random House, 1982).

occasion, and stick to your decision. No more than two beers or two cocktails a day is a reasonable limit. You have proven to yourself that you can control your drinking if you set a target such as this and consistently do not exceed it.

2. **Learn to say no.** Many people have "just one more" drink because others in the group are, or because someone puts pressure on them, not because they really want a drink. When you reach the sensible limit you have set for yourself, politely but firmly refuse to exceed it. If you are being the generous host, pour yourself a glass of water or juice "on the rocks." Nobody will notice the difference.

3. **Drink slowly.** Never gulp down a drink. Choose your drinks for their flavor, not their "kick," and savor the taste of each sip.

4. **Dilute your drinks.** If you prefer cocktails to beer, try having long drinks. Instead of downing your gin or whiskey neat or nearly so, drink it diluted with a mixer such as tonic, water, or soda water, in a tall glass. That way you can enjoy both the flavor and the act of drinking but you will take

---

ALCOHOL ABUSE: ARE YOU DRINKING TOO MUCH?

1. When you are holding an empty glass at a party, do you always actively look for a refill instead of waiting to be offered one?

2. If given the chance, do you frequently pour out a more generous drink for yourself than seems to be the "going" amount for others?

3. Do you often have a drink or two when you are alone, either at home or in a bar?

4. Is your drinking ever the direct cause of a family quarrel, or do quarrels often seem to occur, if only by coincidence, when you have had a drink or two?

5. Do you feel that you must have a drink at a specific time every day — right after work, for instance?

6. When worried or under unusual stress, do you almost automatically take a stiff drink to "settle your nerves?"

7. Are you untruthful about how much you have had to drink when questioned on the subject?

8. Does drinking ever cause you to take time off work, or to miss scheduled meetings or appointments?

9. Do you feel physically deprived if you cannot have at least one drink every day?

10. Do you sometimes crave a drink in the morning?

11. Do you sometimes have "mornings after" when you cannot remember what happened the night before?

Evaluation

You should regard a "yes" answer to any one of the above questions as a warning sign. Do not increase your consumption of alcohol. Two "yes" answers suggest that you already may be becoming dependent on alcohol. Three or more "yes" answers indicate that you may have a serious problem, and you should get professional help.

Figure 13.2 • *American Medical Association questionnaire on drinking.*

longer to finish each drink. Also, you can make your two-drink limit last all evening or switch to the mixer by itself.

5. **Do not drink on your own.** Make a point of confining your drinking to social gatherings. You may have a hard time resisting the urge to pour yourself a relaxing drink at the end of a hard day, but many formerly heavy drinkers have found that a soft drink satisfies the need as well as alcohol did and that it was just a habit. What may help you really unwind, even with no drink at all, is a comfortable chair, loosened clothing, and perhaps a soothing audiotape, television program, or good book to read.

Treatment of Addiction

Treatment of alcoholism and other drug addictions seldom is accomplished without professional guidance and support. The first step is to recognize the reality of the problem. The questionnaire given in Figure 13.3 will help you recognize possible addictive behavior in yourself or someone you know. If your answers to more than half of these questions are positive, you may have a problem and should speak to your doctor or contact the local mental health clinic for a referral (see the Yellow Pages in your phone book).

DO'S AND DON'TS WHEN YOUR DATE DRINKS

- **Don't** make excuses for his/her behavior, no matter how embarrassing.
- **Don't** allow embarrassment to put you in a situation with which you are uncomfortable.
- **Do** be sure that body language and tone of voice match verbal messages you send.
- **Do** make your position clear. "No!" is much more effective than "Please stop!" or "Don't!"
- **Do** make it clear that you will call the police if rape is attempted.
- **Do** leave as quickly as you can, without your date. **Don't** stop to argue. Intoxicated people can't listen to reason.
- **Do** call a cab, a friend, or your parents. **Don't** ride home with your date.

Source: "Sexuality Under the Influence of Alcohol." *Human Sexuality Supplement to Current Health*, 2 (October 1990), p. 3.

● Sexually Transmitted Diseases

Sexually transmitted diseases (STDs) have reached epidemic proportions in the United States. Of the more than 25 known STDs, some are still incurable. The American Social Health Association stated that 25% of all Americans will acquire at least one STD in their lifetime. Each year more than 12 million people are newly infected with STDs, including 4.6 million cases of chlamydia, 1.8 million of gonorrhea, 1 million of genital warts, half a million cases of herpes, and almost 100,000 cases of syphilis. Attracting most of the attention because of its life-threatening potential were more than 74,180 new cases of AIDS in the United States in 1995.

Chlamydia

Chlamydia is a bacterial infection that spreads during vaginal, anal, or oral sex, or from the vagina to a newborn baby during childbirth. Chlamydia can damage the reproductive system seriously.

This disease is considered to be a major factor in male and female infertility. Because it may have no symptoms, three of four people don't have any symptoms until the infection has become quite serious. According to the Centers for Disease Control, about 20% of all college students have chlamydia.

When symptoms are present, they tend to mimic other STDs, so the disease can be mistreated. Symptoms of serious infection include abdominal pain, fever, nausea, vaginal bleeding, and arthritis. Chlamydia can be treated successfully with oral antibiotics but will not reverse any damage done already to the reproductive system.

Gonorrhea

One of the oldest STDs, **gonorrhea**, also is caused by a bacterial infection. Gonorrhea is transmitted through vaginal, anal, and oral sex.

TERMS

Sexually transmitted diseases (STDs) Communicable diseases spread through sexual contact.

Chlamydia A sexually transmitted disease caused by a bacterial infection that can cause significant damage to the reproductive system.

Gonorrhea Sexually transmitted disease caused by a bacterial infection.

COULD YOU BE AN ADDICT?

Directions

The following test, designed by Dr. Lawrence J. Hatterer, is not a way to diagnose whether you are in the early, middle, or chronic stage of addictive disease. It is meant merely to help you understand addictive behavior better so you can recognize it in yourself or perhaps in people you know.

1. I am a person of excesses. I can't regulate what I do for pleasure and often use a substance or indulge in an activity heavily to get high.

2. I am an extremely self-involved person. People tell me I am into myself too much.

3. I am compulsive. I must have what I want when I want it, regardless of the consequences.

4. I am excessively dependent on or independent of others.

5. I am preoccupied. I spend a lot of time thinking or fantasizing about a particular activity or substance. Also, I will work my day around doing it or go to pains to make sure it's available.

6. I deny that I do this, and lie about it to others who ask me.

7. I have been involved in this behavior for at least a year.

8. I've told myself I could easily stop, even though I've shown no signs of slowing down.

9. Once I start indulging in this behavior or substance, I find I have trouble stopping.

10. One or more members of my family also are involved in some kind of excessive behavior or substance abuse.

11. I find I gravitate mostly toward people who have the same behavior or take the same substance as I do.

12. I seem to be developing a tolerance of the behavior or substance. I have had a need to steadily increase the amounts I take or the time I spend doing it.

13. I have found that my excessive use of highs has, in fact, only made my problems worse.

14. If someone tries to keep me from obtaining the substance or practicing the activity, I get angry and reject or abuse that person.

15. I experience withdrawal symptoms if I cannot indulge in the substance or activity.

16. This has gotten in the way of my functioning. I have missed something important — days at work, time with my friends, family, children — because of it.

17. The substance/activity is destroying my home life. I know I am hurting those closest to me.

18. I have failed in many goals in life, lost money, given up many social and occupational contacts, all because of my excessive behavior.

19. I have tried to stop or cut down on my excesses but have been unsuccessful.

20. I have physically endangered myself or others in accidents that were a direct result of my excessive behavior.

Evaluation

If you answer "yes" to half or more of the questions, you may have a problem with addictive disease and should seek immediate professional help. For a referral, contact your local mental health clinic (look in the Yellow Pages) or speak to your doctor.

Used by permission from *McCall's* magazine. Copyright © 1986 by the McCall Publishing Company.

Figure 13.3 • *Questionnaire on addiction.*

Typical symptoms in men include a puslike secretion from the penis and painful urination. Most infected women don't have any symptoms until the infection is fairly serious. At this stage, women develop fever, severe abdominal pain, and pelvic inflammatory disease (see below).

If untreated, gonorrhea can produce infertility, widespread bacterial infection, heart damage, arthritis in men and women, and blindness in children born to infected women. Gonorrhea is treated successfully with penicillin and other antibiotics.

Pelvic Inflammatory Disease

Each year approximately 750,000 women have **pelvic inflammatory disease (PID)**. This disease usually is caused by chlamydia and gonorrhea.

Typical symptoms of PID are fever, nausea, vomiting, chills, spotting between menstrual periods, heavy bleeding during periods, and pain in the lower abdomen during sexual intercourse, between menstrual periods, or urination. Many women do not know they have PID because they have no symptoms.

PID often develops when the STD spreads to the fallopian tubes, uterus, and ovaries. If the woman becomes pregnant, she may have an ectopic or tubal pregnancy. The pregnancy destroys the embryo and can kill the patient.

PID is treated with antibiotics, bed rest, and sexual abstinence. Further, surgery may be required to remove infected or scarred tissue or to repair or remove the fallopian tubes or uterus.

Genital Warts

Genital warts are caused by viral infection. They show up anywhere from 1½ to 8 months after exposure. These warts may be flat or raised and usually are found on the penis or around the vulva and the vagina, but they also can appear in the mouth, throat, rectum, on the cervix, or around the anus.

Of sexually active people in the United States, 20% to 30% are infected with the virus that causes this STD. In some cities, nearly half of all sexually active teenagers have genital warts. Similar to chlamydia, the virus is spread through vaginal, anal, or oral sex, or from the vagina to a newborn baby.

Health problems associated with genital warts include increased risk for cancers of the cervix, vulva, and penis, and enlargement and spread of the warts leading to obstruction of the urethra, vagina,

and anus. Babies born to infected mothers commonly develop warts over their bodies; therefore, Cesarean sections are recommended.

Treatment requires completely removing all warts. This can be done by freezing them with liquid nitrogen, dissolving them with chemicals, or removing them through electrosurgery or laser surgery. Infected patients may have to be treated more than once because genital warts can recur.

Herpes

Herpes also is caused by a viral infection (herpes simplex virus types I and II). Sores appear on the mouth, genitals, rectum, or other parts of the body. The symptoms usually disappear within a few weeks, causing some people to believe they are cured. Herpes is presently incurable, though, and its victims do remain infected. Repeated outbreaks are common.

Herpes is highly contagious and can be transmitted through simple finger contact from the mouth to the genitals. Victims are most contagious during an outbreak. In conjunction with the sores, victims usually have mild fever, swollen glands, and headaches.

Syphilis

Another common type of STD, also caused by bacterial infection, is **syphilis**. Approximately 3 weeks after infection, a painless sore appears where the bacteria entered the body. This sore disappears on its own in a few weeks. If untreated, more sores may appear within 6 months of the initial outbreak but again will disappear by themselves.

A latent stage, during which the victim is not contagious, may last up to 30 years, lulling victims into thinking they are healed. During the last stage of the disease, some people develop paralysis, crippling, blindness, heart disease, brain damage and

---

TERMS

Pelvic inflammatory disease (PID) An overall designation referring to the effects of chlamydia and gonorrhea.

Genital warts Sexually transmitted disease caused by a viral infection.

Herpes A sexually transmitted disease caused by a viral infection (herpes simplex virus types I and II).

Syphilis A sexually transmitted disease caused by a bacterial infection.

insanity, and they even may die as a direct result of the disease. One of the oldest known STDs, syphilis used to end up killing its victims. Penicillin and other antibiotics now are used to treat it.

HIV and AIDS

AIDS is the most frightening of all STDs because it is fatal and has no known cure (and no cure on the horizon). AIDS — which stands for **acquired immunodeficiency syndrome** — is the end stage of infection by the **human immunodeficiency virus** (HIV).

HIV is a chronic infectious disease that spreads among individuals who choose to engage in risky behavior such as unprotected sex or the sharing of hypodermic needles. When a person becomes infected with HIV, the virus multiplies, attacks, and destroys white blood cells. These cells are part of the immune system, and their function is to fight off infections and diseases in the body.

As the number of white blood cells killed increases, the body's immune system gradually breaks down or may be destroyed completely. Without the immune system, a person becomes susceptible to **opportunistic infections** or cancers.

HIV is a progressive disease. At first, people who become infected with HIV may not know they are infected. An incubation period of weeks, months, or years may go by during which no symptoms appear. The virus may live in the body 10 years or longer before symptoms emerge.

As the infection progresses to the point at which certain diseases develop, the person is said to have AIDS. HIV itself doesn't kill. Nor do people die of AIDS. AIDS is the term used to define the final stage of HIV infection. Death is caused by a weakened immune system that is unable to fight off these opportunistic diseases.

Earliest symptoms of AIDS include unexplained weight loss, constant fatigue, mild fever, swollen lymph glands, diarrhea, and sore throats. Advanced symptoms include loss of appetite, skin diseases, night sweats, and deterioration of the mucous membranes.

Most of the illnesses AIDS patients develop are harmless and rare in the general population but are fatal to AIDS victims. The two most common fatal conditions in AIDS patients are *pneumocystis carinii pneumonia* (a parasitic infection of the lungs) and *kaposis sarcoma* (a type of skin cancer). The AIDS virus also may attack the nervous system, causing brain and spinal cord damage.

VANESSA WAS IN A FATAL CAR ACCIDENT LAST NIGHT. ONLY SHE DOESN'T KNOW IT YET.

Drug and alcohol use can make people more willing to have unplanned and unprotected sex, thereby, risking HIV infection.
Photo courtesy of the National Institute on Drug Abuse, U.S. Department of Health & Human Services.

On the average, the individual develops the symptoms that fit the case definition of AIDS about 7 to 8 years following infection. From that point on, the person may live another 2 to 3 years. In essence, from the point of infection, the individual may endure a chronic disease 8 to 10 years.

The only means to determine whether someone has HIV is through an HIV antibody test. Being HIV-positive does not necessarily mean the person has AIDS. Several years may go by before the person develops the diseases that fit the case definition of AIDS.

Upon HIV infection, the immune system's line of defense against the virus is to form antibodies that bind to the virus. On the average, the body takes 3 months to manufacture enough antibodies to show up positive in an HIV antibody test. Sometimes this may take 6 months or longer.

If HIV infection is suspected, a prudent waiting period of 3 to 6 months is suggested prior to testing. During this time, and from there on, individuals should refrain from further endangering themselves and others through risky behaviors. Some people choose to be tested to be reassured that their risky behaviors are acceptable. Even if the test turns up negative for HIV, this does not represent a "license" to continue risky behaviors.

No one has to become infected with HIV. Once infected with HIV, a person never will become uninfected. There is no second chance. Everyone must protect himself or herself against this chronic disease. No one should be so ignorant as to believe that it can never happen to him or her!

before the present relationship and still doesn't know of the infection, (d) may not be honest with you and chooses not to tell you about the infection, or (e) is shooting up drugs and becomes infected. In any of these cases, HIV can be passed on to you.

Because your future and your life are at stake, and because you may never know if your partner is infected, you should give serious and careful consideration to postponing sex until you believe you have found a lifetime monogamous relationship. In doing so, you will not have to live with the fear of catching HIV or other STDs or deal with an unplanned pregnancy.

As strange as this may seem to some, many people postpone sexual activity until they are married. This is the best guarantee against HIV. Young people should understand that married life will provide plenty of time for fulfilling and rewarding sex.

If you choose to delay sex, do not let peers pressure you into having sex. Some people would have you believe you are not a real man or woman if you don't have sex. Manhood and womanhood are not proven during sexual intercourse but, instead, through mature, responsible, and healthy choices.

Other people lead you to believe that love doesn't exist without sex. Sex in the early stages of a relationship is not the product of love but is simply the fulfillment of a physical, and often selfish, drive. A loving relationship develops over a long time with mutual respect for each other.

Teenagers are especially susceptible to peer pressure leading to premature sexual intercourse. The result: more than a million teen pregnancies per year and a 43% pregnancy rate for all girls at least once as a teenager. Too many young people wish they had postponed sex and silently admire those who do. Sex lasts only a few minutes. The consequences of irresponsible sex may last a lifetime. And in some cases, they are fatal!

Then there are those who enjoy bragging about their sexual conquests and mock people who choose to wait. In essence, many of these conquests are only fantasies expounded in an attempt to gain popularity with peers.

Sexual promiscuity never leads to a trusting, loving, and lasting relationship. Mature people respect others' choices. If someone does not respect your choice to wait, he or she certainly does not deserve your friendship or, for that matter, anything else.

There is no greater sex than that between two loving and responsible individuals who mutually trust and admire each other. Contrary to many beliefs, these relationships are possible. They are built upon unselfish attitudes and behaviors.

As you look around, you will find that many people have these values. Seek them out and build your friendships and future around people who respect you for what you are and what you believe. You don't have to compromise your choices or values. In the end you will reap the greater rewards of a choice and lasting relationship, free of AIDS and other STDs.

Also, be prepared so that you will know your course of action before you get into an intimate situation. Look for common interests, and work together toward them. Express your feelings openly: "I'm not ready for sex; I just want to have fun and kissing is fine with me." If your friend does not accept your answer and is not willing to stop the advances, be prepared with a strong response. Statements like "Please stop" or "Don't!" are for the most part ineffective. Use a firm statement such as: "No, I'm not willing to do it" or "I've already thought about this and I'm not going to have sex." If this still does not work, it is effective to label the behavior as rape and say: "This is rape and I'm going to call the police."

STD Risk Reduction

What about those who do not have — or do not desire — a monogamous relationship? Some other things can be done to lower, but never completely eliminate, the risk for developing STDs in general:

1. Plan before you get into a sexual situation. Determine the conditions under which you will allow sex to take place. Take a few moments now and ask yourself: "Am I willing to have sex with this person?" If you decide to have sex, practice safer sex. There is no reason to accept anything else. You will feel better about yourself.

2. Know your partner. The days are gone when anonymous bathhouse or singles-bars sex is safe. Limit your sexual relationships, and always practice safer sex.

TERMS

Monogamous A sexual relationship in which two people have sexual relations only with each other.

3. Discuss STDs with the person you are contemplating having sex with before you do so. Talking about STDs might be awkward, but the short-lived embarrassment of addressing intimate questions can keep you from contracting or spreading disease. If you do not know the person well enough to address this issue, or you are uncertain about the answers, do not have sex with this individual.

4. Limit the number of sexual partners you have. Having one partner lowers your chance of infection. The more partners you have, the greater is your chance for infection.

5. If you are sexually promiscuous, consider having periodic physical checkups. Getting exposed to an STD by a person who does not have any symptoms and who is unaware of the infection is easy. Sexually promiscuous men and women between ages 15 and 35 are considered to be in a particularly high-risk group for developing STDs.

6. Use "barrier" methods of contraception to help prevent the disease from spreading. Condoms, diaphragms, the contraceptive sponge, and spermicidal suppositories, foams, and jellies can all deter the spread of certain STDs. Spermicidal agents may act as a disinfectant as well. Many physicians are especially encouraging promiscuous teenagers to use condoms. Traditionally, teenagers do not use any birth-control methods at all and remain at high risk for STDs. Take a few minutes at this time and list at least three ways that you may bring up the subject of condom use with your partner. Also, think of ways that you might convince a person to use one. If your partner refuses to use one, your answer should be quite simple: "No condom, no sex."

7. Negotiate safer sex. Focus on the problem and not the person. Describe your feelings about the problem and use "I" instead of "you." For example, you may say: "I'm feeling awkward and uncomfortable. The only way I can feel comfortable is by using a condom." You also can offer options and provide alternative solutions to your partner. You may indicate: "We can work this out together. Let's go for a drive and get a condom with a spermicide agent. We'll feel better about what we're doing."

8. Be responsible enough to abstain from sexual activity if you know you have an infection. Go to a physician or clinic for treatment, and ask your doctor when you can safely resume sexual activity. Abstain until it is safe. Just as you want to be protected in a sexual relationship, you should want to protect your partner as well.

If you are diagnosed with an STD and you believe you know the person who gave it to you, think of ways that could bring up the subject of STDs with this person. You need to take responsibility and discuss this matter with your partner. Hopefully, as a result of your conversation, medical treatment can be initiated and others can be protected from infection as well.

9. Urinate immediately following sexual intercourse. This is not a reliable method, but it may help (especially men) flush bacteria and viruses from the urinary tract.

10. Thoroughly wash immediately after sexual activity. Washing with hot, soapy water will not guarantee safety against STDs, but it can prevent you from spreading certain germs on your fingers and may wash away bacteria and viruses that have not entered the body yet.

11. If you suspect your partner is infected with a STD, ask. He or she may not even be aware of the infection, so look for signs of infection, such as sores, redness, inflammations, a rash, growths, warts, or discharge. If you are unsure, abstain.

12. Consider abstaining from sexual relations if you have any kind of an illness or disease, even a common cold. Any kind of illness makes you more susceptible to other illnesses, and lower immunity can make you extra vulnerable to STDs. The same holds true for times when you are under extreme stress, when you are fatigued, and when you are overworked. Drugs and alcohol also can lower your resistance to disease.

13. Wear loose-fitting clothes made from natural fibers. Tight-fitting clothing made from synthetic fibers (especially underwear and nylon pantyhose) can create conditions that encourage the growth of bacteria and actually can aggravate STDs.

HIV Risk Reduction

Based upon recommendations from health experts, observing the following precautions can reduce your risk for getting HIV, and subsequently AIDS:

1. Postpone sex until you and your uninfected partner are prepared to enter into a lifetime

monogamous relationship. In his book, *What You Can Do to Avoid AIDS*, Earvin "Magic" Johnson stated:[2]

> But if I had known what I do now when I was younger, I would have postponed sex as long as I could, and I would have tried to have it the first time with somebody that I knew I wanted to spend the rest of my life with. I certainly want my children to postpone sex. Now the rest of my life may be a lot shorter than I thought it was going to be, and I may not be around to see my son, Andre, grow up and to see what happens to the baby Cookie and I are having in the summer of '92, and, of course, I may not have the long life I want with Cookie.

2. Unless you are in a monogamous relationship and you know your partner is not infected (which you may never know for sure), practice safer sex every single time you have sex. This means you should use a latex condom from start to finish for each sexual act. If you think your partner should use a condom but refuses to do so, say no to sex with that person.

   Many experts believe greater protection can be obtained by placing a small amount of the spermicide nonoxynol–9 inside the condom at its tip and then lubricating the outside with additional spermicide. Nonoxynol–9 is used to kill the man's sperm for birth control purposes. In test tubes, it has been shown to kill STD germs and HIV. This spermicide, however, should not be used in place of a condom because it will not offer the same protection as the condom does by itself.

3. Avoid having multiple and anonymous sexual partners. Keep in mind that anyone you have sex with could be infected with HIV.

4. Don't have sexual contact with anyone who does not practice safer sex.

5. Avoid sexual contact with anyone who has had sex with people at risk for getting HIV, even if they now are practicing safer sex.

6. Don't have sex with prostitutes.

7. If you do have sex with someone who might be infected with HIV or whose history is unknown to you, avoid exchange of body fluids.

8. Don't share toothbrushes, razors, or other implements that could become contaminated with blood with anyone who is, or who might be, infected with HIV.

9. Be cautious regarding procedures such as acupuncture, tattooing, and ear piercing, in which needles or other nonsterile instruments may be used again and again to pierce the skin or mucous membranes. These procedures are safe if proper sterilization methods or disposable needles are followed. Before undergoing the procedure, ask what precautions are being taken.

10. If you are planning to undergo artificial insemination, insist on frozen sperm obtained from a laboratory that tests all donors for infection with HIV. Donors should be tested twice before accepting the sperm — once at the time of donation and again a few months later.

11. If you know you will be having surgery in the near future, and if you are able, consider donating blood for your own use. This will eliminate completely the already small risk of contracting HIV through a blood transfusion. It also will eliminate the more substantial risk for contracting other blood-borne diseases, such as hepatitis, from a transfusion.

Avoiding of risky behaviors that destroy quality of life and life itself are critical components of a healthy lifestyle. Learning the facts so you can make responsible choices can protect you and those around you from startling and unexpected conditions. Using alcohol in moderation (or not at all), avoiding other drugs, and preventing sexually transmitted diseases are essential in averting both physical and psychological damage.

Notes

1. American Medical Association, *Family Medical Guide* (New York: Random House, 1982).

2. E. M. Johnson, *What You Can Do to Avoid AIDS* (New York: Random House, 1992).

Suggested Readings

"Addiction." *Aerobics News*. Dallas: Institute for Aerobics Research, July 1987.

American Medical Association. *Family Medical Guide*. New York: Random House, 1982.

Bennett, E. G., and D. Woolf (Editors). *Substance Abuse*. Albany, NY: Delmar Publishers, 1991.

Carroll, C. R. *Drugs in Modern Society*. Dubuque, IA: Wm. C. Brown Publishers, 1995.

Channing L. Bete Co. *About AIDS and Shooting Drugs*. South Deerfield, MA: Author, 1986.

Goldberg, R. *Drugs Across the Spectrum*. Englewood, CO: Morton Publishing, 1997.

Hafen, B. Q., A. L. Thygerson, and K. J. Frandsen. *Behavioral Guidelines for Health & Wellness*. Englewood, CO: Morton Publishing, 1988.

Schlaadt, R. G., and P. T. Shannon. *Drugs*. Englewood Cliffs, NJ: Prentice Hall, 1994.

Healthy Lifestyle Issues and Wellness Guidelines for the Future

14

*B*etter health, higher quality of life, and longevity are the three most vital benefits derived from a lifetime physical fitness program. Physical fitness in itself does not always lower the risk for chronic diseases and ensure better health, but the importance of a healthy lifestyle is one means to attain the highest potential for total well-being.

In addition to the wellness issues already discussed, three factors that are a part of daily living and may influence your well-being directly are: (a) spirituality, (b) exercise and aging, and (c) health-promoting behaviors. These components of wellness are the focus of this chapter.

Guidelines for preventing consumer fraud and selecting a health/fitness club also are presented in this last chapter. Further, you will have the

Objectives

- Define spiritual well-being and its relationship to a healthy lifestyle.
- Describe the relationship between fitness and aging.
- Learn guidelines for preventing consumer fraud.
- Understand factors to consider when selecting a health/fitness club.
- Know how to select appropriate exercise equipment.
- Become acquainted with the Prevention Index, a measure of the effort the American people are making to prevent disease and improve total well-being.
- Review health/fitness accomplishments and chart a wellness program for the future.

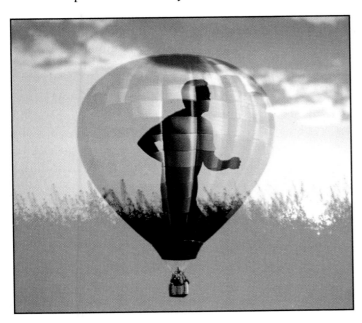

opportunity to determine how well you are achieving your wellness objectives. Finally, you will receive instructions to help you chart a personal wellness program for the future.

● Spiritual Well-Being

The National Interfaith Coalition on Aging defines spiritual well-being as *an affirmation of life in a relationship with God, self, community, and environment that nurtures and celebrates wholeness* (see Figure 14.1). Because this definition encompasses Christians and non-Christians alike, it assumes that all people are spiritual in nature. Spiritual health provides a unifying power that integrates the other dimensions of wellness. Basic characteristics of spiritual people include a sense of meaning and direction in life, a relationship to a higher being, freedom, prayer, faith, love, closeness to others, peace, joy, fulfillment, and **altruism.**

Religion has been a major part of cultures since the beginning of time. Although not everyone in the United States claims affiliation with a certain religion or denomination, current surveys indicate that 94% of the U.S. population believes in God or a universal spirit functioning as God.

People, furthermore, believe to a varying extent that (a) a relationship with God is meaningful; (b) God can grant help, guidance, and assistance in

Figure 14.1 ● *Components of spiritual well-being.*

daily living; and (c) mortal existence has a purpose. If we accept any or all of these statements, attaining spirituality will have a definite effect on our happiness and well-being.

The scientific association between **spirituality** and health is more difficult to establish than that of other lifestyle factors such as alcohol use, smoking, physical inactivity, seat belt use, and so on. Several research studies, nonetheless, have reported positive relationships among spiritual well-being, emotional well-being, and life's satisfaction. Further, people who attend church and participate in religious organizations regularly enjoy better health, have a lower incidence of chronic diseases, handle stress more effectively, and seem to live longer.

Although the reasons why religious affiliation enhances wellness are difficult to determine, possible reasons include the promotion of healthy lifestyle behaviors, social support, assistance in times of crisis and need, and counseling to overcome one's weaknesses.

Researchers have found that most successful men and women have strong spiritual values. Furthermore, almost all of these people experienced a crisis early in life. Spiritual beliefs seemed to help them overcome the crisis and aided in developing better coping techniques to deal with future trauma.

Altruism, a key attribute of spiritual people, seems to enhance health and longevity. Altruism is defined as *true concern for the welfare of others* (opposite of egoism) or a sincere desire to serve others above one's personal needs. Altruism has been the focus of several studies in recent years. Researchers believe that doing good for others is good for oneself, especially for the immune system. The health benefits of altruism could be so powerful, researchers at Harvard found, that even just watching films of altruistic endeavors enhances the formation of an immune system chemical that helps fight disease.[1]

In a study of more than 2,700 people in Michigan,[2] the investigators found that people who did regular volunteer work lived longer. People who did not perform regular volunteer work (at least once a week) had a 250% greater mortality risk during the course of the study.

Wellness requires a balance between physical, mental, spiritual, emotional, and social well-being. The relationship between spirituality and wellness, therefore, is meaningful in our quest for a better quality of life. As with other parameters of wellness, optimum spirituality requires development of the spiritual nature to its fullest potential.

● Exercise and Aging

Unlike any prior time in American society, the elderly population constitutes the fastest growing segment. In 1880, less than 3% of the total population, or fewer than 2 million people, was older than 65. By 1980 the elderly population had reached approximately 25 million, more than 11.3% of the population. According to estimates, the elderly will make up more than 20% of the total population by the year 2035.

Historically, older adults have been neglected when developing fitness programs. Nevertheless, fitness is just as important for older people as it is for young people. Although much research remains to be done in this area, studies indicate that older individuals who are physically fit also enjoy better health and a higher quality of life.

The main objective of fitness programs for older adults should be to help them improve their functional health status. This implies the ability to maintain independent living status and avoiding disability. The American Alliance of Health, Physical Education, Recreation and Dance (AAHPERD) defines functional fitness for older adults as *the physical capacity of the individual to meet ordinary and unexpected demands of daily life safely and effectively*.[3] This definition clearly indicates the need for fitness programs that closely relate to activities this population normally encounters. The AAHPERD committee encourages participation in programs that will help develop cardiovascular endurance, localized

Good physical fitness provides freedom to enjoy many of life's recreational and leisure activities.

muscular endurance, muscular flexibility, agility and balance, and motor coordination. A copy of the battery of fitness tests for older adults can be obtained from AAHPERD, Reston, Virginia.

Relationship Between Fitness and Aging

Although previous research studies have documented declines in physiological functioning and motor capacity as a result of aging, no hard evidence at present proves that declines in physical work capacity are related primarily to the aging process. Lack of physical activity — a common phenomenon seen in our society as people age — may be accompanied by decreases in physical work capacity that are greater by far than the effects of aging itself.

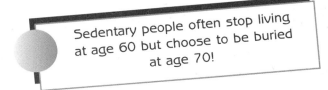

Sedentary people often stop living at age 60 but choose to be buried at age 70!

Data on individuals who have taken part in systematic physical activity throughout life indicate that these groups of people maintain a higher level of functional capacity and do not experience the typical declines in later years. From a functional point of view, the typical sedentary American is about 25 years older than his or her chronological age indicates. Thus, an active 60-year-old person can have a work capacity similar to that of a sedentary 35-year-old.

Unfortunately, unhealthy behaviors precipitate premature aging. For sedentary people, productive life ends at about age 60. Most of these people hope to live to be 65 or 70 and often must cope with serious physical ailments. These people stop living at age 60 but choose to be buried at age 70 (see the theoretical model in Figure 14.2).

Scientists believe a healthy lifestyle allows people to live a vibrant life — a physically, intellectually,

TERMS

Altruism   True concern for the welfare of others.

Spirituality   An affirmation of life that recognizes a higher being and integrates the dimensions of wellness.

Figure 14.2 • *Relationships between physical work capacity, aging, and lifestyle habits.*

emotionally, socially active and functionally independent existence — to age 95. When death comes to active people, it usually is rather quick and not as a result of prolonged illness (see Figure 14.2). Such are the rewards of a wellness way of life.

Physical Training in the Older Adult

The trainability of elderly men and women alike and the effectiveness of physical activity for health enhancement have been demonstrated in prior research. Older adults who increase their level of physical activity experience significant changes in cardiorespiratory endurance, strength, and flexibility. The extent of the changes depends on their initial fitness level and the types of activities selected for their training (walking, cycling, strength training, and so on).

Improvements in maximal oxygen uptake in older adults are similar to those of younger people, although older people seem to require a longer training period to achieve these changes. Declines in endurance (maximal oxygen uptake) per decade of life after age 25 seem to be about 9% for sedentary adults and 5% or less in active people.

Results of a recent study on the effects of aging on the cardiorespiratory system of male exercisers versus nonexercisers showed that the maximal oxygen uptake of regular exercisers was almost twice that of the nonexercisers (see Table 14.1).[4] Between ages 50 and 68 the study revealed a decline in maximal oxygen uptake of only 13% in the active group, compared to 41% in the inactive group. These changes indicate that about one-third of the loss in maximal oxygen uptake results from aging and two-thirds of the loss comes from inactivity. Blood pressure, heart rate, and body weight also were remarkably better in the exercising group.

In strength development older adults can increase their strength levels, but the amount of muscle hypertrophy achieved decreases with age. Strength gains close to 200% have been found in previously inactive adults over age 90.[5] In terms of body composition, inactive adults continue to gain body fat after age 60 despite the tendency toward lower body weight.

Older adults who wish to initiate or continue an exercise program are encouraged strongly to have a complete medical exam, including a stress electrocardiogram test (see Chapter 9). Recommended activities for older adults include calisthenics, walking, jogging, swimming, cycling, and water aerobics.

Isometric and other intense weight-training exercises should be avoided. Activities that require all-out effort or require participants to hold their breath (valsalva maneuver) tend to lessen blood flow to the heart and cause a significant increase in blood pressure and the load placed on the heart. Older adults should participate in activities that require continuous and rhythmic muscular activity (about 50% to 70% of functional capacity). These activities do not

Table 14.1 *Effects of Physical Activity and Inactivity on Older Men*

	Exercisers	Non-exercisers
Age (yrs)	68.0	69.8
Weight (lbs)	160.3	186.3
Resting heart rate (bpm)	55.8	66.0
Maximal heart rate (bpm)	157.0	146.0
Heart rate reserve* (bpm)	101.2	80.0
Blood pressure (mm Hg)	120/78	150/90
Maximal oxygen uptake (ml/kg/min)	38.6	20.3

* Heart rate reserve = maximal heart rate − resting heart rate.

From "The Effect of Physical Activity on Aerobic Power in Older Men (A Longitudinal Study)," by F. W. Kash, J. L. Boyer, S. P. Van Camp, L. S. Verity, and J. P. Wallace, *Physician and Sports Medicine* 18:4 (1990), 73–83.

cause large increases in blood pressure or place an intense overload on the heart.

The Prevention Index

The Prevention Index is an annual measure of the effort adults in the U.S. are making to prevent disease and accidents and to promote good health and longevity. This nationwide index of the American public, commissioned by *Prevention Magazine*, has been developed from information collected by Louis Harris and Associates in two national surveys:

1. Self-reported practice of preventive health and safety behaviors based on a national probability sample of 1,250 adults in the continental United States 18 years of age and older.

2. Ratings on the relative importance of each of these behaviors for preventing disease and disability in the general population (on a scale of 1 to 10), as determined by a sample of 103 representative experts in disease prevention and health promotion.

In the Harris national probability survey of adults, 21 of the behaviors were selected for inclusion in the Prevention Index according to the following criteria:

1. A documented relationship between the health behavior and disease or disability, as published in the professional literature.

2. Behaviors that are relevant to the entire adult population.

3. Behaviors that individuals can control or affect (thus the exclusion of important environmental determinants of health such as exposure to air pollution or industrial toxins).

Currently accepted standards of practice for each behavior were determined by thorough review of the professional literature and consultation with experts. In the case of continuous variables (for example, moderate alcohol consumption, exercise, frequency of dental examination), practice was ascertained by the prevailing consensus in the relevant professional literature and from personal consultation with researchers and spokespersons of professional organizations. For behaviors with no clear consensus on a minimum compliance level (for example, taking steps to control stress or restricting cholesterol intake), practice was defined in terms of

always engaging in the behavior (taking steps to control stress) or trying a lot (restricting cholesterol intake). The 1996 percentages of the adult population practicing these 21 major health-promoting behaviors are given in Table 14.2.[6]

A detailed description of the development and computation of the Prevention Index and related analyses is presented in the technical report, "The Prevention Index: A Report Card on the Nation's Health," available from *Prevention Magazine*. You can score your own prevention profile by taking the test provided in Figure 14.3.

Quackery and Fraud

The rapid growth in fitness and wellness programs during the last three decades has spurred the promotion of fraudulent products that deceive consumers into "miraculous," quick, and easy ways toward

Table 14.2 *1996 Prevention Index Results*

Health-Promoting Behavior	% of Adults Practicing
1. Annual blood pressure test	85
2. Annual dental exam	75
3. Limit sodium in the diet	48
4. Limit fat in the diet	52
5. Consume adequate fiber	57
6. Limit cholesterol in the diet	45
7. Adequate vitamins/minerals	58
8. Limit sugar in the diet	37
9. Maintain proper weight	19
10. Frequent strenuous exercise	40
11. Do not smoke	72
12. Control stress	69
13. Sleep 7–8 hours per night	59
14. Socialize regularly	83
15. Drink alcohol moderately	90
16. Wear seat belts	73
17. Obey speed limit	48
18. Avoid driving after drinking	84
19. Smoke detector in home	93
20. Avoid smoking in bed	92
21. Avoid home accidents	80
Average	**65**

Data from Consumers' Survey conducted for *Prevention Magazine* by Louis Harris & Associates. *Summary Report — The Prevention Index 1996: A Report Card on the Nation's Health* (Emmaus, PA: *Prevention Magazine*, 1996).

total well-being. Quackery and fraud have been defined as the *conscious promotion of unproven claims for profit*.

Today's market is saturated with "special" foods, diets, supplements, pills, cures, equipment, books, and videos that promise quick, dramatic results. Advertisements for these products often are based on testimonials, unproven claims, secret research, half-truths, and quick-fix statements that the uneducated consumer wants to hear. In the meantime, the organization or enterprise making the claims stands to make a large profit from the consumers' willingness to pay for astonishing and spectacular solutions to problems related to their unhealthy lifestyle.

Television, magazine, and newspaper advertisements are not necessarily reliable. For instance, one piece of equipment sold through television and newspaper advertisements promised to "bust the gut" through 5 minutes of daily exercise that appeared to target the abdominal muscle group. This piece of equipment consisted of a metal spring attached to the feet on one end and held in the hands on the other end. According to handling and shipping distributors, the equipment was "selling like hotcakes," and companies could barely keep up with the consumer's demands.

> Quick-fix, miraculous, special, secret, mail orders only, money-back guarantee, and testimonials often are used in advertisements of fraudulent promotions.

Three problems became apparent to the educated consumer. First, there is no such thing as spot-reducing; therefore, the claims could not be true. Second, 5 minutes of daily exercise burn hardly any calories and, therefore, have no effect on weight loss. Third, the intended abdominal (gut) muscles were not really involved during the exercise. The exercise engaged mostly the gluteal and lower back muscles. This piece of equipment now can be found at garage sales for about a tenth of its original cost!

Although people in the United States tend to be firm believers in the benefits of physical activity and positive lifestyle habits as a means to promote better health, most do not reap these benefits because they simply do not know how to put into practice a sound fitness and wellness program that will give

them the results they want. Unfortunately, many uneducated wellness consumers are targets of deception by organizations making fraudulent claims for their products.*

Even though deceit is all around us, we can protect ourselves from consumer fraud. The first step, of course, is education. You have to be an informed consumer of the product you intend to purchase. If you do not have or cannot find the answers, seek the advice of a reputable professional. Ask someone who understands the product but does not stand to profit from the transaction. As examples, a physical educator or an exercise physiologist can advise you regarding exercise equipment; a registered dietitian can provide information on nutrition and weight control programs; a physician can offer advice on nutritive supplements. Also, be alert to those who bill themselves as "experts." Look for qualifications degrees, professional experience, certifications, reputation.

Another clue to possible fraud is that if it sounds too good to be true, it probably is. Quick-fix, miraculous, special, secret, mail orders only, money-back guarantee, and testimonials often are heard in advertisements of fraudulent promotions. When claims are made, ask where the claims are published. Newspapers, magazines, and trade books are apt to be unreliable sources of information. Refereed scientific journals are the most reliable sources of information. When a researcher submits information for publication in a refereed journal, at least two qualified and reputable professionals in the field conduct blind reviews of the manuscript. A blind review means the author does not know who will review the manuscript and the reviewers do not know who submitted the manuscript. Acceptance for publication is based on this input and relevant changes.

● Health/Fitness Club Memberships

As you follow a lifetime wellness program, you may want to consider joining a health/fitness facility. Or, if you have mastered the contents of this book and your choice of fitness activity is one you can pursue on your own (walking, jogging, cycling), you may

---

*If you have questions or concerns about a health product, you may write to the National Council Against Health Fraud (NCAHF), P. O. Box 1276, Loma Linda, CA 92354. The purpose of this organization is to monitor deceitful advertising, investigate complaints, and offer the public information regarding fraudulent health claims.

THE PREVENTION INDEX

Please carefully check "YES" or "NO" to each of the following questions.

Yes   No

☐ ☐ 1   Do you have a blood pressure reading at least once a year?

☐ ☐ 2. Do you go to the dentist at least once a year for treatment or a checkup?

☐ ☐ 3. Do you avoid eating too much salt or sodium?

☐ ☐ 4. Do you avoid eating too much fat?

☐ ☐ 5. Do you eat enough fiber from whole grains, cereals, fruits, and vegetables?

☐ ☐ 6. Do you avoid eating too many high cholesterol foods, such as eggs, dairy products, and fatty meats?

☐ ☐ 7. Do you get enough vitamins and minerals in your diet?

☐ ☐ 8. Do you avoid getting too much sugar and sweet food?

☐ ☐ 9. Is your body weight within the recommended range for your sex, height, and bone structure?

☐ ☐ 10. Do you exercise strenuously (that is, so you breathe heavily and your heart and pulse rate are accelerated for a period lasting at least 20 minutes) 3 days or more a week?

☐ ☐ 11. Do you smoke cigarettes now?

☐ ☐ 12. Do you consciously take steps to control or reduce stress in your life?

☐ ☐ 13. Do you usually sleep a total of 7 to 8 hours during each 24-hour day? (If you usually sleep either more or less than this, please mark "no.")

☐ ☐ 14. Do you socialize with close friends, relatives, or neighbors at least once a week?

☐ ☐ 15. In general, when you drink alcoholic beverages, do you consume fewer than 14 drinks per week and fewer than two on any single day? (Mark "yes" only if the answer to both parts of this question is "yes." If you never drink at all, also mark "yes." A "drink" means a drink with a shot of hard liquor, a can or bottle of beer, or a glass of wine.)

☐ ☐ 16. Do you wear a seat belt all the time when you are in the front seat of a car?

☐ ☐ 17. Do you drive at or below the speed limit all the time? (If you don't drive, please mark "yes.")

☐ ☐ 18. Do you ever drive after drinking? (If you don't drink, please mark "no.")

☐ ☐ 19. Do you have a smoke detector in your home?

☐ ☐ 20. Does anyone in your household smoke in bed?

☐ ☐ 21. Do you take any special steps or precautions to avoid accidents in and around your home?

Interpreting The Prevention Index (PI)

The correct answer for questions 11, 18, and 20 is "no." The correct answer for all other questions is "yes." Add up your total number of correct responses. Then divide that number by 21 to obtain the percentage of the 21 Prevention Index behaviors that you practice.

$$\text{PI} = \frac{\text{Number of correct answers}}{21} = \frac{}{21} = \boxed{}$$

RATINGS

Prevention Index	Category
90>	Excellent
70–89	Good
60–69	Average
<59	Poor

Figure 14.3 • *Index to disease and accident prevention.*

not need to join a health club. Barring injuries, you may continue your exercise program outside the walls of a health club for the rest of your life. You also can conduct strength training and stretching programs within the walls of your own home (see Chapters 4 and 5).

To stay up to date on fitness and wellness developments, you probably should buy a reputable and updated fitness/wellness book every 4 to 5 years. You also might subscribe to a credible health, fitness, nutrition, or wellness newsletter (see Table 14.3) to stay current.

If you are contemplating membership in a fitness facility:

● Examine all exercise options in your community: health clubs/spas, YMCAs, gyms, colleges, schools, community centers, senior centers, and the like.

● Check to see if the facility's atmosphere is pleasurable and nonthreatening to you. Will you feel comfortable with the instructors and other people who go there? Is it clean and well kept up? If the answer is no, this may not be the right place for you.

● Analyze costs versus facilities, equipment, and programs. Take a look at your personal budget. Will you really use the facility? Will you exercise there regularly? Many people obtain memberships and permit dues to be withdrawn automatically from a local bank account, yet seldom attend the fitness center.

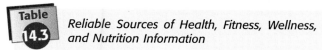

Table 14.3 Reliable Sources of Health, Fitness, Wellness, and Nutrition Information

Newsletter	Yearly Issues	Approx. Annual Cost
Consumer Reports Health Letter P.O. Box 56356 Boulder, CO 80323–2148	12	$24
Executive Health's Good Health Report P.O. Box 8880 Chapel Hill, NC 27515	12	$34
Tufts University Diet & Nutrition Letter P.O. Box 57857 Boulder, CO 80322–7857	12	$20
University of California Berkeley *Wellness Letter* P.O. Box 420148 Palm Coast, FL 32142	12	$20

● Find out what types of facilities are available: running track, basketball/tennis/racquetball courts, aerobic exercise room, strength training room, pool, locker rooms, saunas, hot tubs, handicapped access, and so on.

● Check the aerobic and strength training equipment available. Does the facility have treadmills, bicycle ergometers, Stair Masters, cross-country skiing simulators, free weights, Universal Gym, Nautilus? Make sure the facilities and equipment meet your activity interests.

● Consider the location. Is the facility close, or do you have to travel several miles to get there? Distance often discourages participation.

● Check on times the facility is accessible. Is it open during your preferred exercise time (for example, early morning or late evening)?

● Work out at the facility several times before becoming a member. Are people standing in line to use the equipment, or is it readily available during your exercise time?

● Inquire about the instructors' qualifications. Do the fitness instructors have college degrees or professional certifications from organizations such as the American College of Sports Medicine (ACSM) or the International Dance Exercise Association (IDEA)? These organizations have rigorous standards to ensure professional preparation and quality of instruction.

● Consider the approach to fitness (including all health-related components of fitness). Is it well-rounded? Do the instructors spend time with members, or do members have to seek them out constantly for help and instruction?

● Ask about supplementary services. Does the facility provide or contract out for regular health and fitness assessments (cardiovascular endurance, body composition, blood pressure, blood chemistry analysis)? Are wellness seminars (nutrition, weight control, stress management) offered? Do these have hidden costs?

● Purchasing Exercise Equipment

A final consideration is that of purchasing your own exercise equipment. The first question you need to ask yourself is: Do I really need this piece of equipment? Most people buy on impulse because of television advertisements or because a salesperson convinced them it is a great piece of equipment that will do wonders for their health and fitness. With some creativity, you can implement an excellent and comprehensive exercise program with little, if any, equipment (see Chapters 3, 4, and 5).

Many people buy expensive equipment only to find they really do not enjoy that mode of activity. They do not remain regular users. Stationary bicycles (lower body only) and rowing ergometers were among the most popular pieces of equipment in the 1980s. Most of them now are seldom used and have become "fitness furniture" somewhere in the basement.

Exercise equipment does have its value for people who prefer to exercise indoors, especially during the winter months. It supports some people's motivation and adherence to exercise. The convenience of having equipment at home also allows for flexible scheduling. You can exercise before or after work or while you watch your favorite television show.

If you are going to purchase equipment, the best recommendation is to actually try it out several times before buying it. Ask yourself several questions: Did you enjoy the workout? Is the unit comfortable? Are you too short, tall, or heavy for it? Is it stable, sturdy, and strong? Do you have to assemble the machine? If so, how difficult is it to put together? How durable is it? Ask for references — people or clubs that have used the equipment extensively. Are they satisfied? Have they enjoyed the activity (the equipment)? Talk with professionals at colleges, sportsmedicine clinics, or health clubs.

Another consideration is to look at used units for signs of wear and tear. Quality is important. Cheaper brands may not be durable, so your investment would be wasted.

Finally, watch out for expensive gadgets. Monitors that provide exercise heart rate, work output, caloric expenditure, speed, grade, and distance may help motivate you, but they are expensive, need repairs, and do not enhance the actual fitness benefits of the workout. Look at maintenance costs and check for service personnel in your community.

● The Future

The main objective of this book is to provide the information and experiences necessary to implement your personal fitness and wellness program. If you have implemented the programs in this book, including exercise, you should be convinced that a wellness lifestyle is the only way to attain a higher quality of life.

Most people who engage in a personal fitness and wellness program experience this new quality of life after only a few weeks of training and practicing healthy lifestyle patterns. In some cases, however, especially individuals who have led a poor lifestyle for a long time, a few months may be required to establish positive habits and feelings of well-being. In the end, though, everyone who applies the principles of fitness and wellness will reap the desired benefits.

Self-Evaluation

Throughout this course you may have had an opportunity to assess various fitness and wellness components and write behavioral objectives to improve your quality of life. You now should take the time to evaluate how well you have achieved your own objectives. First of all, assess how well you accomplished your goals for the five dimensions of wellness. Use the form provided in Figure 1.23 in Chapter 1. Second, if time allows and facilities and technicians are available, reassess the health-related components of physical fitness. If you are unable to reassess these components, determine subjectively how well you accomplished your objectives. You will find a self-evaluation form in Figure A.1 of Appendix A.

Behavioral Objectives for the Future

The real challenge will come now that you are about to finish this course: a lifetime commitment to fitness and wellness. Adhering to a program in a structured setting is a lot easier, but from now on you will be on your own. Realizing that you may not have achieved all of your objectives during this course, or perhaps you need to reach beyond your current achievements, a final assignment will help you chart the future. You can do this by referring to the Wellness Scale provided in Figure 14.4. This guide provides a list of various wellness components, each illustrating a scale from poor to excellent. Using the Wellness Scale, rate yourself for each component according to the following instructions:

1. Indicate with an "I" (I = Initial) the category from poor to excellent where you stood on each

Name:_____ Course:_____ Section: _____ Date:_____

Wellness Components	Wellness Rating				
	Poor	Fair	Average	Good	Excellent
Cardiorespiratory Endurance					
Muscular Strength/Endurance					
Muscular Flexibility					
Body Composition					
Nutrition					
Cardiovascular Disease Prevention					
Cancer Prevention					
Stress Control					
Tobacco Use					
Substance Abuse Control*					
Sexuality*					
Accident Prevention and Personal Safety					
Spirituality*					
Health Education					

*These components are personal, and you are not required to reveal this information. If you think that counseling is necessary, you are encouraged to seek professional help.

Figure 14.4 ● *Wellness Scale.*

component at the beginning of the semester. For example, if at the start of this course, you rated poor in cardiorespiratory endurance, place an "I" under the poor column for this component.

2. Mark with a "C" (C = Current) a second column (between poor and excellent) to indicate where you stand on each component at the current time. If your level of cardiorespiratory endurance improved to average by the end of the semester, write a "C" under this column. If you were not able to work on a given component, simply make a "C" out of the "I."

3. Select one or two components you intend to work on in the next 2 months. Developing new behavioral patterns takes time, and trying to work on too many components at once most likely will lower your chances for success. Start with components in which you think you will have a high chance for success.

   Next, place a "G" (G = Goal) under the Intended Objectives column to accomplish by the end of this period. If your goal in the next 2 months is to achieve a "good" level of cardiorespiratory endurance, place a "G" under the good column for this component in the Wellness Scale.

After you have completed the previous exercise, use Figure 14.5 to write behavioral objectives for the two components you intend to work on during the next 2 months. As you write and work on these objectives, keep in mind the following guidelines:

1. **Set both general and specific objectives.** The general objective is the ultimate goal you intend to achieve. The specific objectives are the steps required to reach this general objective. For example, a general objective might be to achieve recommended body weight. Several specific objectives could be to: (a) lose an average of one pound (or one fat percentage point) per week, (b) monitor body weight before breakfast every morning, (c) assess body composition every two weeks, (d) limit fat intake to less than 30% of total calories, (e) eliminate all pastries from the diet during this time, and (f) exercise in the proper target zone for 40 minutes, five times per week.

2. **Whenever possible, set objectives (general and specific) that are measurable.** For example, "to lose weight" is not measurable. In the previous general objective, recommended body weight

implies lowering your body weight (fat) to the recommended percent body fat standards given in Chapter 6. If this person is a 19-year-old female, the high fitness recommended fat percent would be in the range of 17% to 27%.

   To be more descriptive, the general objective could be reworded as: Reduce body weight to 22% body fat. The sample specific objectives given in Item 1 also are measurable. For instance, you can figure out easily whether you are losing a pound (a percentage point) per week. You could conduct a nutrient analysis to assess the average fat intake, or you can monitor your weekly exercise sessions to make sure you are meeting this specific objective.

3. **Make objectives realistic.** If you currently weigh 170 pounds and your target weight at 22% is 120 pounds, implementing a weight loss program to lose 50 pounds in 2 months would be unsound if not impossible. This program would not allow implementation of adequate behavior modification techniques and ensure weight maintenance at the target weight.

4. **Write either short-term or long-term objectives.** If the general objective is to attain recommended body weight and you are 50 pounds overweight, setting a general short-term objective of losing 10 pounds and writing specific objectives to accomplish this goal is best. Then the task will not seem as overwhelming and will be easier to do.

5. **Set a specific date to achieve your objective.** To simply state "I will lose weight" is not time-specific. It is much easier to work toward a deadline.

6. **Educate yourself about the objective you plan to work on.** You cannot lose weight if you do not know the principles governing weight loss and maintenance. This is the reason only three in 10 individuals achieve the target weight loss and only one in those three is able to keep it off thereafter.

7. **Think positive, and reward yourself for your accomplishments.** As difficult as some tasks may seem, where there's a will, there's a way. If you prepare a plan of action according to these guidelines, you should be able to achieve your objective. Reward yourself for your accomplishments. Buy yourself new clothing, exercise shoes,

BEHAVIORAL OBJECTIVES

Select two components from the Wellness Scale and write general objectives to achieve in 2 months. Then write the specific objectives that will lead to accomplishment of the general objectives.

General Objective: _____

Specific Objectives: _____

1. _____
2. _____
3. _____
4. _____
5. _____
6. _____
7. _____
8. _____

General Objective: _____

Specific Objectives: _____

1. _____
2. _____
3. _____
4. _____
5. _____
6. _____
7. _____
8. _____

Figure 14.5 • *Behavioral objectives for the future.*

or something special you have wanted for some time.

8. **Seek support from those around you.** Losing weight is difficult if you share meal planning and cooking with a roommate who enjoys foods that are high in fat and sweets. It can be even worse if the roommate also has a weight problem and does not desire or have the willpower to lose weight. Surround yourself with people who will help and encourage you along the way. If necessary, plan and prepare your own meals.

9. **Recognize that you will face obstacles and make mistakes.** Making mistakes is human and does not mean failure. Failure comes only to those who give up. Use your mistakes and learn from them by creating a plan that will help you get around self-defeating behaviors in the future.

10. **Monitor your progress regularly.** You will not always be meeting the specific objectives. If you are not, you will need to evaluate your objectives and perhaps make changes in the general or the specific objectives, or both. People are different, and you may not be able to progress as fast as someone else. Be flexible with yourself, and reconsider your plan of action.

● Fitness/Wellness Challenge for the Future

Throughout this book you have been provided with comprehensive guidelines to implement a healthy lifestyle program. Implementing such a program will allow you to enjoy a healthier, longer, and better life. Though most of the factors that lead to disease and illness are within our control, some are genetically or environmentally related. Your first challenge, therefore, is to follow these guidelines to help you prevent disease.

The process of change is never easy. Lifestyle behaviors are developed over many years. For most, to improve functional capacity and quality of life requires change in behaviors, which takes time and an ongoing, conscious effort.

For instance, for someone who has not been on a regular aerobic program, the process of starting and adhering to exercise requires knowledge (exercise prescription guidelines), commitment, support, action, and perseverance. Although health and self-esteem benefits can be reaped immediately upon the start of exercise, considerable improvements in fitness may take months or longer.

Prior to her marriage a young lady who never had been on a jogging program became convinced that aerobic exercise would improve her fitness and help her maintain recommended body weight. Her fiancé believed in fitness and had been jogging regularly for several years. An exercise prescription was written, and they started jogging together.

Exercise helped accomplish her goals through her first two pregnancies. The feeling of being physically fit was a reward in itself, but being able to jog 2 consecutive miles was seldom truly enjoyable. With young children at home, the couple was forced to take turns jogging so that one always could be home. Her jogging program consisted of a 20-minute jog: 1 mile out and 1 mile back.

One day 25 minutes went by and she had not returned home. At 30 minutes, there was a knock on the door: "Honey, I feel great, I'll be back in 10 minutes." This same event was repeated at 40 and 50 minutes. That young lady had jogged for a full 60 minutes for the first time in her life, and the experience was genuinely joyful. That day, this lady finally reached "the top of the mountain" and experienced the joy of being physically fit. Jogging became as easy as a "bird in flight." She has not stopped jogging in more than 20 years! It wasn't easy at first, but knowledge, commitment, support, action, and perseverance paid off.

Fitness and healthy lifestyle habits lead to improved health, quality of life, and wellness.

Fitness also was the factor that led to improvements in other wellness components in the lives of this couple (continuing health education, proper nutrition, stress reduction, and chronic disease prevention). Fitness is the daily "bread and butter" that enhances their quality of life. Their children now also follow the parents' active lifestyle. This has prompted the parents to say: "The family that exercises together stays together."

Perhaps the new quality of life that fitness provided was explained best by the late Dr. George Sheehan, cardiologist, avid runner, and health and fitness promoter, when he wrote:

> For every runner who tours the world running marathons, there are thousands who run to hear the leaves and listen to the rain, and look to the day when it is all suddenly as easy as a "bird in flight." For them, sport is not a test but a therapy, not a trial but a reward, not a question but an answer.[7]

If you have read and successfully completed all of the assignments set out in this book, including a regular exercise program, you should be convinced of the value of exercise and healthy lifestyle habits in helping achieve a new quality of life.

The real challenge will come now: a lifetime commitment to fitness and wellness. To make the commitment easier, enjoy yourself and have fun along the way. Implement your program based on your interests and what you enjoy doing most. Then, adhering to your new lifestyle will not be difficult.

Your activities over the last few weeks or months may have helped you develop positive "addictions" that will carry on throughout life. If you truly experience the feelings Dr. Sheehan expressed, there will be no looking back. If you don't get there, you won't know what it's like. Fitness and wellness is a process, and you need to put forth a constant and deliberate effort to achieve and maintain a higher quality of life. Improving the quality of your life, and most likely your longevity, is in your hands. Only you can take control of your lifestyle and thereby reap the benefits of wellness.

Notes

1. E. R. Growald and A. Lusks. "Beyond Self," *American Health,* March 1988, pp. 51-53.
2. Growald and Lusks.
3. W. Osness, M. Adrian, B. Clark, W. W. K. Hoeger, D. Raab, and R. Wiswell. "The AAHPERD Fitness Task Force, History and Philosophy," *Journal of Physical Education, Recreation and Dance* 60:3 (1989), 64-65.
4. F. W. Kash, J. L. Boyer, S. P. Van Camp, L. S. Verity, and J. P. Wallace. "The Effect of Physical Activity on Aerobic Power in Older Men (A Longitudinal Study)," *The Physician and Sports Medicine,* 18:4 (1990), 73–83.
5. W. S. Evans. "Exercise, Nutrition and Aging," *Journal of Nutrition,* 122 (1992), 796–801.
6. Prevention Magazine. *The Prevention Index 1996: A Report Card on the Nation's Health* (Emmaus, PA: Prevention Magazine, 1996).
7. Human Relations Media, "What is Fitness?" *Dynamics of Fitness: The Body in Action* (Pleasantville, NY: Author, 1980).

Suggested Readings

Clark, B., W. Osness, W. W. K. Hoeger, M. Adrian, D. Raab, and R. Wiswell. "Tests for Fitness in Older Adults: AAHPERD Fitness Task Force." *Journal of Physical Education, Recreation, and Dance* 60:3 (1989), 66-71. A copy of the battery of tests can be obtained from AAHPERD.

Food and Drug Administration (FDA). "Foods, Drugs or Frauds." *FDA Consumer,* May 1985.

Hafen, B. Q., and W. W. K. Hoeger. *Wellness: Guidelines for a healthy Lifestyle.* Englewood, CO: Morton Publishing, 1998.

Hagberg, J. M., J. E. Graves, and M. Limacher et al. "Cardiovascular Responses of 70–79 Year Old Men and Women to Exercise Training." *Journal of Applied Physiology,* 66 (1989), 2589-2594.

Health Quackery. *Consumer Reports Books.* Mount Vernon, NY: Consumer's Union, 1980.

Hoeger, W. W. K., and S. A. Hoeger. *Principles and Labs for Physical Fitness and Wellness.* Englewood, CO: Morton Publishing, 1997.

Levy, M., and J. Shafran. *Gym Psych: The Insider's Guide to Health Clubs.* New York: Fawcett Columbine, 1986.

Physical Fitness and Wellness Profile

Fill out the following profile as you obtain the results for each fitness and wellness component. Attempt to determine the fitness components (cardio-respiratory endurance, muscular strength/endurance, muscular flexibility, and body composition) during the first two or three weeks so you may proceed with your exercise program. After determining each component, discuss with your instructor the objectives to be accomplished and the date of completion.

Name: _____   Course: _____   Section: _____

| Item | Pre-Assessment | | | Objective[a] | Post-Assessment | | |
	Date	Test Results	Classification		Date	Test Results	Classification
Cardiorespiratory Endurance							
Muscular Strength							
Muscular Flexibility							
Body Composition							
Cardiovascular Risk							
Cancer Risk							
Lung							
Colon-Rectum							
Skin							
Breast[b]							
Cervical[b]							
Endometrial[b]							
Prostate[c]							
Testicular[c]							
Pancreatic							
Kidney & Bladder							
Esophageal & Stomach							
Ovarian[b]							
Thyroid							
Leukemia							
Lymphomas							
Stress							
Life Exp. Survey							
Vulnerability Scale							
Tobacco Use[d]							

Instructor's Signature: _____

Student's Signature: _____

[a] Indicate specific objective and date of completion.
[b] Women only
[c] Men only
[d] For test results indicate type and amount smoked; for classification indicate smoker, ex-smoker, nonsmoker.

Figure A.1 • *Personal Fitness and Wellness Profile.*

Nutritive Value of Selected Foods

Code	Food	Amount	Weight gm	Calories	Protein gm	Fat gm	Sat. Fat gm	Cholesterol mg	Carbohydrate gm	Calcium mg	Iron mg	Sodium mg	Vit A I.U.	Thiamin (Vit B₁) mg	Riboflavin (Vit B₂) mg	Niacin mg	Vit C mg
1.	Almond Joy, candy bar	1.5 oz.	42	227	2.5	12	10.2	0	28	3	1.2	0	0	0.00	0.00	0.0	0
2.	Almonds, shelled	1/4 c	36	213	6.6	19	1.4	0	9	83	1.7	2	0	0.09	0.33	1.3	0
3.	Apple, raw, unpared	1 med	150	80	0.3	1	0.0	0	20	10	0.4	1	120	0.04	0.03	0.1	6
4.	Apple juice, canned or bottled	1/2 c	124	59	0.1	0	0.0	0	15	8	0.7	1	0	0.01	0.03	0.1	1
5.	Apple Pie, McDonald's	1	307	260	2	15	10.0	6	30	8	0.48	240	0	0.06			
6.	Applesauce, canned, sweetened	1/2 c	128	116	0.3	0	0.0	0	31	5	0.7	3	50	0.02	0.01	0.0	2
7.	Apricots, canned, heavy syrup	3 halves; 1 3/4 tbsp. liq.	85	73	0.5	0	0.0	0	19	9	0.3	1	1,480	0.02	0.02	0.3	3
8.	Apricots, dried, sulfured, uncooked	10 med halves	35	91	1.8	0	0.0	0	23	23	1.9	9	3,820	0.00	0.06	1.2	4
9.	Apricots, raw	3 (12 per lb)	114	55	1.1	0	0.0	0	14	18	0.5	1	2,890	0.06	0.04	0.6	11
10.	Arby Q, Arby's	1	190	389	18	15	5.5	29	48	84	6.1	1,268	0	0.27	0.41	9.2	0
11.	Arby Sauce, Arby's	.5 oz.	14	15	0	0	0.0	0	3	0	0.2	113	1	0.00	0.00	0.0	16
12.	Asparagus, cooked green spears	4 med	60	12	1.3	0	0.0	0	2	13	0.4	1	540	0.10	0.11	0.8	15
13.	Avocado, raw	1/2 med	120	185	2.4	19	3.2	0	7	11	0.6	4	310	0.12	0.22	1.7	12
14.	Bacon, cooked, drained	2 slices	15	86	3.8	8	2.7	30	1	2	0.5	153	0	0.08	0.05	0.8	0
15.	Bacon, lettuce, tomato sandwich	1	130	327	11.6	19	4.7	21	31	84	2.5	661	426	0.42	0.28	4.1	10
16.	Bagel	1 3 1/2 in.	68	180	7.0	0	0.2	0	35	20	2.1	124	0	0.26	0.20	2.4	1
17.	Banana, raw	1 sm (7 1/4")	140	81	1.0	0	0.0	0	21	8	0.7	1	180	0.05	0.06	0.7	10
18.	Banana, nut bread	1 slice	50	169	3.0	8	1.5	33	22	18	0.9	172	49	0.09	0.09	0.8	1
19.	BBQ Sauce, McDonald's	1.12 oz.	32	50	0	0.6	0.2	0	12	0.0	0.0	350	200	0.00	0.00	0.0	2.4
20.	Beans, green snap, cooked	1/2 c	65	16	1.0	0	0.0	0	3	32	0.4	4	340	0.05	0.06	0.3	8
21.	Beans, lentils	1/4 c	50	53	3.9	0	0.0	0	10	12	1.0	0	10	0.03	0.04	0.4	8
22.	Beans, lima (Fordhook), froz., cooked	1/2 c	85	84	6.0	0	0.0	0	17	40	2.1	1	240	0.15	0.08	1.1	15
23.	Beans, red kidney, cooked	1 c	185	218	14.4	1	0.0	0	40	70	4.4	6	10	0.20	0.11	1.3	0
24.	Beans, refried	1/2 c	145	148	9.0	1	0.2	0	25	71	2.6	614	0	0.07	0.08	0.7	9
25.	Bean sprouts, mung, raw	1/2 c	52	18	2.0	0	0.0	0	4	10	0.7	3	10	0.07	0.07	0.4	10
26.	Beef, chuck, cooked	3 oz.	85	212	25.0	12	7.8	80	0	11	3.1	43	20	0.05	0.19	3.8	0
27.	Beef, corned, canned	3 oz.	85	163	21.0	10	8.0	70	0	22	5.0	802	0	0.02	0.27	3.9	0
28.	Beef, ground, lean	3 oz.	85	186	23.3	10	5.0	81	0	10	3.0	57	20	0.08	0.20	5.1	0
29.	Beef, lite roast deluxe, Arby's	1	182	294	18	10	3.5	42	33	156	3.0	826	200	0.27	0.52	8.4	8
30.	Beef, meatloaf	1 piece	111	246	20.0	15	6.1	125	6	37	2.4	434	181	0.08	0.23	4.1	1
491.	Beef, meatloaf, traditional Healthy Choice	1	340	320	16.0	8	4.0	35	46	40	1.8	460	750	0.00	0.00	0.0	54
31.	Beef N' Cheddar, Arby's	1	194	508	25	27	7.7	52	43	180	4.1	1,166	0	0.42	0.67	9.8	1
32.	Beef, round steak, cooked, trimmed	3 oz.	85	222	24.3	13	6.0	77	0	10	3.0	60	20	0.07	0.20	4.8	0
33.	Beef, rump roast	3 oz.	85	177	24.7	9	4.0	80	0	10	3.1	61	10	0.06	0.19	4.4	0
34.	Beef, sirloin, cooked	3 oz.	85	329	19.6	27	13.0	77	0	9	2.5	48	50	0.05	0.15	4.0	0
493.	Beef, sirloin tips, Healthy Choice	1	334	280	23.0	8	0.0	65	30	20	2.7	370	3,500	0.15	0.17	5.0	42
500.	Beef stroganoff, Weight Watchers	1	238	290	22.0	9	4.0	25	26	8	2.7	600	300	0.23	0.26	4.0	4
35.	Beef, T-bone steak	3 oz.	85	403	16.7	37	15.6	66	0	7	2.2	40	23	0.07	0.14	3.5	0
36.	Beef, thin, sliced	3 oz.	85	105	18.5	3	1.4	36	0	11	1.8	1,409	0	0.01	0.16	4.5	0
37.	Beer	12 fl. oz.	360	151	1.1	0	1.1	0	14	18	0.0	25	0	0.01	0.11	2.2	0
38.	Beer, light	12 fl. oz.	354	96	0.7	0	0.0	0	4	17	0.1	10	0	0.03	0.10	1.3	0
39.	Beets, red, canned, drained	1/2 c	80	32	0.8	0	0.0	0	8	15	0.6	164	15	0.01	0.02	0.1	2
40.	Beet greens, cooked	1/2 c	73	13	1.3	0	0.0	0	2	72	1.4	55	3,700	0.05	0.11	0.2	11
41.	Biscuits, baking powder	1 med	35	114	2.5	6	1.1	0	18	60	0.8	272	0	0.06	0.06	0.7	0
42.	Blueberries, fresh cultivated	1/2 c	73	45	0.5	0	0.0	0	11	10	0.8	1	75	0.02	0.05	0.4	10
43.	Bologna	1 slice (1 oz.)	28	86	3.4	8	3.0	15	1	2	0.5	369	0	0.05	0.06	0.7	0
44.	Bologna, turkey	2 slices	57	113	7.8	9	3.0	56	1	47	0.9	498	0	0.03	0.09	2.1	0
45.	Bouillon, broth	1 cube	4	5	0.8	0	0.0	0	0	0	0.0	960	0	0.00	0.00	0.0	0
46.	Brandy	1 oz.	28	69	0.0	0	0.0	0	0	0	0.0	1	0	0.00	0.00	0.0	0
47.	Bread, corn	1 slice	78	161	5.8	6	0.1	0	23	94	0.9	490	120	0.10	0.15	0.5	1
48.	Bread, cracked wheat	1 slice	25	65	2.3	1	0.2	0	12	16	0.7	106	0	0.10	0.10	0.8	0

Code	Food	Amount	Weight gm	Calories	Protein gm	Fat gm	Sat. Fat gm	Cholesterol mg	Carbohydrate gm	Calcium mg	Iron mg	Sodium mg	Vit A I.U.	Thiamin (Vit B_1) mg	Riboflavin (Vit B_2) mg	Niacin mg	Vit C mg
49.	Bread, French enriched	1 slice	35	102	3.2	1	0.2	0	19	15	0.8	203	0	0.10	0.08	0.9	0
50.	Bread, oatmeal	1 slice	25	65	2.1	1	0.2	0	12	15	0.7	124	0	0.12	0.07	0.9	0
51.	Bread, pita pocket	1 piece	60	165	6.2	1	0.1	0	33	49	1.5	339	0	0.27	0.13	2.3	0
52.	Bread, pumpernickel	1 slice	32	80	2.9	1	0.2	0	15	23	0.9	277	0	0.11	0.17	1.1	0
53.	Bread, rye (American)	1 slice	25	61	2.3	0	0.0	0	13	19	0.4	139	0	0.05	0.02	0.4	0
54.	Bread, white enriched	1 slice	25	68	2.2	1	0.2	0	13	21	0.6	127	0	0.06	0.05	0.6	0
55.	Bread, whole wheat	1 slice	25	61	2.6	1	0.6	0	12	25	0.8	132	0	0.06	0.03	0.7	0
56.	Broccoli, cooked drained	1 sm stalk	140	36	4.3	0	0.0	0	6	123	1.1	14	3,500	0.13	0.28	1.1	126
57.	Broccoli, raw	1 sm stalk	114	38	4.1	0	0.0	0	7	117	1.3	17	2,835	0.10	0.23	0.9	125
58.	Brownies, with nuts	1	20	95	1.3	6	2.3	18	11	9	0.4	51	20	0.05	0.05	0.3	0
59.	Brussels sprouts, froz., cooked, drained	1/2 c	78	28	3.2	0	0.0	0	5	25	0.8	8	405	0.06	0.11	0.5	63
60.	Bulgur, wheat	1 c	135	227	8.4	1	0.0	0	47	27	1.8	809	0	0.07	0.04	3.2	0
61.	Burrito, bean	1	166	307	12.5	9.5	3.6	14	45	173	2.4	983	283	0.15	0.22	2.3	5
62.	Burrito, combination, Taco Bell	1	175	404	21.0	16	5.9	17	43	91	3.7	300	1,666	0.34	0.31	4.6	15
482.	Burrito, 7 layer, Taco Bell	1	234	458	14.0	20	5.9	17	55	85	2.3	983	1,485	0.00	0.00	0.0	5
483.	Burrito, 7 layer light, Taco Bell	1	276	440	19.0	9	3.5	8	67	250	4.5	1,430	1,750	0.00	0.00	0.0	5
63.	Butter	1 tsp	5	36	0.0	4	0.4	12	0	1	0.0	46	160	0.00	0.00	0.0	0
64.	Buttermilk, cultured	1 c	245	88	8.8	0	1.3	5	12	296	0.1	319	10	0.10	0.44	0.2	2
65.	Cabbage, boiled, drained wedge	1/2 c	85	16	0.9	0	0.0	0	3	36	0.3	10	100	0.02	0.02	0.1	21
66.	Cabbage, raw chopped	1/2 c	45	11	0.6	0	0.0	0	3	22	0.2	9	60	0.03	0.03	0.2	21
67.	Cake, angel food, plain	1 piece	60	161	4.3	0	0.0	0	36	5	0.1	170	0	0.01	0.08	0.1	1
68.	Cake, carrot	1 piece	96	385	4.2	21	4.1	74	48	44	1.3	279	75	0.11	0.12	0.9	4
69.	Cake, cheesecake	1 piece (3½")	85	257	4.6	16	9.0	150	24	48	0.4	189	216	0.03	0.11	0.4	0
70.	Cake, chocolate, w/icing	1 piece	69	235	3.0	8	3.6	37	40	41	1.4	181	100	0.07	0.10	0.6	0
71.	Cake, coffee	1 piece	72	230	4.5	7	2.5	47	38	44	1.2	310	120	0.14	0.15	1.3	0
72.	Cake, devil's food, iced	1 piece	99	365	4.5	16	5.0	68	55	69	1.0	233	160	0.02	0.10	0.2	0
73.	Cake, pound	1 piece	30	120	2.0	5	1.0	32	15	20	0.5	98	200	0.05	0.06	0.5	0
74.	Cake, white, choc. icing	1 piece	71	268	3.5	11	3.7	2	48	35	0.3	162	40	0.19	0.14	1.6	0
75.	Candy, hard	1 oz.	28	109	0.0	0	0.0	0	28	6	0.5	9	0	0.00	0.00	0.0	0
76.	Cantaloupe	1/4 melon 5" diam.	239	35	2.0	0	0.0	0	10	20	0.4	17	4,620	0.06	0.04	0.6	45
77.	Caramel (candy, plain or choc.)	1 oz.	28	113	1.1	3	1.6	0	22	42	0.8	64	0	0.01	0.05	0.1	0
78.	Carrots, cooked, drained	1/2 c	73	23	0.7	0	0.0	0	5	24	0.4	10	7,615	0.04	0.04	0.4	5
79.	Carrots, raw	1 carrot 7½" long	81	30	0.8	0	0.0	0	7	27	0.5	34	7,930	0.04	0.04	0.4	6
80.	Cashew, roasted, unsalted	2 oz.	57	326	9.2	27	5.4	0	16	23	2.3	10	0	0.24	0.10	1.0	0
81.	Cauliflower, cooked, drained	1/2 c	63	14	1.5	0	0.0	0	3	13	0.5	6	40	0.06	0.05	0.4	35
82.	Celery, green, raw, long	1 outer stalk 8"	40	7	0.4	0	0.0	0	2	16	0.1	50	110	0.01	0.01	0.1	4
83.	Cereal, All-Bran	1/4 c	21	53	3.0	1	0.1	0	16	17	3.4	242	947	0.28	0.33	3.8	11
84.	Cereal, Alpha Bits	1 c	28	111	2.2	1	0.0	0	25	8	1.8	219	1,875	0.40	0.40	5.0	0
85.	Cereal, Bran	1/2 c	30	72	3.8	1	0.0	0	22	25	3.0	247	2,000	1.00	0.80	3.0	0
86.	Cereal, Cheerios	1 c	23	89	3.4	2	1.2	0	16	38	3.6	246	949	0.32	0.32	4.0	20
87.	Cereal, Corn Chex	1 c	28	111	2.0	0	0.0	0	25	3	1.8	271	75	0.40	0.07	5.0	12
88.	Cereal, Corn Flakes	1 c	25	97	2.0	0	0.0	0	21	3	0.6	251	180	0.29	0.55	2.9	15
89.	Cereal, Cream of Wheat	1 c	244	140	3.6	1	0.1	0	29	54	10.9	5	0	0.24	0.07	1.5	9
90.	Cereal, Frosted Mini-Wheats	4 biscuits	31	111	3.2	0	0.0	0	26	10	2.0	9	2,050	0.40	0.50	5.5	0
91.	Cereal, Fruit & Fibre w/dates	1 c	56	180	6.0	2	0.3	0	42	20	9.0	340	3,780	0.75	0.85	10.0	16
92.	Cereal, Granola, Nature Valley	1/2 c	57	252	5.8	10	7.0	0	38	36	1.9	116	41	0.20	0.10	0.4	0
93.	Cereal, Grape Nuts	1/2 c	57	202	6.6	0	0.0	0	47	22	2.5	394	3,815	0.80	0.80	10.0	0
94.	Cereal, Life	1 c	44	162	8.1	1	0.1	0	32	154	11.6	229	0	0.95	1.00	11.6	0
95.	Cereal, Nutri-Grain Wheat	1 c	44	158	3.8	1	0.1	0	37	12	1.2	299	2,915	0.60	0.70	7.7	23
96.	Cereal, Oatmeal, quick, cooked	1/2 c	120	66	2.4	1	0.2	0	12	11	0.7	262	0	0.10	0.03	0.1	0
97.	Cereal, Raisin Bran	1 c	49	160	4.0	1	0.2	0	40	25	24.0	293	2,500	0.51	0.57	6.7	0
98.	Cereal, Rice Krispies	3/4 c	22	85	1.4	0	0.0	0	19	3	1.4	255	971	0.30	0.30	3.8	11
99.	Cereal, Shredded Wheat	1 c	19	65	2.1	0	0.0	0	11	8	0.6	1	0	0.06	0.05	0.9	0

Code	Food	Amount	Weight gm	Calories	Protein gm	Fat gm	Sat Fat gm	Cholesterol mg	Carbohydrate gm	Calcium mg	Iron mg	Sodium mg	Vit A I.U.	Thiamin (Vit B₁) mg	Riboflavin (Vit B₂) mg	Niacin mg	Vit C mg
100.	Cereal, Special K	1 c	21	83	4.2	0	0.0	0	16	6	3.4	199	1,430	0.30	0.30	3.8	11
101.	Cereal, Sugar Corn Pops	1 c	28	108	1.4	0	0.0	0	26	1	1.8	103	1,875	0.40	0.40	5.0	15
102.	Cereal, Sugar Frosted Flakes	1 c	35	133	1.8	0	0.0	0	32	1	2.2	284	2,315	0.50	0.50	6.2	19
103.	Cereal, Sugar Smacks	1 c	37	141	2.7	1	0.1	0	32	4	2.4	100	2,500	0.49	0.57	6.7	20
104.	Cereal, Total	1 c	33	116	3.3	1	0.1	0	26	56	21.0	409	8,845	1.70	2.00	23.3	70
105.	Cereal, Wheat Chex	1 c	46	169	4.5	1	0.2	0	38	18	7.3	308	0	0.60	0.17	8.1	24
106.	Cereal, whole wheat, cooked	1/2 c	123	55	2.2	0	0.0	0	12	9	0.06	260	0	0.08	0.03	0.8	0
107.	Cereal, whole wheat flakes, ready-to-eat	1 c	30	106	3.1	1	0.0	0	24	12	2.0	310	1,410	0.35	0.42	3.5	11
108.	Cereal, 40% Bran Flakes	1 c	39	125	4.9	1	0.1	0	31	19	11.2	363	2,610	0.51	0.59	6.9	0
109.	Cereal, 100% Bran	1/2 c	33	89	4.2	2	0.3	0	24	23	4.1	229	0	0.80	0.90	10.4	31
110.	Champagne	4 oz.	113	87	0.2	0	0.1	0	2	6	0.4	7	0	0.00	0.01	0.1	0
111.	Cheese, American	1 oz. slice	28	100	6.0	8	5.6	27	0	188	0.1	307	343	0.01	0.10	0.0	0
112.	Cheese, bleu	1 oz.	28	100	6.0	8	5.3	25	1	89	0.1	510	204	0.01	0.11	0.3	0
113.	Cheese, cheddar	1 oz.	28	114	7.0	9	6.0	30	0	204	0.2	171	300	0.01	0.11	0.0	0
114.	Cheese, cottage, 2%	1/2 c	113	103	15.5	2	1.4	10	4	78	0.2	459	79	0.03	0.21	0.2	0
115.	Cheese, cottage, creamed	1/2 c	105	112	14.0	5	6.4	15	3	99	0.3	241	180	0.03	0.26	0.1	0
116.	Cheese, creamed	1 oz.	28	99	6.0	8	3.0	31	1	167	0.3	71	320	0.02	0.14	0.3	0
117.	Cheese, feta	1 oz.	28	75	4.5	6	4.2	25	1	140	0.2	316	180	0.04	0.23	0.3	0
118.	Cheese, monterey jack	1 oz.	28	106	6.9	9	5.4	26	0	212	0.2	152	405	0.00	0.11	0.3	0
119.	Cheese, mozzarella, skim	1 oz.	28	80	7.6	5	3.1	15	1	207	0.1	150	216	0.01	0.10	0.0	0
120.	Cheese, parmesan	1 tbsp	5	23	2.1	2	1.0	4	0	69	0.1	93	45	0.00	0.02	0.0	0
121.	Cheese, ricotta, part skim	1 oz.	28	39	3.2	2	1.4	9	1	77	0.1	35	160	0.01	0.05	0.2	0
122.	Cheese, souffle	1 portion	110	240	10.9	19	9.5	189	7	221	1.1	400	880	0.06	0.26	0.2	0
123.	Cheese, swiss	1 oz.	28	107	8.0	8	5.0	26	1	272	0.1	74	360	0.01	0.10	0.2	0
124.	Cheese puffs, Cheetos	1 oz.	28	158	2.2	10	4.8	5	14	17	0.4	344	130	0.01	0.03	0.2	2
125.	Cheeseburger, McDonald's		115	321	15.2	16	6.7	40	29	170	2.9	736	353	0.30	0.24	4.4	41
126.	Cherries	10	75	47	0.9	0	0.0	0	12	15	0.3	8	450	0.20	0.24	1.6	5
127.	Chicken, BK Broiler sandwich, Burger King	1 sandwich	168	379	24.0	18	3.0	53	31	48	2.3	764	350	0.42	0.22	9.2	5
128.	Chicken Breast Filet, Arby's	1	204	445	22	23.0	3.0	45	52	72	1.9	958	0	0.23	0.58	9.0	5
129.	Chicken breast, roast w/skin	1	98	193	29.2	8	2.1	83	0	14	1.0	69	91	0.07	0.12	12.5	0
501.	Chicken burrito w/vegetables, Weight Watchers	1	216	330	15.0	14	4.0	65	36	56	2.3	800	190	0.52	0.39	5.9	3
484.	Chicken cacciatore, Budget Gourmet	1	312	300	20.0	13	0.0	60	27	150	1.8	810	200	0.23	0.51	5.0	21
496.	Chicken cacciatore, Lean Cuisine	1	308	280	22.0	7	2.0	45	31	40	1.4	570	500	0.22	0.17	6.0	9
130.	Chicken chow mein	1 c	250	255	31.0	11	3.6	75	10	58	2.5	718	250	0.08	0.23	4.3	10
488.	Chicken chow mein, Healthy Choice	1	241	220	18.0	3	0.8	45	31	20	1.4	440	405	0.15	0.14	4.0	4
497.	Chicken chow mein, Lean Cuisine	1	255	240	14.0	5	1.0	30	34	40	1.1	530	300	0.15	0.17	5.0	6
502.	Chicken chow mein, Weight Watchers	1	255	200	12.0	2	0.5	25	34	40	0.7	430	1,500	0.00	0.00	0.0	36
131.	Chicken club sandwich, Wendy's	1	220	520	30	25	6.0	75	44	120	9.6	980	100	0.60	0.45	16.0	9
132.	Chicken Cordon Bleu, Arby's	1	225	518	30	27	5.3	92	52	204	2.1	1,463	0	0.42	0.68	10.2	5
133.	Chicken, drumstick, Kentucky Fried	1	54	136	14.0	8	2.2	73	2	20	0.9	320	30	0.04	0.12	2.7	0
134.	Chicken, drumstick, roasted	1	52	112	14.1	6	1.6	48	0	6	0.7	47	52	0.04	0.11	3.1	0
135.	Chicken McNuggets	6	111	329	19.5	21	5.2	64	15	11	1.3	521	92	0.16	0.14	7.7	2
136.	Chicken Nuggets, Wendy's	6 pc.	94	280	14	20	5.0	50	12	48	0.48	600	0	0.09	0.11	6.0	0
137.	Chicken, patty sandwich	1	157	436	24.8	23	6.1	68	34	44	1.9	2,732	47	0.13	0.26	9.2	4
138.	Chicken, wing, Kentucky Fried	1	45	151	11.0	10	2.9	70	4	0	0.6	300	0	0.03	0.07	0.0	0
139.	Chicken, roast	3 oz.	85	141	27.0	3	0.4	45	0	10	1.2	54	51	0.03	0.09	9.9	0

Code	Food	Amount	Weight gm	Calories	Protein gm	Fat gm	Sat Fat gm	Cholesterol mg	Carbohydrate gm	Calcium mg	Iron mg	Sodium mg	Vit A I.U.	Thiamin (Vit B_1) mg	Riboflavin (Vit B_2) mg	Niacin mg	Vit C mg
140.	Chicken, roast, light meat without skin	3 oz.	85	149	24.0	5	0.8	50	0	11	1.5	54	127	0.06	0.19	4.7	0
	dark meat without skin																
141.	Chicken, Roast Deluxe, Arby's		195	276	24	7	1.7	33	33	156	1.9	777	200	0.44	0.80	9.4	7
510.	Chicken, Rotisserie, dark w/skin Kentucky Fried	1/4 chicken	146	333	30.0	24	6.6	163	1	10	0.2	980	75	0.00	0.00	0.0	1
511.	Chicken, Rotisserie, light w/skin Kentucky Fried	1/4 chicken	176	335	40.0	19	5.4	157	1	10	0.2	1,100	75	0.00	0.00	0.0	1
142.	Chicken Sandwich, breaded Wendy's		208	450	26	20	4.0	60	44	120	9.6	740	100	0.45	0.36	14.0	6
143.	Chicken Sandwich, Grilled, Wendy's		177	290	24	7	1.0	60	35	120	2.4	670	100	0.38	0.27	10.0	6
144.	Chicken Sandwich, McChicken		187	415	19	19	9.0	50	39	180	1.8	830	100	0.90	0.18	9.0	2.4
485.	Chicken, Teriyaki, Budget Gourmet		340	360	20.0	12	0.0	55	44	80	1.4	610	1,500	0.15	0.34	6.0	12
145.	Chili con carne	1 c	255	339	19.1	16	5.8	28	31	82	4.3	1,354	150	0.08	0.18	3.3	8
146.	Chocolate fudge	1 oz.	28	115	0.6	3	2.1	1	21	22	0.3	54	0	0.01	0.03	0.1	0
147.	Chocolate, milk	1 oz.	28	147	2.0	9	3.6	5	16	65	0.3	27	80	0.02	0.10	0.1	0
148.	Chocolate, milk w/almonds	1 oz.	28	150	2.9	10	4.4	5	15	61	0.6	23	30	0.03	0.13	0.3	9
149.	Clam, canned, drained	3 oz.	85	83	13.0	2	0.2	50	2	46	3.5	750	93	0.01	0.09	0.9	2
150.	Cocoa, hot, with whole milk	1 c	250	218	9.1	9	6.1	33	26	298	0.8	123	318	0.10	0.44	0.4	0
151.	Cocoa, plain, dry	1 tbsp	5	14	0.9	1	0.0	0	3	7	0.6	0	0	0.01	0.02	0.1	2
152.	Coconut, shredded, packed	1/2 c	65	225	2.3	23	20.0	0	6	8	1.1	165	0	0.03	0.01	0.3	0
153.	Cod, batter fried	3.5 oz.	100	199	19.6	10	3.9	55	8	80	0.5	100	2	0.02	0.02	1.8	0
154.	Cod, cooked	3 oz.	85	144	24.3	4	1.5	60	0	27	0.9	63	150	0.06	0.09	2.7	0
155.	Cod, poached	3.5 oz.	100	94	20.9	1	0.3	60	0	29	0.5	110	2	0.08	0.08	3.0	0
156.	Coffee	3/4 cup	180	1	0.0	0	0.0	0	0	1	0.2	2	0	0.00	0.00	0.1	0
157.	Coleslaw	1 c	120	173	1.6	17	1.0	5	6	53	0.5	144	190	0.06	0.06	0.4	35
158.	Collards, leaves without stems, cooked, drained	1/2 c	95	32	3.4	1	2.0	0	5	178	0.8	28	7,410	0.01	0.19	1.2	72
159.	Cookies, chocolate chip, homemade	2 2¼" diam.	20	103	1.0	6	1.7	14	12	7	0.4	70	20	0.02	0.02	0.2	0
160.	Cookies, fig bars	4 bars	56	210	2.0	4	1.0	27	42	40	1.4	180	31	0.08	0.07	0.7	0
161.	Cookies, oatmeal raisin	2" diam.	26	122	1.5	5	1.3	1	18	9	0.6	74	20	0.04	0.04	0.5	0
162.	Cookies, peanut butter, homemade	2 cookies	24	123	2.0	7	2.0	11	14	10	0.5	71	12	0.03	0.03	0.9	0
163.	Cookies, sandwich, all	4 cookies	40	195	2.0	8	2.0	0	29	12	1.4	189	0	0.90	0.07	0.8	0
164.	Cookies, shortbread	4 cookies	32	155	2.0	8	2.9	27	20	13	0.8	123	40	0.10	0.09	0.9	0
165.	Cookies, vanilla	5 1¾" diam.	20	93	1.0	3	0.8	10	15	8	0.1	50	25	0.00	0.01	0.0	0
166.	Cookies, vanilla wafers	10 wafers	40	185	2.0	7	1.8	25	29	16	0.8	150	70	0.07	0.10	1.0	0
167.	Corn, boiled on cob	1 ear 5" long	140	70	2.5	1	0.0	0	16	2	0.4	1	310	0.09	0.08	1.1	7
168.	Corn, canned, drained	1/2 c	83	70	2.2	1	0.0	0	16	4	0.4	195	290	0.03	0.04	0.8	4
169.	Corn chips	1 oz.	28	155	2.0	9	1.8	0	16	35	0.5	233	110	0.04	0.05	0.4	1
170.	Cornmeal, degermed, yellow, enriched, cooked	1/2 c	120	60	1.3	0	0.0	0	13	1	0.5	264	70	0.07	0.05	0.6	0
171.	Crab, canned	1 c	135	135	23.0	3	0.5	135	1	61	1.1	1,350	70	0.11	0.11	2.6	0
172.	Crackers, cheese	10 crackers	10	50	1.0	3	0.9	6	5	11	0.4	112	25	0.05	0.04	0.4	0
173.	Crackers, graham	2 squares	14	55	1.1	1	0.3	0	10	6	0.2	95	0	0.01	0.03	0.2	0
174.	Crackers, Ritz	1 cracker	3	15	0.2	1	0.2	0	2	3	0.1	30	0	0.01	0.01	0.1	0
175.	Crackers, Ryewafers, whole grain	2 crackers	14	55	1.0	1	0.3	0	10	7	0.5	115	0	0.06	0.03	0.5	0
176.	Crackers, saltines	4 squares	11	48	1.0	1	0.3	0	8	2	0.1	123	0	0.00	0.00	0.1	0
177.	Crackers, soda	1	3	13	0.3	0	0.1	0	2	1	0.1	39	0	0.02	0.01	0.1	0
178.	Crackers, Triscuits	1	5	23	0.4	1	0.3	0	3	0	0.0	0	0	0.00	0.00	0.0	0
179.	Crackers, Wheat Thins	1	2	9	0.2	0	0.1	0	1	1	0.1	17	0	0.01	0.01	0.1	0

Code	Food	Amount	Weight gm	Calories	Protein gm	Fat gm	Sat. Fat gm	Cholesterol mg	Carbohydrate gm	Calcium mg	Iron mg	Sodium mg	Vit A I.U.	Thiamin (Vit B₁) mg	Riboflavin (Vit B₂) mg	Niacin mg	Vit C mg
180.	Cranberry juice	1 c	253	145	0.1	0	0.0	0	36	8	0.4	5	5	0.02	0.02	0.1	90
181.	Cream, light coffee or table	1 tbsp	15	20	0.5	2	0.5	5	1	16	0.0	7	70	0.00	0.02	0.0	0
182.	Cream, heavy whipping	1 tbsp	15	53	0.3	6	1.3	12	1	11	0.0	5	230	0.00	0.02	0.0	0
183.	Croissant		57	235	4.7	12	4.0	13	27	20	2.1	452	50	0.17	0.13	1.3	0
184.	Croissants (Sara Lee)	1 roll	18	59	1.6	2	0.3	0	8	22	0.6	105		0.14	0.09	0.8	0
185.	Croissan'wich, egg, cheese Burger King	1 sandwich	110	315	13.0	20	7.0	222	19	112	1.8	607	500	0.22	0.37	1.4	0
186.	Cucumbers, raw pared	9 sm slices	28	4	0.3	0	0.0	0	1	7	0.3	2	70	0.01	0.01	0.1	3
187.	Danish, Apple, McDonald's	1	115	390	6	17	11.0	25	51	7	1.0	370	0	0.30	0.18	2.0	15
188.	Danish, Cinnamon Raisin	1	110	440	6	21	13.0	34	58	48	0.12	430	0	0.30	0.27	3.0	4
189.	Dates hydrated	5	46	110	0.9	0	0.0	0	29	24	1.2	1	20	0.04	0.04	0.9	0
190.	Doughnut, plain	1	42	164	1.9	8	2.0	19	22	17	0.6	210	30	0.07	0.07	0.5	0
191.	Doughnut, yeast raised	1	27	235	4.0	13	5.2	21	26	17	1.4	222	2	0.28	0.12	1.8	0
192.	Dressing, Bleu cheese	1 tbsp	15	77	0.7	8	1.9	4	1	12	0.0	8	32	0.00	0.02	0.0	0
193.	Dressing, French	1 tbsp	16	83	0.1	9	1.4	0	1	2	0.1	184	0	0.00	0.00	0.0	0
194.	Dressing, French, low cal	1 tbsp.	15	24	0.0	2	0.2	0	2	6	0.1	306	0	0.00	0.00	0.0	0
195.	Dressing, Italian	1 tbsp.	15	69	0.1	9	1.3	0	2	1	0.0	73	29	0.00	0.00	0.0	0
196.	Dressing, Italian, low cal	1 tbsp.	15	10	0.0	1	0.0	0	1	1	0.0	136	1	0.00	0.00	0.0	1
197.	Dressing, Ranch style	1 tbsp.	15	54	0.4	6	0.9	6	2	15	0.0	65	36	0.01	0.02	0.0	0
198.	Dressing, Thousand island	1 tbsp.	15	60	0.2	6	1.0	4	2	2	0.1	110	75	0.00	0.01	0.0	1
199.	Dressing, Thousand island, low cal	1 tbsp.	15	25	0.1	2	0.2	2	3	2	0.1	153	70	0.00	0.00	0.0	0
200.	Egg, hard cooked	1 large	50	72	6.0	5	1.6	212	1	24	1.0	113	520	0.05	0.13	0.0	0
201.	Egg, fried with butter		46	95	5.4	7	2.4	240	1	28	0.9	162	320	0.04	0.13	0.0	0
202.	Egg McMuffin		138	327	18.5	15	5.9	259	31	226	2.9	885	591	0.47	0.44	3.8	1
203.	Egg salad sandwich		111	325	10.0	19	3.9	215	28	95	2.5	461	242	0.29	0.29	2.1	0
204.	Egg, scrambled, with milk, butter	1 egg	64	95	6.0	7	3.0	244	0	54	0.9	176	510	0.04	0.18	0.0	0
205.	Egg, white	1 large	33	17	3.6	0	0.0	0	0	3	0.0	48	0	0.00	0.09	0.0	0
206.	Egg, yolk, raw	1 yolk	17	63	2.8	5	1.6	212	0	26	1.0	8	390	0.04	0.07	0.0	0
207.	Enchilada, beef		200	487	21.8	23	8.8	63	26	425	2.9	262	595	0.02	0.27	3.5	5
208.	Enchilada, cheese		230	632	25.3	34	17.6	82	31	876	2.6	596	1,672	0.13	0.40	1.2	15
209.	Figs, dried	1 large	21	60	1.0	0	0.0	0	15	26	0.6	1	20	0.16	0.17	3.9	0
210.	Filet of Fish, McDonald's		131	402	15.0	23	7.9	43	34	105	1.8	709	152	0.28	0.28	3.9	4
489.	Fish, fillet, florentine, Healthy Choice		273	220	26.0	7	3.0	65	13	150	0.7	590	2,500	0.15	0.34	2.0	1
211.	Fish sandwich, Wendy's		182	460	16	25	5.0	55	42	120	1.8	780	0	0.60	0.45	4.0	1
494.	Fish, Sole Au Gratin, Healthy Choice		312	270	16.0	5	0.0	55	40	80	1.1	470	0	0.23	0.17	1.6	6
212.	Fish, sticks	2	56	140	12.0	6	1.6	52	8	22	0.6	106	40	0.06	0.10	1.2	0
213.	Flounder	3 oz.	85	171	25.5	7	1.0	60	0	21	1.2	201	0	0.06	0.06	2.1	3
214.	Flour, all purpose enriched	1 c	125	455	13.0	1	0.0	0	95	20	3.6	3	0	0.55	0.33	4.4	0
215.	Flour, whole wheat	1 c	120	400	16.0	2	0.0	0	85	49	4.0	4	0	0.66	0.14	5.2	0
216.	Frankfurter, cooked		57	176	7.0	16	5.6	45	1	4	1.1	627	0	0.09	0.11	1.5	0
217.	Frankfurter, turkey, cooked		45	102	6.4	8	2.7	39	1	58	0.8	454	60	0.04	0.08	1.7	0
218.	French Dip, Arby's		154	368	22	15	5.6	43	35	60	2.8	1,018	0	0.20	0.50	8.4	0
219.	French toast	1 piece	65	123	4.9	4	1.1	73	15	79	1.1	189	285	0.15	0.17	1.1	5
220.	Fries, Curly, Arby's	1 small	99	337	4	18	7.4	0	43	24	1.1	167	0	0.06	0.07	2.0	15
221.	Fruit cocktail	1 c	245	91	1.0	0	0.0	0	24	22	1.0	12	370	0.05	0.02	1.2	7
222.	Fruit cocktail, juice pack	1 c	248	115	1.1	0	0.0	0	29	20	0.5	10	380	0.03	0.04	1.0	5
223.	Grapefruit, raw white	1/2 med	301	56	1.0	0	0.0	0	15	22	0.5	1	10	0.05	0.04	1.0	52
224.	Grapefruit juice, unsweet. canned	1/2 c	124	50	0.6	0	0.0	0	12	11	0.2	1	10	0.05	0.03	0.3	46
225.	Grapes, seedless, European	10 grapes	50	34	0.3	0	0.0	0	9	6	0.2	2	50	0.03	0.03	0.2	2
226.	Grape juice, unsweetened bottled	1/2 c	127	84	0.3	0	0.0	0	21	14	0.4	3	0	0.05	0.03	0.2	0
227.	Gravy, beef, homemade	1 tbsp	17	19	0.3	2	1.0	1	1	1	0.1	49	0	0.01	0.01	0.2	0

Code	Food	Amount	Weight gm	Calories	Protein gm	Fat gm	Sat. Fat gm	Cholesterol mg	Carbohydrate gm	Calcium mg	Iron mg	Sodium mg	Vit A I.U.	Thiamin (Vit B₁) mg	Riboflavin (Vit B₂) mg	Niacin mg	Vit C mg
228.	Haddock, fried (dipped in egg, milk, bread crumbs)	3 oz.	85	141	17.0	5	1.0	54	5	33	0.9	150	0	0.03	0.06	2.7	3
229.	Halibut, broiled with buter or margarine	3 oz.	85	144	21.0	6	2.1	55	0	15	0.6	114	570	0.03	0.06	7.2	1
230.	Ham (cured pork)	3 oz.	85	318	20.0	26	9.4	77	0	9	2.6	48	0	0.43	0.20	3.8	0
231.	Ham, lunch meat	1 slice	28	37	5.5	1	0.5	13	.3	2	0.2	405	0	0.26	0.06	1.4	7
508.	Hamburger, Arch Deluxe, McDonalds	1	242	560	27.0	32	11.0	90	42	120	3.0	960	650	0.40	0.43	7.5	3
509.	Hamburger, Arch Deluxe w/bacon, McDonalds	1	253	610	31.0	36	13.0	105	42	120	3.7	1,190	650	0.40	0.43	7.5	3
232.	Hamburger, Big Classic, Wendy's	1	251	480	27	23	7.0	75	44	180	4.2	850	300	0.45	0.27	7.0	12
233.	Hamburger, Big Mac	1	204	581	25.1	36	12.0	85	40	207	5.0	999	388	0.49	0.39	7.3	3
234.	Hamburger bun	1 bun	40	129	3.7	2	1.0	0	23	61	1.3	271	2	0.22	0.15	1.8	0
235.	Hamburger, Jr. Bacon Cheeseburger, Wendy's	1	170	440	22	25	8.0	65	33	240	3.0	870	300	0.45	0.27	6.0	9
236.	Hamburger, McDonald's	1	99	257	13.0	9	3.7	26	30	63	3.0	526	231	0.23	0.23	5.1	2
237.	Hamburger, Mclean Deluxe	1	206	320	22	10	5.0	60	35	180	2.4	670	500	0.38	0.36	7.0	6
238.	Hamburger, Mclean Deluxe, w/cheese	1 burger	219	370	24	14	8.0	75	35	240	2.4	890	750	0.38	0.36	7.0	6
239.	Hamburger, Quarter pounder	1 burger	160	427	24.6	24	9.1	80	29	98	4.3	718	115	0.35	0.32	7.2	3
240.	Hamburger, Quarter pounder, with cheese	1 burger	186	525	29.6	32	12.8	107	31	255	4.8	1,195	640	0.37	0.41	7.1	3
241.	Hamburger, Wendy's	1	219	440	26	23	7.0	75	36	120	3.6	850	300	0.38	0.18	7.0	9
242.	Ham N' Cheese, Arby's	1	169	355	25	14	5.1	55	35	204	1.8	1400	0	0.83	0.40	7.8	0
243.	Honey	1 tbsp	21	64	0.0	0	0.0	0	17	1	0.1	1	0	0.00	0.01	0.1	0
244.	Honeydew melon	1 slice (1/10 melon)	129	45	0.6	0	0.0	0	12	8	0.1	13	25	0.10	0.02	0.8	32
245.	Horsey Sauce, Arby's	.5 oz.	14	55	0	5	2.0	0	3	24	0.0	105	0	0.00	0.00	0.0	0
246.	Hotcakes w/Margarine & Syrup, McDonald's	1 serving	174	440	8	12	5.0	8	74	120	1.2	685	200	0.30	0.36	3.0	0
247.	Hotdog bun	1 bun	40	115	3.3	2	1.0	0	20	54	1.2	241	2	0.20	0.13	1.6	0
248.	Ice cream, vanilla	1/2 c	67	135	3.0	7	4.4	27	14	97	0.1	42	295	0.03	0.14	0.1	1
249.	Ice cream cone	1 small	115	185	4.3	5	2.2	24	30	183	0.1	109	218	0.06	0.36	0.4	1
250.	Ice cream cone, Dairy Queen	medium	142	230	6.0	7	4.6	15	35	200	0.0	150	300	0.09	0.26	0.0	0
251.	Ice cream cone, hot fudge sundae	1	164	357	7.0	11	5.4	27	58	215	0.6	170	233	0.07	0.31	1.1	2
252.	Ice milk, vanilla	1/2 c	61	100	3.0	3	1.8	13	15	102	0.1	45	140	0.04	0.15	0.1	1
253.	Instant breakfast, whole milk	1 c	281	280	15.0	8	5.1	33	34	301	8.0	286	2,057	0.39	0.46	5.2	29
254.	Instant breakfast, skim milk	1 c	282	216	15.4	0	0.0	4	35	312	8.0	292	1,635	0.39	0.41	5.2	29
255.	Jams or preserves	1 tbsp	7	18	0.0	0	0.0	0	5	1	0.1	1	1	0.00	0.00	0.0	0
256.	Jelly	1 tbsp	18	49	0.0	0	0.0	0	13	4	0.3	3	0	0.00	0.01	0.0	1
257.	Kale, fresh cooked, drained	1/2 c	55	22	2.5	0	0.0	0	3	103	0.9	24	4,565	0.06	0.10	0.9	51
258.	Kiwi fruit, raw	1 med	76	46	1.0	0	0.0	0	11	20	0.3	4	65	0.02	0.04	0.4	75
259.	Kool Aid, with sugar	1 c	240	2	0.0	0	0.0	0	25	0	0.0	0	0	0.00	0.00	0.0	6
260.	Lamb leg, roast, trimmed	3 oz.	85	237	22.0	16	7.3	60	0	9	1.4	53	0	0.13	0.23	4.7	0
261.	Lamb loin chop, broiled, lean	3 oz.	84	183	25.0	8	3.4	78	0	16	1.7	70	7	0.10	0.23	5.7	0
490.	Lasagna, Healthy Choice	1	284	260	18.0	5	0.0	20	37	100	2.7	420	750	0.30	0.26	2.0	2
262.	Lasagna, homemade	1 piece	220	357	23.6	18	8.3	50	27	413	2.8	703	1,008	0.19	0.30	3.3	6
498.	Lasagna, Lean Cuisine	1	291	260	19.0	5	2.0	25	34	150	1.8	590	500	0.15	0.25	3.0	6
263.	Lemon juice, fresh	1 tbsp	15	4	0.1	0	0.0	0	1	1	0.0	1	1	0.00	0.00	0.0	7
264.	Lemonade (concentrate)	12 oz.	340	137	0.2	0	0.1	0	36	11	0.6	11	73	0.02	0.07	0.1	13
265.	Lentils, cooked	1/2 c	100	106	8.0	0	0.0	0	19	25	2.1	0	20	0.07	0.06	0.6	0
266.	Lettuce, crisp head	1 c sm chunks	75	10	0.7	0	0.0	0	2	15	0.4	7	250	0.05	0.05	0.2	5
267.	Lettuce, cos or romaine	1 c chopped	55	10	0.7	0	0.0	0	2	37	0.8	5	1,050	0.08	0.04	0.2	10
268.	Liver, beef, fried	1 slice 3 oz.	85	195	22.0	9	2.5	345	5	9	7.5	156	45,390	0.22	3.56	14.0	23
269.	Liverwurst, fresh	1 slice 1 oz.	28	87	5.0	7	3.5	50	1	3	1.5	0	1,800	0.06	0.37	1.6	0

Code	Food	Amount	Weight gm	Calories	Protein gm	Fat gm	Sat. Fat gm	Cholesterol mg	Carbohydrate gm	Calcium mg	Iron mg	Sodium mg	Vit A I.U.	Thiamin (Vit B$_1$) mg	Riboflavin (Vit B$_2$) mg	Niacin mg	Vit C mg
270.	Lobster	1 c	145	138	27.0	2	1.0	293	0	94	1.2	305	0	0.15	0.10	0.0	0
271.	M&M's, chocolate, plain	1 oz.	28	140	1.9	6	3.3	0	19	47	0.5	24	30	0.01	0.07	0.2	0
272.	M&M's, chocolate, w/peanuts	1 oz.	28	145	3.2	7	3.2	0	17	36	0.4	17	15	0.02	0.05	0.9	0
273.	Macaroni, enriched, cooked	1/2 c	70	78	2.4	0	0.0	0	16	6	0.7	1	0	0.10	0.06	0.8	0
274.	Macaroni and cheese	1/2 c	100	215	8.2	11	4.0	21	20	181	0.9	543	430	0.10	0.20	0.9	0
275.	Margarine	1 tsp	5	34	0.0	4	0.7	2	0	1	0.0	46	160	0.00	0.00	0.0	0
276.	Mars bar	1 bar	50	240	4.0	11	4.8	0	30	85	0.6	85	1	0.02	0.16	0.5	*
277.	Matzo	1 piece	30	117	3.0	0	0.0	0	25	*	*	0	*	*	*	*	*
278.	Mayonnaise	1 tsp	5	36	0.0	4	0.7	3	0	1	0.0	28	13	0.00	0.00	0.0	0
513.	Mayonnaise, light	1 tsp.	5	17	0.0	0	0.3	2	1	0	0.0	30	0	0.00	0.00	0.0	0
507.	Milk, 1% fat	1 c	244	102	8.0	3	1.6	10	12	300	0.1	123	720	0.09	0.41	0.2	2
279.	Milk, chocolate, 2%	1 c	250	180	8.0	5	3.1	17	26	284	0.6	151	143	0.05	0.41	0.3	2
280.	Milk, evaporated whole	1/2 c	126	172	9.0	10	5.8	40	13	329	0.2	149	405	0.09	0.43	0.2	2
281.	Milk, lowfat 2%	1 c	244	121	8.0	5	2.9	18	12	295	0.1	121	695	0.20	0.40	0.2	2
282.	Milk shake, chocolate	1 (10 fluid oz.)	340	433	11.5	13	7.8	45	70	383	1.1	328	312	0.15	0.83	0.5	0
283.	Milk shake, Frosty, Wendy's	16 oz.	324	460	13	13	7.0	55	76	480	1.0	260	500	0.14	1.08	0.8	4
284.	Milk shake, strawberry	1 (10 fluid oz.)	340	383	11.4	10	6.0	37	64	384	0.4	281	418	0.12	0.61	0.5	3
285.	Milk shake, vanilla, McDonald's	1 c	289	323	10	8	5.1	29	52	346	0.2	250	346	0.09	0.66	0.6	2
286.	Milk, skim	1 c	245	85	8.0	1	0.3	4	12	301	0.1	126	745	0.09	0.34	0.2	2
287.	Milk, whole 3.5% fat	1 c	244	149	8.0	8	5.1	33	11	290	0.1	119	380	0.03	0.39	0.2	1
288.	Milky Way bar	1 bar	60	260	3.2	9	5.4	14	43	86	0.5	140	125	0.01	0.15	0.0	0
289.	Molasses, medium	1 tbsp	20	50	0.0	0	0.0	0	13	33	0.9	3	0	0.01	0.01	0.0	0
290.	Muffin, apple bran, fat free, McDonald's		75	180	5	0	0.0	0	40	48	0.7	200	0	0.15	0.18	2.0	0
291.	Muffin, blueberry	1	45	135	3.0	5	1.5	19	20	54	0.9	198	40	0.10	0.11	0.9	1
292.	Muffin, bran	1	45	125	3.0	6	1.4	24	19	60	1.4	189	230	0.11	0.13	1.3	3
293.	Muffin, cornmeal	1	45	145	3.0	5	1.5	23	21	66	0.9	169	80	0.11	0.11	0.9	0
294.	Muffin, English, plain	1	57	140	4.5	1	0.3	0	26	96	1.7	378	0	0.26	0.18	2.1	0
295.	Muffin, English w/butter	1	63	186	5.0	5	2.3	15	30	117	1.5	310	164	0.28	0.49	2.6	1
296.	Mushrooms, fresh cultivated	1/2 c sliced	35	12	1.0	0	0.0	0	2	4	0.5	4	0	0.04	0.12	2.4	0
297.	Mustard greens, cooked drained	1/2 c	70	16	1.7	0	0.0	0	3	96	1.2	13	4,060	0.05	0.10	0.4	33
298.	Noodles, egg, enriched cooked	1/2 c	80	100	3.3	1	0.0	0	19	8	0.7	2	55	0.11	0.07	1.0	0
299.	Nuts, brazil	1 oz. (6-8 nuts)	28	185	4.1	19	4.8	0	3	53	1.0	0	0	0.27	0.03	0.5	1
300.	Nuts, pecans	1 oz.	28	195	2.6	20	1.4	0	4	21	0.7	0	40	0.24	0.04	0.3	1
301.	Nuts, walnuts	1 oz. (14 halves)	28	185	4.2	18	1.8	0	5	28	0.9	1	10	0.09	0.04	0.3	0
302.	Oil, corn	1 tbsp.	15	125	0.0	14	1.9	0	0	0	0.0	0	0	0.00	0.00	0.0	0
303.	Oil, olive	1 tbsp.	15	125	0.0	14	1.3	0	0	0	0.0	0	0	0.00	0.00	0.0	0
304.	Oil, safflower	1 tbsp.	15	125	0.0	14	2.0	0	0	0	0.0	0	0	0.00	0.00	0.0	0
305.	Oil, soybean	1 tsp.	5	44	0.0	5	0.0	0	0	0	0.0	0	0	0.00	0.00	0.0	0
306.	Okra, cooked, drained	1/2 c	80	23	1.6	0	0.9	0	5	74	0.4	2	390	0.11	0.15	0.7	16
307.	Olives, black, ripe	10 extra large	55	61	0.5	7	1.0	0	1	40	0.8	385	30	0.00	0.00	0.0	0
308.	Onions, mature, cooked, drained	1/2 c sliced	105	31	1.3	0	0.0	0	7	25	0.4	8	40	0.03	0.03	0.2	8
309.																	
310.	Onion rings, fried	3	30	122	1.6	8	2.3	0	11	9	0.5	113	68	0.08	0.04	1.1	0
311.	Onion rings (Brazier) Dairy Queen	1 serving	85	360	6.0	17	6.0	15	33	20	0.4	125	0	0.09	0.00	0.4	2
312.	Orange juice, froz., reconstituted	1/2 c	125	61	0.9	0	0.0	0	15	13	0.1	1	270	0.12	0.02	0.5	60
313.	Orange, raw (medium skin),	1 med	180	64	1.3	0	0.0	0	16	54	0.5	1	260	0.13	0.05	0.5	66
314.	Oysters, Eastern, breaded, fried	1 oyster	45	90	5.0	5	1.4	35	5	49	3.0	70	220	0.07	0.10	1.3	4
315.	Oysters, raw, Eastern	1/2 c (6-9 med)	120	79	10.0	2	1.3	60	4	113	6.6	145	370	0.17	0.22	3.0	0
316.	Pancakes	6" diam x 1/2" thick	73	169	5.2	10	1.0	36	25	74	0.9	310	90	0.12	0.16	0.9	0
317.	Pancakes, buckwheat	4 in. diam.	27	55	2.0	2	0.9	20	6	59	0.4	125	17	0.04	0.05	0.2	0
318.	Pancakes w/butter, syrup	1 large	100	250	4.0	5	1.9	24	47	1	1.1	535	160	0.13	0.18	1.1	2
319.	Papaya, raw	1/2 med	227	60	0.9	0	0.0	0	15	31	0.5	5	2,660	0.06	0.06	0.5	85

Code	Food	Amount	Weight gm	Calories	Protein gm	Fat gm	Sat. Fat gm	Cholesterol mg	Carbohydrate gm	Calcium mg	Iron mg	Sodium mg	Vit A I.U.	Thiamin (Vit B₁) mg	Riboflavin (Vit B₂) mg	Niacin mg	Vit C mg
320.	Parsnips, cooked	1 large 9" long	160	106	2.4	1	0.0	0	24	72	1.0	13	50	0.11	0.13	0.2	16
503.	Pasta primavera, Weight Watchers	1	238	260	15.0	11	0.8	5	22	300	1.8	800	1,750	0.23	0.26	3.0	18
321.	Peaches, canned, heavy syrup	half 2⅛ tbsp liq.	96	75	0.4	0	0.0	0	19	4	0.3	2	410	0.01	0.02	0.6	3
322.	Peaches, canned, juice pack	half	77	34	0.5	0	0.0	0	9	5	0.2	3	147	0.01	0.01	0.5	3
323.	Peaches, raw, peeled	2¾" diam.	175	58	0.9	0	0.0	0	15	14	0.8	2	2,030	0.03	0.08	1.5	11
324.	Peanut butter	2 tbsp	32	188	8.0	16	1.0	0	6	18	0.6	194	0	0.04	0.04	4.8	0
325.	Peanut butter, jam sandwich	1	100	340	11.4	14	2.6	0	45	87	2.3	414	1	0.32	0.22	5.3	0
326.	Peanuts, roasted	1 oz.	28	166	7.0	14	1.0	0	5	21	0.6	119	0	0.09	0.04	4.9	0
327.	Pears, canned, heavy syrup	half 2¼ tbsp liq.	103	78	0.2	0	0.0	0	20	5	0.2	1	0	0.01	0.02	0.1	1
328.	Pears, canned, juice pack	half	77	38	0.3	0	0.0	0	10	7	0.2	3	3	0.01	0.01	0.2	1
329.	Pears, raw	1 pear	180	100	1.1	1	0.0	0	25	13	0.5	2	30	0.03	0.07	0.2	7
330.	Peas, canned, drained	1/2 c	85	75	4.0	0	0.0	0	14	22	1.6	200	585	0.08	0.05	0.7	7
331.	Peas, frozen, cooked drained	1/2 c	80	55	4.1	0	0.0	0	10	15	1.5	92	480	0.22	0.07	1.4	11
332.	Peppers, sweet, raw	1 pepper 3¼" x 3" diam.	200	36	2.0	0	0.0	0	8	15	1.1	21	690	0.13	0.13	0.8	210
333.	Pickles, dill	1 large 4" long	135	15	0.9	0	0.0	0	3	35	1.4	1,928	140	0.00	0.03	0.0	8
334.	Pickles, sweet	1 large 3" long	35	51	0.2	0	0.0	0	13	4	0.4	0	30	0.00	0.01	0.0	2
335.	Pie, Apple	1 piece (3½")	118	302	2.6	13	3.5	120	45	9	0.4	355	40	0.02	0.02	0.5	1
336.	Pie, Apple, fried	1 pie	85	255	2.2	14	5.8	14	32	12	0.9	326	15	0.09	0.06	1.0	1
337.	Pie, Blueberry	1 piece (3½")	158	380	4.0	17	4.0	0	55	26	2.1	423	140	0.17	0.14	1.7	6
338.	Pie, Cherry	1 piece (3½")	118	308	3.1	13	5.0	137	45	17	0.4	355	40	0.02	0.02	0.5	1
339.	Pie, Cherry, fried	1 pie	85	250	2.0	14	5.8	13	32	11	0.7	371	95	0.06	0.06	0.6	1
340.	Pie, Chocolate cream	1 piece (1/6 pie)	175	311	7.4	13	4.5	15	42	160	1.1	427	170	0.15	0.30	1.1	1
341.	Pie, Lemon meringue	1 piece (1/6 pie)	140	355	4.7	14	3.5	137	53	25	1.4	395	330	0.10	0.14	0.8	4
342.	Pie, Pecan	1 piece (1/6 pie)	138	583	6.3	24	3.9	13	92	35	1.9	304	206	0.22	0.17	1.1	0
343.	Pie, Pumpkin	1 (3½")	114	241	4.6	13	3.0	70	28	58	0.6	244	2,810	0.03	0.11	0.6	0
344.	Pineapple, canned, heavy syrup	1/2 c	128	95	0.4	0	0.0	0	25	14	0.4	2	65	0.10	0.03	0.3	9
345.	Pineapple, canned, juice pack	1/2 c	125	75	0.5	0	0.0	0	20	17	0.3	1	24	0.12	0.24	0.3	12
346.	Pineapple, raw	1/2 c diced	78	41	0.3	0	0.0	0	11	13	0.4	1	55	0.07	0.03	0.2	13
347.	Pizza, cheese, thin 'n crispy, Pizza Hut	1/2 10" pie	*	450	25.0	15	7.0	125	54	450	4.5	1,200	750	0.30	0.51	5.0	1
348.	Pizza, Cheese, Thick 'n Chewy, Pizza Hut	1/2 10" pie	*	560	34.0	14	6.0	110	71	500	5.4	1,100	1,000	0.68	0.68	7.0	1
504.	Pizza, Cheese, Weight Watchers	1	164	300	22.0	7	3.0	35	37	450	1.4	630	1,000	0.30	0.51	3.0	12
505.	Pizza, deluxe comb. Weight Watchers	1	200	330	26.0	10	3.0	25	35	350	1.8	650	1,750	0.30	0.51	3.0	21
506.	Pizza, Pepperoni, Weight Watchers	1	171	320	26.0	10	3.0	35	31	400	1.8	710	1,000	0.23	0.51	3.0	15
480.	Pizza, pepperoni, pan, Pizza Hut	2 pieces	211	540	29.0	22	9.2	42	62	520	6.3	1,127	500	0.63	0.49	5.4	8
481.	Pizza, supreme, pan, Pizza Hut	2 pieces	255	589	32.0	30	13.8	48	53	500	5.0	1,363	600	0.81	0.80	6.0	10
349.	Plums, Japanese and hybrid, raw	1 plum 2⅛" diam.	70	32	0.3	0	0.0	0	8	8	0.3	1	160	0.02	0.02	0.3	4
350.	Popcorn, cooked, oil	1 c	11	55	0.9	3	0.5	0	6	3	0.3	86	20	0.01	0.02	0.1	0
351.	Popcorn, popped, plain, large kernel	1 c	6	12	0.8	0	0.0	0	5	1	0.2	0	0	0.00	0.01	0.1	0
352.	Pork, roast, trimmed	2 slices 3 oz.	85	179	24.0	8	2.2	65	0	11	3.1	863	0	0.55	0.22	4.3	0
353.	Pork, sausage, cooked	1 sm link	17	72	2.8	6	2.1	13	0	0	0.3	221	0	0.00	0.00	0.0	0
354.	Potato, au gratin	1/2 c	245	228	5.6	10	6.3	12	32	203	0.8	1,076	380	0.05	0.20	2.3	8
355.	Potato, baked in skin	1 potato 2⅓ x 4¼"	202	145	4.0	0	0.0	0	33	14	1.1	6	0	0.15	0.07	2.7	31
356.	Potato chips	10 chips	20	114	1.1	8	2.1	0	10	8	0.4	150	0	0.04	0.01	1.0	3
357.	Potato, French fried long	10 strips 3½-4"	78	214	3.4	10	1.7	0	28	12	1.0	5	0	0.10	0.06	2.4	16
358.	Potato, hashbrowns, McDonald's	1 patty	55	144	1.4	9	3.0	4	15	5	0.4	325	6	0.06	0.01	0.8	4
359.	Potato, mashed, milk added	1/2 c	105	69	2.2	1	0.4	8	14	25	0.4	316	20	0.09	0.06	1.1	11

Code	Food	Amount	Weight gm	Calories	Protein gm	Fat gm	Sat. Fat gm	Cholesterol mg	Carbohydrate gm	Calcium mg	Iron mg	Sodium mg	Vit A I.U.	Thiamin (Vit B₁) mg	Riboflavin (Vit B₂) mg	Niacin mg	Vit C mg
360.	Potato salad w/eggs, mayo	1/2 c	125	179	3.4	10	7.8	85	14	24	0.8	662	262	0.10	0.08	1.1	12
361.	Potato, hash brown	1/2 c	78	170	2.5	9	3.5	0	22	12	1.2	27	0	0.09	0.02	1.9	5
362.	Pretzel, thin, twists	1 oz.	28	113	2.8	1	0.3	0	23	8	0.6	456	0	0.09	0.07	1.2	0
363.	Prunes, dried "softenized" without pits	5 prunes	61	137	1.1	0	0.0	0	36	26	0.1	4	860	0.05	0.09	0.9	2
364.	Prune juice, canned or bottled	1/2 c	128	99	0.5	0	0.0	0	24	18	5.3	3	0	0.02	0.02	0.5	3
365.	Pudding, chocolate, canned	5 oz.	142	205	3	11	9.5	1	30	74	1.2	285	155	0.04	0.17	0.6	0
366.	Pudding, tapioca, canned	5 oz.	142	160	3	5	4.8	1	28	119	0.3	252	5	0.03	0.14	0.4	0
367.	Pudding, vanilla, canned	5 oz.	142	220	2	10	9.5	1	33	79	0.2	305	1	0.03	0.12	0.6	0
368.	Quiche, Lorraine	1 piece	242	825	18	66	31.9	392	40	290	1.9	898	2,250	0.15	0.44	1.7	1
369.	Raisins, unbleached, seedless	1 oz.	28	82	0.7	0	0.0	0	22	18	1.0	8	10	0.03	0.02	0.1	1
370.	Raspberries, fresh	1 c	123	60	1.1	1	0.0	0	14	27	0.7	0	80	0.04	0.11	1.1	31
371.	Raspberries, frozen	1 c	250	255	1.7	1	0.0	0	62	38	1.6	3	75	0.05	0.11	1.5	41
495.	Ravioli, baked cheese, Lean Cuisine	1	241	240	13.0	8	3.0	55	30	200	1.4	590	300	0.06	0.25	1.2	36
372.	Rice, brown, cooked	1/2 c	96	116	2.5	1	0.0	0	25	12	0.5	275	0	0.09	0.02	1.3	0
373.	Rice, white enriched, cooked	1/2 c	103	113	2.1	0	0.0	0	25	11	0.9	384	0	0.12	0.01	1.1	0
374.	Rice, wild, cooked	1/2 c	100	92	3.6	0	0.0	0	19	5	1.1	2	0	0.11	0.16	1.6	0
375.	Roast beef sand., regular, Arby's	1	155	383	22	18	7.0	43	35	72	3.2	936	0	0.28	0.50	11.0	9
376.	Roast beef sub, Arby's	1	305	623	38	32	11.5	73	47	492	5.2	1,847	500	0.56	0.76	14.2	9
377.	Roll, hard, white	1 roll	50	155	5	2	0.0	0	30	24	1.4	313	0	0.20	0.12	1.7	0
378.	Reuben sandwich	1	237	488	28.7	28	10.4	85	30	364	5.3	1,685	461	0.25	0.44	3.9	12
379.	Salad, caesar side, Wendy's	1	130	160	10	6	1.0	10	18	96	1.2	700	1,250	0.23	0.27	2.0	24
380.	Salad, chef, Burger King	1 serving	273	178	17	9	4.0	103	7	128	1.6	568	4,750	0.35	0.26	3.6	15
381.	Salad, chef, McDonald's	1	265	170	17	9	4.0	111	8	180	1.0	400	5,000	0.30	0.27	4.0	21
382.	Salad, chicken, Burger King	1 serving	258	142	20	4	1.0	49	8	32	1.3	443	4,600	0.14	0.17	8.5	20
383.	Salad, chicken w/celery	1/2 c	78	266	10.5	25	4.1	48	1	16	0.7	199	153	0.03	0.08	3.3	1
384.	Salad, deluxe Garden, Wendy's	1	271	110	7	5	1.0	0	9	240	1.0	380	3,000	0.15	0.36	1.2	36
385.	Salad, garden, Arby's	1	330	117	7	5	2.7	12	11	192	1.1	134	4,900	0.17	0.20	1.2	52
386.	Salad, grilled Chicken, Wendy's	1	338	200	25	8	1.0	55	9	240	1.8	690	3,000	0.23	0.36	8.0	36
387.	Salad, tuna	1 c	205	375	33	19	3.3	80	19	31	2.5	877	53	0.06	0.14	13.3	6
388.	Salami, dry	1 oz.	28	128	7.0	11	1.6	24	0	4	1.0	349	0	0.10	0.07	1.5	0
389.	Salmon, broiled with butter or margarine	3 oz.	85	156	23.0	6	2.2	53	0	0	0.9	99	150	0.15	0.06	8.4	0
390.	Salmon, canned Chinook	3 oz.	85	179	16.6	12	0.8	30	0	131	0.7	105	197	0.03	0.01	6.2	0
514.	Salsa	1 tbsp.	15	5	0.0	0	0.0	0	1	1	0.1	100	115	0.01	0.06	0.05	5
391.	Sardines, canned drained	1 oz.	28	58	7.0	3	1.0	20	0	124	0.8	233	60	0.01	0.06	1.5	0
392.	Sauerkraut, canned	1/2 c	118	21	1.2	0	0.0	0	5	43	0.6	878	60	0.04	0.05	0.3	17
393.	Sausage biscuit w/egg, McDonald's	1	175	505	19	33	20.0	260	33	120	2.4	1,210	300	0.45	0.36	4.0	0
394.	Sausage McMuffin, McDonald's	1	135	345	15	20	11.0	57	27	240	1.8	770	200	0.53	0.27	5.0	0
395.	Sausage McMuffin, w/Egg	1	159	430	21	25	14.0	270	27	300	2.4	920	500	0.53	0.45	5.0	0
396.	Sausage, smoked link, pork	1	68	265	15	25	7.7	46	1	20	0.8	1,020	0	1.04	0.29	5.0	14
397.	Scallops, breaded, cooked	6 pieces	90	195	15	10	2.5	70	10	39	2.0	298	105	0.11	0.11	1.6	0
398.	Sherbet	1/2 c	97	135	1.1	2	1.3	7	29	52	0.2	44	92	0.02	0.04	0.1	2
399.	Shrimp, boiled	3 oz.	85	99	18.0	1	0.1	128	1	99	2.7	0	60	0.00	0.03	1.5	0
400.	Shrimp, fried	7 medium	85	200	16.0	10	2.5	168	11	61	2.0	384	130	0.06	0.09	2.8	0
487.	Shrimp, linguini, Budget Gourmet	1	284	330	15.0	15	0.0	75	33	10	3.6	1,250	1,000	0.30	0.17	3.0	2
401.	Snickers bar	1 bar	61	290	6.6	4	5.4	0	37	70	0.5	170	25	0.03	0.11	1.8	0
402.	Soda pop, cola	12 oz.	369	144	0.0	0	0.0	0	37	27	0.0	30	0	0.00	0.00	0.0	0
403.	Soda pop, diet	12 oz.	340	2	0.1	0	0.0	0	0	13	0.1	31	0	0.00	0.00	0.0	0
404.	Soda pop, Ginger ale	12 oz.	366	113	0.1	0	0.0	0	29	8	0.1	45	0	0.00	0.00	0.0	0
405.	Soda pop, lemon-lime	12 oz.	340	138	0.0	0	0.0	0	35	8	0.2	38	0	0.00	0.00	0.0	0

Name: _____

Day	Calories	Protein (gm)	Fat (gm)	Sat. Fat (gm)	Chol-esterol (mg)	Carbo-hydrates (gm)	Calcium (mg)	Iron (mg)	Sodium (mg)	Vit. A (I.U.)	Thiamin Vit. B1 (mg)	Riboflavin Vit. B2 (mg)	Niacin (mg)	Vit. C (mg)
One														
Two														
Three														
Totals														
Average[a]														
Percentages[b]														
Recommended Dietary Allowances*														
Men 15–18 yrs.[c]	See below[d]	See	<30%[e]	<10%[e]	<300[e]	58%>[e]	1,200	12	2,400[e]	5,000	1.5	1.8	20	60
Men 19–24 yrs.			<30%[e]	<10%[e]	<300[e]	58%>[e]	1,200	10	2,400[e]	5,000	1.5	1.7	19	60
Men 25–50 yrs.			<30%[e]	<10%[e]	<300[e]	58%>[e]	800	10	2,400[e]	5,000	1.5	1.7	19	60
Men 51+ yrs.			<30%[e]	<10%[e]	<300[e]	58%>[e]	800	10	2,400[e]	5,000	1.2	1.4	15	60
Women 15–18 yrs.			<30%[e]	<10%[e]	<300[e]	58%>[e]	1,200	15	2,400[e]	4,000	1.1	1.3	15	60
Women 19–24 yrs.			<30%[e]	<10%[e]	<300[e]	58%>[e]	1,200	15	2,400[e]	4,000	1.1	1.3	15	60
Women 25–50 yrs.			<30%[e]	<10%[e]	<300[e]	58%>[e]	800	15	2,400[e]	4,000	1.1	1.3	15	60
Women 51+ yrs.			<30%[e]	<10%[e]	<300[e]	58%>[e]	800	10	2,400[e]	4,000	1.0	1.2	13	60
Pregnant			<30%[e]	<10%[e]	<300[e]	58%>[e]	1,200	30	2,400[e]	4,000	1.5	1.6	17	70
Lactating			<30%[e]	<10%[e]	<300[e]	58%>[e]	1,200	15	2,400[e]	6,000	1.6	1.8	20	95

[a]Divide totals by 3 or number of days assessed.
[b]Percentages: Protein and Carbohydrates = multiply average by 4, divide by average calories, and multiply by 100. Fat and Saturated Fat = multiply average by 9, divide by average calories, and multiply by 100.
[c]Use Table 8.1 (Chapter 8) for all categories.
[d]Protein intake should be .8 grams per kilogram of body weight. Pregnant women should consume an additional 15 grams of daily protein, while lactating women should have an extra 20 grams.
[e]Based on recommendations by nutrition experts.
*Adapted from Recommended Dietary Allowances, © 1989, by the National Academy of Sciences, National Academy Press, Washington, D.C.

Figure B.2 • *Three-day nutritional analysis.*

Date: _____

Name: _____   Age: _____   Weight: _____

Sex: Male–M, Female–F (Pregnant–P, Lactating–L, Neither–N)

Activity Rating: Sedentary (limited physical activity)   = 1
                     Moderate physical activity   = 2
                     Hard labor (strenuous physical activity   = 3

Number of days to be analyzed: _____   Day: _____

No.	Code*	Food	Amount
1			
2			
3			
4			
5			
6			
7			
8			
9			
10			
11			
12			
13			
14			
15			
16			
17			
18			
19			
20			
21			
22			
23			
24			
25			
26			
27			
28			
29			
30			
31			

*When done, to advance to the next day or end, type 0 (zero).

Figure B.3 ● *Daily nutrient intake form for computer software use (make additional copies as necessary).*

Health Protection Plan for Environmental Hazards, Crime Prevention, and Personal Safety*

APPENDIX

C

*Questionnaire published by the Preventive Medicine Institute/Strang Clinic. New York, 1982.
Reproduced with permission.

Personal Environment

In addition to environmental problems in the community at large there are also important problems in our own immediate environment that affect our health, well-being, and comfort. These are problems we can control and improve ourselves.

The following self-assessment relates to environmental hazards dealing with water, wastes, noise and air pollution in our everyday lives.

All "no" answers are a cue to ACTION.

Concerning AIR POLLUTION, do you...?	YES	NO
...Know the optimal conditions for temperature, humidity and air movement in your home?	○	○
...Change the air filters once a year in your air conditioners or forced air heating systems?	○	○
...Are your work areas ventilated so that fumes and dusts do not accumulate?	○	○
...Do your throat or nasal passages feel moist and clear in the morning (not dry or stuffy)?	○	○
...Know what to do when the weather report says the quality of the air is unsatisfactory?	○	○
...Know what a "killer smog" is?	○	○
...If you smoke, do you avoid smoking in a bedroom or areas where children play?	○	○

RISK FACTORS:

- *Bronchitis, asthma, emphysema, and heart disease are all aggravated by air pollution.*
- *Chronic exposure to dusts of metal or wood are risk factors for cancer of the respiratory passages.*
- *Children of cigarette smokers have a higher than usual incidence of respiratory infections.*
- *Many so-called allergies of the sinuses and upper respiratory tract are really due to air pollution.*

AWARENESS COUNTS:

- **The optimal air comfort levels are 66-68°F temperature, 30-40% humidity, and air movement at 20-50 feet per minute. Lower humidity will lead to dryness of the respiratory passages, increase skin evaporation and make your home feel colder than it is.**
- **When the air quality is reported as "unsatisfactory" people with heart and lung disease should stay indoors.**
- **"Killer smog" refers to trapped air which cannot rise, with no available dispersing breeze, which accumulates industrial, auto and heating combustion products into a suffocating density. This may be fatal to those with cardiopulmonary disease, and uncomfortable for everyone.**

Concerning WATER...?	YES	NO
...Have you checked your home drinking water in the last year for clarity, color and taste?	○	○
...If you shake up a glass of tap water does it remain clear (not foamy or frothy)?	○	○
...Do you have a screen filter on your water tap?	○	○
...Do you check restaurant water and ice for clarity and cleanliness?	○	○
...Do you know the common water-borne diseases?	○	○
...Do you know what kind of water purification tablets are best for traveling?	○	○
...Do you take care when traveling in developing countries or in un-settled areas to drink bottled water, or coffee, tea, or soup made with boiling water, and to avoid ice cubes?	○	○
...Do you think all wilderness water is safe?	○	○
...Do you know what source of water is almost always safe to drink?	○	○

Concerning WASTE...?	YES	NO
...Do you place ordinary kitchen waste in plastic bags for disposal?	○	○
...Do you know what kinds of wastes require special handling?	○	○
...Are your garbage cans free from bad odors?	○	○
...Is your sink or toilet bowl free from bad odors or back up of waste water in your drain?	○	○
...If you live in a home with a septic tank do you know its location?	○	○
...Do you know the last time the septic tank was cleaned?	○	○

RISK FACTORS: WATER AND WASTE

- *Diseases associated with water and waste include: typhoid fever, cholera, hepatitis, poliomyelitis, E. coli dysentery and amoebic dysentery.*
- *Very hard water containing large amounts of magnesium can cause diarrhea in children. It is difficult to wash with, and will cause deposits in water pipes.*
- *Chlorine is commonly used for water purification. An excess is harmful since it may be converted into chloroform, a toxic chemical.*
- *The presence of water supplies in proximity to industrial plants is a cause for concern since there are many instances of toxic chemicals leaking into local water supplies in this country.*

AWARENESS COUNTS: WATER

- All water taps should have screen filters to trap particulate material which may accidentally enter the water supply. These should be removed and cleaned regularly.
- Frothy water is due to detergents leaking into the water supply and this can cause intestinal upsets.
- Cloudy water may be due only to rusty pipes and while it may stain kitchen utensils it is not harmful; but turbid water with an odor may be due to seepage of sewage or industrial wastes into the water supply and this can be dangerous to health. Every state has a water supply agency that can give you information on the condition of your local water supply. However, if your water comes from a well, no one is checking it for purity. <u>You</u> must take the initiative and find out from the state agency how this can be done.
- The best type of water purification tablets is the iodine-releasing variety rather than the chlorine type. These are obtainable from your local pharmacy. Use these only if traveling in an area where bottled water is not available.
- Not all wilderness water is pure. It may come from springs which have toxic chemicals, or be contaminated by animal use upstream. If purified water is not available, the safest water to drink is rain water. (Make sure it is stored in a clean container.)

AWARENESS COUNTS: WASTE

- Plastic bags for disposal of ordinary wastes have the advantage of keeping your garbage containers, indoor and outdoor, clean and free of odors. This helps prevent fly, roach, and rodent infestation, and the accidental contamination of food.
- Aerosol cans, solvents, and fuels should not be placed in plastic bags, and should not be disposed of with household wastes because of the hazards of fire and explosion; your local waste disposal service should be contacted regarding special handling.
- Bad odors or backup of waste water into your sink, tub, or toilet is a serious matter since this is untreated sewage and poses a health hazard. There may be an obstruction in the sewage system; check with your plumber first. If you have a septic tank, it may have to be cleaned. The frequency of cleaning of septic tanks depends on size and use. Three to four years of regular use is an average duration of time before cleaning is necessary.
- It's important to know the location of your septic tank and also those of your neighbors in relationship to your well water supply. There should be a distance of 100 feet between the septic tank and well. Your board of health can give you additional information about specific conditions in your area.

Concerning NOISE...?	YES	NO
...Do you know how to tell if you are in an environment which could damage your hearing?	○	○
...Do you know that permanent hearing loss can occur with a single exposure to a painfully loud noise?	○	○
...Are you aware of the other effects on your health that noise can have other than hearing loss?	○	○
...Do you know the accidents that can occur due to noise causing "warning concealment"?	○	○
...Are you aware of "slow reaction time" as a noise associated danger?	○	○
...Do you know what age group is especially susceptible to noise induced hearing loss?	○	○

RISK FACTORS:

NOISE

- *Noise hazards can lead not only to permanent hearing damage, but it has been established that noise can cause personality disorders, increase aggressive behavior and have an aggravating effect on headaches, hypertension, and peptic ulcers. It also lowers work efficiency and interferes with sleep patterns.*

AWARENESS COUNTS:

- *If you are in a noisy environment several hours a day where you have to raise your voice to be heard, you are in an area of potential danger for hearing loss. Noise that is painfully loud, such as pneumatic hammers or amplified rock music, has the greatest potential to damage hearing.*

- *The age group in which there is particular susceptibility to hearing loss is adolescence.*

- *It is particularly important to sleep in a quiet environment; use rugs, drapes, double windows, and finally ear plugs if necessary, to obliterate disturbing sound. (Cotton makes a poor plug unless saturated with wax or vaseline. Sponge plastic ear plugs are better.)*

- *Pleasant background music can sometimes be used to mask disturbing sounds. However, background noise can conceal safety warnings, or lead to slow reaction time and thus contribute to accidents.*

FOLLOW-THROUGH

For information on all environmental hazards, write to:

The U.S. Environmental Protection Agency
Office of Public Affairs (A-107) Washington, D.C. 20460

For information about noise hazards, write to:

The National Information Center for Quiet
P.O. Box 57171 Washington, D.C. 20037

Crime Prevention
Through your own efforts, you can learn to reduce the opportunity and temptation for the criminal by accepting the responsibility to do everything possible for the protection of your personal well being and property. All "no" answers are a cue to ACTION.

To protect yourself, do you...?	YES	NO
...Always us a peephole or chain lock to identify your visitor?	○	○
...Watch out for suspicious people or cars in your neighborhood?	○	○
...Make an effort to get better acquainted with your neighbors, especially if you live in a large apartment building?	○	○
...Avoid resisting the orders of a robber or purse snatcher?	○	○
...List only your last name and initials in the phone directory and on the mailbox?	○	○
...Always lock your doors during the day, even if you are at home?	○	○
...Leave lights on doors you will be using when you return after dark?	○	○
...Always have your key in your hand when you return home so you can open the door immediately?	○	○

RISK FACTORS:
PROTECTING YOURSELF

- *Women alone and the elderly are at highest risk at being victims of crime.*
- *People who are disabled are more vulnerable to crime.*
- *Certain areas of every large city are high crime areas and should be avoided if possible.*

AWARENESS COUNTS:

- List only your last name and initial in the phone directory and on the mailbox, particularly if you are a woman living alone.
- Always have your key ready when you return home.
- Always ask a visitor to identify himself before you let him in.
- Use automatic timers to turn on lights, radio, etc.
- If a window or lock has been forced or broken while you were out, use a neighbor's phone to call the police and wait outside until they arrive.
- Be cautious of unidentified phone callers. Hang up immediately if the caller will not identify himself.
- When traveling about at night, try to have a companion with you.
- Remember to ask for identification *before* you let repairmen, meter readers, or any other stranger into your home.

To protect yourself, do you...?	YES	NO
...Make specal plans for your home when you are away on vacation?	O	O
...Avoid leaving a key under the doormat or in any accessible area?	O	O
...Have you made sure that your door (s) have sturdy locks?	O	O
...Check all windows and doors regularly for security?	O	O
...Stop newspaper and milk deliveries when you go on vacation?	O	O
...Keep especially valuable items in a safety deposit box away from home?	O	O

RISK FACTORS:
PROTECTING YOUR HOME

- Those at higher risk of home crime are people who leave their homes unattended for long periods of time and those who are nighttime travellers.
- Most crime takes place under cover of darkness.
- Letting mail and newspapers accumulate at your door announces the vulnerability of your home.

AWARENESS COUNTS:

- **Keep your doors locked at all times.**
- **Have lights on an automatic timer while you are away.**
- **An alarm system is a useful crime deterrent.**
- **Make sure windows are secured.**
- **Make sure doorways and hallways are well lighted.**
- **Leave a radio on (a radio uses little electricity and gives the impression that your home is occupied).**

About Locks: Doors should be equipped with either a drop-bolt or dead-bolt lock. Do not use spring locks on any outside door. Spring locks work simply by closing the door and can be easily opened with a plastic card. Drop-bolt or dead-bolt locks can only be unlocked with a key.

FOLLOW-THROUGH

Check with your local police department about joining the Operation Identification Program. You are provided with a sticker to display on your home and your valuable property is engraved with a non-removable code number. The police have a registered list of this property and statistics show that burglars avoid such homes because marked items are difficult to dispose of. Many police departments have crime prevention units and will give you personal advice.

Many states make available the Federal Crime Insurance Program – it provides federal crime insurance against burglary and robbery losses – rates depend upon the crime rate in the area where your home is located. For more information write to:

Federal Crime Insurance, P.O. Box 11033
Washington, D.C. 20014 Toll Free (800) 638-8780

Review your homeowner's insurance coverage to make sure you have adequate coverage.

Personal Safety

While not all accidents are preventable, many are. Failure to take simple precautionary measures increases the risk of an avoidable accident. See if you can identify safety problem areas.
All "yes" answers are a cue to Action.

Concerning PERSONAL SAFETY,	YES	NO
...Have you had any accidents in the past years which could have been prevented?	○	○
...If yes, where did this occur? at home?	○	○
in your automobile?	○	○
at work?	○	○

To ensure your SAFETY AT HOME,	YES	NO
...Do you fail to go through your dwelling, room by room, deliber-ately looking for safety hazards once a year?	○	○
...Does your dwelling have fewer than two means of escape in the event of an emergency?	○	○

	YES	NO
...If you smoke, do you ever smoke in bed?	○	○
...Do you fail to keep a first aid kit, smoke alarm and fire extinguisher at home?	○	○
...Are there loose electrical wiring or fixtures around your home?	○	○
...Are carpets put down without non-skid backings?	○	○
...Are poisons and pills in areas within reach of pre-school children?	○	○

In the BATHROOM, do you fail to...	YES	NO
...Check the temperature of bath or shower water with your hand first?	○	○
...Make sure electrical appliances are never used near water?	○	○
...Use non-skid paste-ons or rubber mats for bathtub and shower surfaces?	○	○

In the KITCHEN, do you fail to...	YES	NO
...Store knives with points away from the hand, or in special holders?	○	○
...Keep curtains away from the cook-ing range?	○	○
...Keep electrical appliances away from water?	○	○
...Keep floors clean of grease and dirt?	○	○
...Are you currently exposed to any of the material listed below?	○	○
dust (such as wood, leather, heavy metals, dyestuff)?	○	○
petroleum products?	○	○
radiation?	○	○
solvents?	○	○
...If yes to any of the above...was your exposure usually indoors?	○	○

	YES	NO
...Did your exposure occur for an equiv-alent of at least one eight hour day per week for a period of five years?	○	○
...If yes to dust, chemicals or petroleum products, was your skin or clothing regularly contacted by these materials?	○	○

To ensure your SAFETY IN YOUR AUTOMOBILE, do you...?	YES	NO
...Neglect to <u>always</u> fasten your seat belts?	○	○
...Ever drink alcoholic beverages before driving?	○	○
...Drive even when you are sleepy?	○	○
...Drive more than <u>40%</u> of the time in the dark?	○	○
...Have you received more than <u>one</u> moving traffic violation this past year?	○	○
...Have you had more than <u>one</u> acci-dent this past year?	○	○

RISK FACTORS: PERSONAL SAFETY

- Accidents are the leading cause of death among those under 44 years old.

- Accidents are the fourth most common cause of death in this country ranking behind heart disease, cancer and stroke.

AWARENESS COUNTS:

- It is especially important that potential problem areas at home, on the road, and at work be identified so that you can create a relatively accident free environment. Improving your accident-prone behavior is the only way to decrease your risk of accidents.
- Your home or apartment should be regularly checked for safety hazards: ■ Slippery stairways
  - Unfastened carpets ■ Faulty fixtures or outlets ■ Store poisons, firearms in safe place
  - Have safety guard rails on upper level windows ■ Place smoke detectors in strategic areas
  - Have emergency numbers posted by the phone ■ Fire strikes more than 1,500 homes every day.
- Automobile accidents take more lives each year than any other type of accident or illness. Many of these can be prevented: ■ Make sure your car is in safe running condition, especially brakes and tires
  - Wear seat belts at <u>all</u> times. ■ Never drive while drinking. ■ Never drive while sleepy. ■ Always lock your car.

To ensure your SAFETY AT WORK,	YES	NO	
...Does your place of work fail to have regular safety checks?	○	○	
...Does your place of work fail to have regular emergency drills such as fire drills?	○	○	
...Does your place of work fail to have a current fire emergency plan?	○	○	
...Does your place of work fail to have rules governing the use of machinery and protective equipment?	○	○	
...Have you ever worked at a job where you were exposed to: asbestos? ○○ chemicals? ○○ coal dust? ○○			

RISK FACTORS:
SAFETY AT WORK

- 13,000 accidental deaths per year occur on the job and over 2 million people are disabled or injured.
- Almost 30 billion dollars per year and about 25 million work days are lost due to accidents at work.

AWARENESS COUNTS:

- Know where fire extinguishers are located.
- Is there a fire emergency plan in your office?
- Know the mandatory safety standards which apply to your business or industry.
- Use all protective clothing required.
- Know the names and hazards of <u>all</u> materials you are exposed to.

FOLLOW-THROUGH

For information regarding safety procedures and requirements <u>on the job</u> write to:
The U.S. Department of Labor, Washington, D.C. 20212

Or get in touch with the Department of Labor office in your region. Or write to:
The National Institute for Occupational Safety and Health, Post Office Building, Cincinnati, Ohio 45202

For information regarding the safety of consumer products, write to:
U.S. Consumer Product Safety Commission Office of Washington, D.C. 20207

For information regarding all kinds of accidents, write to:
The National Safety Council, 444 N. Michigan Avenue, Chicago, Illinois 60611

Preventive Medicine Institute /Strang Clinic   55 East 34 Street • New York, N.Y. 10016 • (212) 683-1000

Blood Pressure Assessment*

Blood pressure is assessed with a sphygmomanometer and a stethoscope. The sphygmomanometer consists of an inflatable bladder contained within a cuff and a mercury gravity manometer or an aneroid manometer from which the pressure is read (see Figure 8.12 and 8.13 in Chapter 8). The appropriate size cuff must be selected to get accurate readings. The size is determined by the width of the inflatable bladder, which should be about 40 percent of the circumference of the midpoint of the arm.

Measurement of blood pressure is usually done in the sitting position, with the forearm and the manometer at the same level as the heart. Initially, record the pressure from each arm, and subsequent pressures from the arm with the highest reading. Apply the cuff approximately one inch above the antecubital space (natural crease of the elbow), with the center of the bladder applied directly over the medial (inner) surface of the arm. Apply the stethoscope head firmly, but with little pressure, over the brachial artery in the antecubital space. The arm should be slightly flexed and placed on a flat surface. Inflate the bladder, while feeling the radial pulse, to about 30 to 40 mm Hg above the disappearance of the pulse.

Do not overinflate the cuff, as it may cause blood vessel spasm, resulting in higher blood pressure readings. Release the pressure at a rate of 2 mm Hg per second. As the pressure is released, determine the systolic blood pressure at the point where the initial pulse sound is heard. Determine the diastolic pressure at the point where the sound disappears. Make the recordings to the nearest 2 mm Hg (even numbers), expressed as systolic over diastolic pressure (for example, 124/80).

When taking more than one reading, completely deflate the bladder and allow at least one minute before making the next recording. Note whether the pressure was recorded from the left or the right arm. Resting blood pressure ratings are given in Table D.1.

In some cases, the loudness of the pulse sounds decreases in intensity (point of muffled sounds) and can still be heard at a lower pressure (50 or 40 mm Hg) or even all the way down to zero. In this situation, record the diastolic pressure at the point where there is a clear/definite change in the loudness of the sound (also referred to as fourth phase), and at complete disappearance of the sound (fifth phase) (for example, 120/78/60 or 120/82/0).

Several readings by different people or at different times of the day should be taken to establish the real values. A single reading may not be an accurate value because of the various factors that can affect blood pressure.

 Table D.1 Blood Pressure Ratings in mm Hg

Systolic	Diastolic	Rating*
≤120	≤80	Very Low Risk
121–130	81–89	Low Risk
131–140	90–99	Moderate Risk
141–150	100–105	High Risk
≥151	≥106	Very high Risk

*Ratings expressed in terms of cardiovascular disease risk.

*Recommendations for Human Blood Pressure Determination by Sphygmomanometers. American Heart Association, 1980.

Name: _____   Course: _____   Section: _____

Date	Arm	Blood Pressure	Recorder's Name

Figure D.1 ● *Blood pressure recording form.*

Glossary

A

Accommodating resistance Strength-training program that requires special equipment with mechanical devices that provide variable resistance, with the intent of overloading the muscle group maximally through the entire range of motion.

Acquired immunodeficiency syndrome (AIDS) Virus (HIV) that destroys the immune system.

Addiction Compulsive and uncontrollable behavior(s) or use of substance(s), most frequently drugs.

Adenosine triphosphate (ATP) A high-energy chemical compound used for immediate energy by the body.

Adipose tissue Fat cells.

Aerobic exercise Exercise that requires oxygen to produce the necessary energy (ATP) to carry out the activity.

AIDS See Acquired immunodeficiency syndrome.

Alcohol (drinking alcohol) Known as ethyl alcohol, a depressant drug that affects the brain and slows down central nervous system activity.

Alcoholism Disease in which an individual loses control over drinking alcoholic-containing beverages.

Altruism The act of providing service to others.

Alveoli Air sacs in the lungs where gas exchange (oxygen and carbon dioxide) takes place.

Amenorrhea Cessation of regular menstrual flow.

Amino acids Chemical compounds that contain nitrogen, carbon, hydrogen, and oxygen. Amino acids are the basic building blocks the body uses to build different types of protein.

Amotivational syndrome A condition characterized by loss of motivation, dullness, apathy, and no interest in the future.

Anabolic steroids Synthetic versions of the male sex hormone testosterone which promotes muscle development and hypertrophy.

Anabolism Process whereby simple substances are formed into more complex substances.

Anaerobic exercise Exercise that does not require oxygen to produce the necessary energy (ATP) to carry out the activity.

Aneurysm Weakness in the arterial wall allowing the formation of a balloon-like pouch.

Angina pectoris Chest pain.

Angiogenesis Capillary (blood vessel) formation into cancerous tumors.

Angioplasty A procedure in which a balloon-tipped catheter is inserted to widen the inner lumen of one or more arteries.

Anorexia nervosa An eating disorder characterized by self-imposed starvation to lose and maintain very low body weight.

Anthropometric measurement Measurement of body girths at different sites.

Anticoagulant Any substance that inhibits blood clotting.

Antioxidants Compounds such as the vitamins C, E, beta-carotene (a precursor to vitamin A), and the mineral selenium, which prevent oxygen from combining with other substances to which it may cause damage. Antioxidants are thought to play a key role in the prevention of heart disease and cancer.

Aquaphobic Having a fear of water.

Arrhythmias Irregular heart rhythms.

Arteries Major vessels that carry blood away from the heart to bodily tissues.

Arteriosclerosis Hardening of the arteries.

Atherosclerosis Type of arteriosclerosis characterized by plaque formation or the buildup of fatty tissue in the inner layers of the wall of the arteries.

ATP See Adenosine triphosphate.

Atrophy Decrease in size of a cell.

Autogenic training Stress management technique; a form of self-suggestion wherein an individual is able to place him/herself in an autohypnotic state by repeating and concentrating on feelings of heaviness and warmth in the extremities.

B

Ballistic or dynamic stretching (flexibility) Exercises performed using jerky, rapid, and bouncy movements.

Basal cell carcinoma Type of skin cancer that occurs primarily on the face. It grows slowly and rarely spreads to other parts of the body.

Basal metabolic rate Lowest level of oxygen consumption (uptake) necessary to sustain life.

Behavior modification A process to permanently change destructive or negative behaviors and replace them with positive behaviors that will lead to better health and well-being.

Benign Noncancerous.

Beta-carotene Precursor to vitamin A.

Bioelectrical impedance Technique to assess body composition, including percent body fat, by running a weak electrical current (totally painless) through the body.

Biofeedback Stress management technique; a process in which a person learns to reliably influence physiological responses of two kinds: (a) responses that are not ordinarily under voluntary control or (b) responses that ordinarily are easily regulated but for which regulation has broken down because of trauma or disease.

Blood pressure Pressure of the blood exerted against the walls of the arteries.

BMI *See* Body Mass Index.

Body composition Term used in reference to the fat and nonfat components of the human body. Body composition is important in the assessment of recommended or "ideal" body weight.

Body density Weight of the body per unit volume.

Body Mass Index (BMI) Anthropometric technique used to determine potential risk for disease based on excessive thinness or fatness.

Breathing techniques for relaxation Stress management technique wherein the individual concentrates on "breathing away" the tension and inhaling fresh air to the entire body.

Brown fat cells Cells that produce body heat by burning fat.

Bulimia Eating disorder characterized by a pattern of binge eating and purging to attempt to lose and maintain low body weight.

C

CAD (Coronary artery disease) *See* Coronary heart disease.

Caffeine A central nervous system stimulating drug most frequently found in coffee, tea, and colas.

Calorie (also referred to as "small calorie") The amount of heat necessary to raise the temperature of 1 gram of water 1° C. Short term for *kilocalorie*. Used to measure the energy value of food and cost of physical activity.

Calorimeter Equipment used to measure the caloric value of food or heat production of animals and humans.

Cancer Group of diseases characterized by uncontrolled growth and spread of abnormal cells into malignant tumors.

Capillary Smallest blood vessels carrying oxygenated blood in the body.

Carbohydrate loading Increasing intake of carbohydrates during heavy aerobic training or prior to aerobic endurance events lasting longer than 90 minutes.

Carbohydrates Compounds containing carbon, hydrogen, and oxygen; the major source of energy for the human body.

Carcinogens Substances that contribute to the formation of cancers.

Carcinoma in situ Encapsulated malignant tumor (cancer) that is found at an early stage and has not spread.

Cardiac output Amount of blood ejected by the heart in 1 minute.

Cardiovascular diseases Conditions that affect the heart and the circulatory system (blood vessels). Examples of cardiovascular diseases are coronary heart disease, peripheral vascular disease, congenital heart disease, rheumatic heart disease, atherosclerosis, strokes, high blood pressure, and congestive heart failure.

Cardiorespiratory endurance Ability of the lungs, heart, and blood vessels to deliver adequate amounts of oxygen to the cells to meet the demands of prolonged (aerobic) physical activity.

Catabolism Process whereby complex substances are broken down into simpler substances.

Catecholamines Hormones; include epinephrine and norepinephrine.

Cellulite Term frequently used in reference to fat deposits that "bulge out." These deposits are nothing but enlarged fat cells from excessive accumulation of body fat.

CHD *See* Coronary heart disease.

Chlamydia Sexually transmitted disease caused by a bacterial infection that can cause significant damage to the reproductive system and may occur without symptoms.

Cholesterol A waxy substance that is technically a steroid alcohol found only in animal fats and oil.

Chronic diseases Conditions that develop over a prolonged time, usually associated with unhealthy lifestyle factors (hypertension, atherosclerosis, coronary disease, strokes, diabetes, cancer).

Chronic obstructive pulmonary disease (COPD) An air flow-limiting condition that includes chronic bronchitis and emphysema, among others.

Chronological age Actual age of the individual (*See also* Functional age).

Circuit training Alternating exercises by performing them in sequence of three to six or more.

Cocaine 2-beta-carbomethoxy-3-betabenozoxytropane, the primary psychoactive ingredient derived from coca plant leaves. Also referred to as coke, C, snow, blow, toot, flake, Peruvian lady, white girl, and happy dust.

Coenzyme Nonprotein molecule required in enzyme reactions.

Cold turkey Elimination of a negative behavior all at once.

Complex carbohydrates Carbohydrates formed by three or more simple sugar molecules linked together; also referred to as polysaccharides. Commonly used to designate foods high in starch.

Compound fats A combination of simple fats with other chemicals. Examples are phospholipids, glucolipids, and lipoproteins.

Concentric muscle contraction Shortening of fibers during muscle contraction.

Congenital heart disease Heart defects present at birth.

Cool-down Tapering off an exercise session slowly.

Coronary arteries Arteries that supply the myocardium or heart muscle with oxygen and nutrients.

Coronary heart disease (CHD) Condition caused by obstruction of coronary arteries by plaque formation (*See also* Atherosclerosis).

Cross training Combining two or more activities to achieve a similar training effect.

Cruciferous vegetables Plants that produce cross-shaped leaves (cauliflower, broccoli, cabbage, Brussels sprouts, kohlrabi), which seem to have a protective effect against cancer.

D

Daily values A set of standard nutritive values developed by the FDA (replaces the U.S. RDA).

Dehydration Loss of body water below normal volume.

Deoxyribonucleic acid (DNA) Genetic material, substance of which genes are made.

Derived fats A combination of simple and compound fats.

Diabetes mellitus Condition in which blood glucose is unable to enter cells because the pancreas either totally stops producing insulin or produces an insufficient amount for the body's needs.

Diastolic blood pressure Pressure exerted by the blood against the walls of the arteries during the relaxation phase (diastole) of the heart.

Dietary fiber Fiber in plant foods that cannot be digested by the human body.

Dietary-induced thermogenesis (DIT) Extra amount of heat production caused by metabolism of food.

Disaccharides Simple carbohydrates formed by two monosaccharide units linked together, one of which is glucose. Major disaccharides are sucrose, lactose, and maltose.

Distress Negative stress; unpleasant or harmful stress under which health and performance begin to deteriorate.

DIT *See* Dietary-induced thermogenesis.

DNA *See* Deoxyribonucleic acid.

Duration How long a person exercises.

Dynamic Strength training method referring to a muscle contraction with movement.

Dysmenorrhea Painful menstruation.

E

Eccentric muscle contraction Lengthening of fibers during muscle contraction.

ECG *See* Electrocardiogram.

EKG *See* Electrocardiogram.

Elastic elongation (flexibility) Temporary lengthening of soft tissue (muscles, tendons, and ligaments).

Electrocardiogram (ECG or EKG) Recording of electrical activity of the heart.

Emphysema Pulmonary disease caused by distention (overinflation) of the alveoli.

Endorphines Morphine-like substances released from pituitary gland in the brain during prolonged aerobic exercise. They are thought to induce feelings of euphoria and natural well-being.

Endurance *See* Cardiovascular endurance and muscular endurance.

Energy The ability to do work.

Energy-balancing equation A principle holding that as long as caloric input equals caloric output, the person will not gain or lose weight. If caloric intake exceeds output, the person gains weight; when output exceeds input, the person loses weight.

Enzyme Catalyst that facilitates chemical reactions.

Epidemiology Science that studies the relationship between diverse factors (lifestyle and environmental) and occurrence of disease.

Essential amino acids Amino acids that must be obtained in the diet because they cannot be produced in the body.

Essential fat Minimal amount of body fat needed for normal physiological functions; constitutes about 3% of total fat in men and 12% in women.

Estrogen Female sex hormone; essential for bone formation and bone density conservation.

Eumenorrhea Normal menstrual cycle.

Eustress Positive stress; health and performance continue to improve, even as stress increases.

Exercise A type of physical activity that requires planned, structured, and repetitive bodily movement done to improve or maintain one or more components of physical fitness.

Exercise adherence Initiating and participating in an exercise program for life.

Exercise electrocardiogram An exercise test during which workload is increased gradually (until the subject reaches maximal fatigue) with blood pressure and twelve-lead electrocardiographic monitoring throughout the test.

Exercise intolerance Inability to function during exercise, leading to symptoms such as very rapid or irregular heart rate, labored breathing, nausea, vomiting, light-headedness, headaches, dizziness, pale skin, flushness, excessive weakness, lack of energy, shakiness, sore muscles, cramps, and tightness in the chest.

Exercise tolerance test *See* Exercise electrocardiogram.

F

Fast-twitch fibers Muscle fibers with greater anaerobic potential and fast speed of contraction.

Fatigue Inability to maintain a given workload.

Fats Compounds made by a combination of triglycerides.

Ferritin Iron stored in the body.

Fiber A form of complex carbohydrate made up of plant material that cannot be digested by the human body.

Fight or flight mechanism Physiological response of the body to stress, which prepares the individual to take action by stimulating the vital defense systems.

Fixed resistance Type of exercise in which a constant resistance is moved through a joint's full range of motion.

Flexibility　Ability of a joint to move freely through its full range of motion.

Fraud　*See* Quackery.

Free fatty acids (FFA)　Fatty acids released by the breakdown of triglycerides.

Free radicals　*See* Oxygen free radicals.

Free weights　Barbells and dumbbells.

Frequency　How often a person engages in an exercise session.

Frostbite　Damage to the tissues as a result of prolonged exposure to extreme cold.

Functional age　Physiological age; usually lower than chronological (actual) age in fit people and vice versa in unfit people.

G

Genetics　Science that studies genetic or hereditary conditions.

Genital warts　Sexually transmitted disease caused by a viral infection. Genital warts increase the risk of cervical cancer. Enlargement and spread of the warts leads to obstruction of the urethra, vagina, and anus.

Girth measurements technique　Method of assessing body composition, including percent body fat, by measuring circumferences at various body sites.

Glucose　Blood sugar, type of carbohydrate (monosaccharide), a primary source of energy for the human body.

Glucose intolerance　Inability to metabolize glucose properly.

Glycogen　Form of carbohydrate (polysaccharide) storage in muscle.

Glycolysis　Breakdown of glucose to pyruvic or lactic acid.

Gonorrhea　Sexually transmitted disease caused by a bacterial infection that can lead to pelvic inflammation in women, infertility, widespread bacterial infection, heart damage, arthritis in men and women, and blindness in children born to infected women.

H

HDL　*See* High density lipoprotein.

Health fitness standards　The lowest level that allows a person to sustain moderate to vigorous physical activity without undue fatigue and the ability to closely maintain this level throughout life.

Health promotion　Programs aimed at helping people develop healthy lifestyle behaviors that will lead to a higher state of wellness.

Health-related fitness　Refers to fitness components that, when enhanced, lead to better health (cardiovascular endurance, body composition, muscular strength and endurance, and muscular flexibility).

Heart attack　*See* Myocardial infarction.

Heart rate reserve　The difference between the maximal heart rate and the resting heart rate.

Heat cramps　Muscle cramps caused by heat-induced changes in electrolyte balance in muscle cells.

Heat exhaustion　Heat-related condition; symptoms include fainting, dizziness, profuse sweating, cold clammy skin, headaches, and a rapid, weak pulse.

Heat stroke　Heat-related emergency; symptoms include serious disorientation, warm dry skin, no sweating, rapid full pulse, vomiting, diarrhea, unconsciousness, and high body temperature.

Hemoglobin　Protein-iron compound in red blood cells that transports oxygen in the blood.

Herpes　Sexually transmitted disease caused by viral infection (herpes simplex virus types I and II). Characterized by appearance of sores on mouth, genitals, rectum, or other parts of the body. Has no known cure.

Hidden fat　Fat in food that can not be observed readily (lean meats contain about 30% to 40% fat calories).

High density lipoprotein (HDL)　Cholesterol-transporting molecules in the blood. High HDL-cholesterol (good cholesterol) seems to offer protection against some forms of cardiovascular disease.

High-impact aerobics (HIA)　Form of aerobics in which both feet may be off the floor at the same time momentarily.

HIV　*See* Human immunodeficiency virus.

Human immunodeficiency virus (HIV)　Virus that causes acquired immunodeficiency syndrome (AIDS).

Hydrostatic weighing　Underwater weighing technique to assess body composition, including percent body fat.

Hyperglycemia　Elevated blood sugar (glucose).

Hyperlipidemia　Elevated blood fats or lipids.

Hyperplasia　An increase in the number of cells.

Hypertension　Chronically elevated blood pressure.

Hypertrophy　An increase in the size of the cell (for example, muscle hypertrophy).

Hypoglycemia　Low blood sugar (glucose).

Hypokinetic disease　Condition associated with a lack of physical activity (for example, hypertension, coronary heart disease, obesity, and diabetes).

Hypotension　Low blood pressure.

Hypothermia　A breakdown in the body's ability to generate heat with a drop in temperature below 95°F.

I

Insulin　Hormone secreted by the pancreas that increases the absorption and utilization of glucose by the body.

Intensity　In cardiorespiratory exercise, how hard a person has to exercise to improve or maintain fitness.

Interval training　Method consisting of repeated bouts of exercise with rest intervals between each exercise bout.

Ischemia　Lack of blood flow.

Isokinetic contraction　Muscular contraction at a constant velocity.

Isokinetic training　Strength-training method in which the speed of the muscle contraction is kept constant because the equipment (machine) provides an accommodating resistance to match the user's force (maximal) through the range of motion.

Isometric training　Strength-training method that refers to a muscle contraction producing little or no movement, such as pushing or pulling against immovable objects.

Isotonic training Strength-training method that refers to a muscle contraction with movement, such as lifting an object over the head.

J

Juvenile diabetes (Type I) Insulin-dependent diabetes. *See also* Diabetes mellitus.

K

Kilocalorie A unit to measure heat energy. A kilocalorie (kcal) or large calorie is the amount of heat necessary to raise the temperature of one kilogram of water one degree Centigrade. One kcal equals 1,000 calories.

L

Lactic acid Strong acid, end product of anaerobic glycolysis (metabolism).

Lactovegetarians Vegetarians who also eat foods from the milk group.

LDL *See* Low density lipoprotein.

Lean body mass Body weight without body fat.

Leisure-time physical activity Any activity undertaken during an individual's discretionary time that helps to increase resting energy or caloric expenditure.

Life Experiences Survey Questionnaire used to assess sources of stress in life.

Lipoprotein A simple protein combined with a lipid group.

Locus of control The extent to which a person believes he or she can influence the external environment.

Low density lipoprotein (LDL) Bad cholesterol-transporting molecules in the blood (the "good" cholesterol). It increases the risk for some forms of cardiovascular disease.

M

Malignant Cancerous.

Marijuana A psychoactive drug prepared from a mixture of crushed leaves, flowers, small branches, stems, and seeds from the hemp plant cannabis sativa. Also referred to as pot and grass.

Maximal heart rate (MHR) Highest heart rate for a person, primarily related to age.

Maximal oxygen uptake (VO$_{2max}$) The maximal amount of oxygen that the body is able to utilize per minute of physical activity, commonly expressed in ml/kg/min; the best indicator of cardiovascular or aerobic fitness.

Meditation Stress management technique used to gain control over one's attention, clearing the mind and blocking out the stressor(s) responsible for the increased tension.

Megadose (of vitamins) Large amount of vitamin(s) intake. For most vitamins, a megadose is ten times the RDA or more.

Melanoma Deadliest of all types of skin cancer. Tumors grow rapidly and spread readily to other parts of the body if not treated at an early stage.

Metabolism All energy and material transformations that occur within living cells necessary to sustain life.

Metastasis Movement of bacteria or body cells from one part of the body to another. Often associated with cancer.

METS (metabolic equivalents) A measurement unit of resting energy expenditure. One MET is the equivalent of 3.5 ml/kg/min.

Minerals Inorganic elements found in the body and in food; essential for normal body functions.

Mitochondria Structures within the cells where energy transformations take place.

Mode Form of exercise.

Moderate-impact aerobics (MIA) Form of aerobics in which at least one foot is in contact with the floor or ground at all times.

Moderate physical activity Physical activity that uses 150 calories of energy per day, or 1,000 calories per week.

Monogamous A sexual relationship in which two people have sexual relations only with each other.

Monosaccharides The simplest carbohydrates (sugars) formed by five- or six-carbon skeletons. The three most common monosaccharides are glucose, fructose, and galactose.

Monounsaturated fat Fatty acids with only one double bond found along the carbon atom chain.

Motivation The desire and will to do something.

Motor neurons Nerves traveling from the central nervous system to the muscle.

Motor skill-related fitness Fitness components that, when improved, lead to enhanced athletic performance (agility, balance, coordination, power, reaction time, and speed).

Motor unit The combination of a motor neuron and the muscle fibers that it innervates.

Muscle fiber A muscle cell.

Muscular endurance (localized muscular endurance) The ability of a muscle to exert submaximal force repeatedly over a period of time (for example, 30 repetitions on a bench press exercise). It usually implies a specific muscle group (chest, thighs, abdominals).

Muscular strength The ability of a muscle to exert maximum force against resistance (for example, 1 repetition maximum or 1 RM on the bench press exercise).

Myocardial infarction Heart attack; damaging or death of an area of the heart muscle as a result of an obstructed artery to that area.

Myocardium Heart muscle.

Myoglobin Iron-containing compound that holds oxygen in muscle tissue.

N

Neuron Nerve cell.

Nicotine Poisonous compound found in tobacco leaves.

Nitrosamines Potentially cancer-causing compounds formed when nitrites and nitrates, which are used to prevent the growth of harmful bacteria in processed meats, combine with other chemicals in the stomach.

Nonmelanoma Skin cancer that spreads or grows directly from the original site but does not metastasize to other regions of the body.

Nonessential amino acids Amino acids that can be manufactured in the body, and therefore, do not have to be obtained in the diet.

Nulliparity Never having had a child.

Nutrient density Ratio of nutrients to calories in food.

Nutrient Substance found in food that provides energy, regulates metabolism, and helps with growth and repair of body tissues.

Nutrition Science that studies the relationship of foods to optimal health and performance.

O

Obesity An excessive accumulation of body fat, usually at least 30% above recommended body weight.

Olestra Fat substitute made from sugar and fatty acids; provides no calories to the body because it passes through the digestive system without being absorbed.

Oligomenorrhea Irregular menstrual cycles.

Omega-3 fatty acids Polyunsaturated fatty acids found primarily in cold water seafood and thought to be effective in lowering blood cholesterol and triglycerides.

Oncogenes Part of DNA that initiates cell division.

One repetition maximum (1 RM) The maximal amount of resistance (weight) that an individual is able to lift in a single effort.

Opportunistic infections Diseases that arise in the absence of a healthy immune system that would fight them off in healthy people.

Osteoporosis Softening, deterioration, or loss of total body bone.

Overload principle Key training concept stating that the demands placed on a system (cardiovascular, muscular) must be increased systematically and progressively over time to cause physiologic adaptation (development or improvement).

Overweight An excess amount of weight against a given standard such as height or recommended percent body fat.

Ovolactovegetarians Vegetarians who include egg and milk products in their diet.

Ovovegetarians Vegetarians who allow eggs in their diet.

Oxygen free radicals Substances formed during metabolism, which attack and damage proteins and lipids, in particular the cell membrane and DNA, leading to the development of diseases such as heart disease, cancer, and emphysema. Antioxidants are believed to exert a protective effect by absorbing free radicals before they can cause damage and also by interrupting the sequence of reactions once damage has begun.

P

Pelvic inflammatory disease (PID) An overall designation referring to the effects of chlamydia and gonorrhea.

Percent body fat Ratio of fat in the body to total weight; includes both essential and storage fat. Used in body composition assessment.

Peripheral vascular disease Narrowing of the peripheral blood vessels (excluding cerebral and coronary arteries).

Physical activity Bodily movement produced by skeletal muscles that requires energy expenditure and produces progressive health benefits.

Physical fitness standard General capacity to adapt and respond favorably to physical effort, implying that individuals are physically fit when they can meet the ordinary as well as the unusual demands of daily life safely and effectively without being overly fatigued, and still have energy left for leisure and recreational activities.

Phytochemicals Chemical compounds thought to prevent and fight cancer; found in large quantities in fruits and vegetables.

Plastic elongation (flexibility) Permanent lengthening of soft tissue (capsules, tendons, and ligaments).

Plyometrics Form of aerobics that requires forceful jumps of springing off the ground immediately after landing from a previous jump.

PNF *See* Proprioceptive neuromuscular facilitation.

Polyunsaturated fat Fatty acids with two or more double bonds along the carbon atom chain.

Prevention index Annual measure of the effort Americans are making to prevent disease and accidents and to promote good health and longevity. The index is based on the 21 most significant health-promoting behaviors in the United States.

Progressive muscle relaxation Stress management technique involving progressive contraction and relaxation of muscle groups throughout the body.

Progressive resistance training *See* Strength training.

Proprioceptive neuromuscular facilitation (PNF) Stretching technique in which muscles are stretched out progressively with intermittent isometric contractions.

Protein Complex organic compounds containing nitrogen and formed by combinations of amino acids. The main substances used in the body to build and repair tissues such as muscles, blood, internal organs, skin, hair, nails, and bones; also part of hormones, antibodies, and enzymes.

Q

Quackery (fraud) Conscious promotion of unproven claims for profit.

R

Range of motion Movement around a given joint.

Rate of perceived exertion (RPE) A perception scale to monitor or interpret the intensity of aerobic exercise.

Recommended body weight Body weight at which there seems to be no harm to human health.

Recommended dietary allowances (RDA) Daily recommended intakes of nutrients for normal, healthy people in the United States.

Recovery time Amount of time the heart takes to return to resting heart rate after exercise.

Red muscle fibers (slow-twitch or type I) Muscle fibers with greater aerobic potential and slow speed of contraction.

Repetition (in strength training) The number of times a given resistance is performed (for example, 12 repetitions on the bench press exercise).

Repetition maximum (RM) The most repetitions that can be performed with a specific resistance or weight (for example, 10 RM with 150 pounds) in strength training.

Residual volume Air left in the lungs following complete exhalation.

Resistance Amount of weight lifted in strength training.

Resting metabolism The amount of energy (expressed in milliliters of oxygen per minute or total calories per day) an individual requires during resting conditions to sustain proper body function.

Reverse cholesterol transport A process in which HDL molecules attract cholesterol and carry it to the liver, where it is changed to bile and eventually excreted in the stool.

Ribonucleic acid (RNA) Genetic material involved in formation of cell proteins.

Risk factors Characteristics that predict which people may develop a certain disease.

RNA *See* Ribonucleic acid.

RPE *See* Rate of perceived exertion.

S

Saturated fat Fatty acids with carbon atoms fully saturated with hydrogens; therefore, only single bonds link the carbon atoms on the chain. High intake of saturated fats increases the risk for coronary heart disease.

Serum cholesterol Blood cholesterol level.

Set Number of repetitions in strength training (e.g., 1 set of 12 repetitions).

Setpoint theory Weight control theory indicating that the body has an established weight and strongly attempts to maintain that weight.

Sexually transmitted diseases (STDs) Conditions spread through sexual contact.

Shin Splints Injury to the lower leg characterized by pain and irritation in the shin region or front of the leg.

Side stitch A sharp pain in the side of the abdomen.

Simple carbohydrates Carbohydrates formed by simple or double sugar units with little nutritive value (for example, candy, cakes). Divided into monosaccharides and disaccharides.

Simple fats A glyceride molecule linked to one, two, or three units of fatty acids (monoglycerides, diglycerides, and triglycerides).

Skinfold thickness Technique to assess body composition, including percent body fat, by measuring the thickness of a double fold of skin at different body sites.

Slow-sustained or static stretching Technique whereby the muscles are lengthened gradually through a joint's complete range of motion and the final position is held a few seconds.

Specificity of training Targeting the specific area the person is attempting to improve (aerobic, anaerobic, strength, flexibility).

Sphygmomanometer Equipment used to measure blood pressure; consists of an inflatable bladder contained within a cuff and a mercury gravity manometer or an aneroid manometer from which the pressure is read.

Spiritual well-being An affirmation of life in a relationship with God, self, community, and environment that nurtures and celebrates wholeness.

Spot reducing Theory that wrongly claims that exercising a specific body part (for example, abdominal or midsection of the body) will result in significant fat reduction in that area.

Squamous cell carcinoma Type of skin cancer that grows at a faster rate that basal cell carcinomas and seems to grow on sun-damaged areas. Squamous cell tumors spread to other parts of the body if not treated at an early stage.

STDs *See* Sexually transmitted diseases

Sterols Derived fats, of which cholesterol is the best known example.

Storage fat Body fat in excess of essential fat; stored in adipose tissue.

Strength *See* Muscular strength.

Strength training Conditioning program that requires weights to help increase muscular strength, endurance, power, or body size.

Step aerobics (SA) Form of aerobics using a combination of stepping and arm movements.

Stress test *See* Exercise electrocardiogram.

Stress The mental, emotional, and physiological response of the body to any situation that is new, threatening, frightening, or exciting.

Stress Vulnerability Scale Questionnaire used to identify a number of factors that can help people decrease their vulnerability to stress.

Stressor Reaction of the organism to a stress-causing event.

Stretching Moving the joints beyond the accustomed range of motion.

Stroke volume Amount of blood ejected by the heart in one beat.

Structured Interview Assessment tool used in determining behavioral patterns (Type A and B personality).

Subluxation Partial dislocation of a joint.

Substrate Substance acted upon by an enzyme (examples: carbohydrates and fats).

Synergy A reaction in which the result is greater than the sum of its two parts.

SPF (sun protection factor) Degree of protection offered by ingredients in sunscreen lotion; at least SPF 15 is recommended.

Synergistic action The effect of mixing two or more drugs which can be much greater than the sum of two or more drugs acting by themselves.

Syphilis Sexually transmitted disease caused by bacterial infection. During the last stage of the disease, some people incur paralysis, crippling, blindness, heart disease, brain damage, insanity, and even death.

Systolic blood pressure Pressure exerted by the blood against walls of the arteries during forceful contraction (systole) of the heart.

T

Tar Chemical compound that forms during the burning of tobacco leaves.

Telomerase Enzyme found in cancer cells that allows them to reproduce indefinitely.

Telomeres Strand of molecules found at both ends of chromosome. After many cell divisions, chromosomes eventually run out of telomeres and the cell dies.

Testosterone Male sex hormone.

Thermogenic response The amount of energy required to digest food.

Transfatty acid Solidified fat formed by adding hydrogen to monosaturated and polyunsaturated fats to increase shelf life.

Triglycerides Fats formed by glycerol and three fatty acids.

Tumor suppressor genes Deactivate the process of cell division.

Type A personality Behavior pattern characteristic of a hard-driving, overambitious, aggressive, at times hostile, and overly competitive person.

Type B personality Behavior pattern characteristic of a calm, casual, relaxed, easy-going individual.

Type C personality Behavior pattern of individuals who are just as highly stressed as the Type A but do not seem to be at higher risk for disease than the Type B.

U

Ultraviolet B rays (UVB) Sunrays that cause sunburn and encourage skin cancers.

V

Variable resistance Training using special machines equipped with mechanical devices that provide differing amounts of resistance through the range of motion.

Vasoconstriction Narrowing or clamping down of blood vessels.

Vasodilation Widening or opening up of blood vessels.

Vegans Vegetarians who eat no animal products at all.

Vegetarians Individuals whose diet is of vegetable or plant origin.

Veins Major vessels that carry blood back to the heart.

Very low density lipoprotein (VLDL) Triglyceride, cholesterol and phospholipid-transporting molecules in the blood. Only a small amount of cholesterol is carried by the VLDL molecules.

Vigorous activity Any activity that requires a MET level equal to or greater than 6 METs.

Vitamins Organic substances essential for normal metabolism, growth, and development of the body.

VLDL *See* Very low density lipoprotein.

W

Waist-to-hip ratio Test designed by a panel of scientists appointed by National Academy of Sciences and Dietary Guidelines Advisory Council for U.S. Departments of Agriculture and Health and Human Services to assess potential risk for diseases associated with obesity.

Warm-up Starting a workout slowly.

Weight training A conditioning program that requires weights to help increase muscular strength, endurance, power, and body size.

Weight-regulating mechanism Mechanism located in the hypothalamus of the brain that regulates how much the body should weigh (*See also* Setpoint theory).

Wellness The constant and deliberate effort to stay healthy and achieve the highest potential for well-being. Implies the adoption of healthy lifestyle factors that will decrease the risk for disease and enhance well-being.

White muscle fibers (fast-twitch or type II) Muscle fibers with greater anaerobic potential and fast speed of contraction.

Work Ability to utilize energy.

Workload Given level of exercise intensity or physical performance.

Y

Yellow fat cells Cells used for fat storage (stores of energy in the form of fat).

Yo-yo dieting Constantly losing and gaining weight.

Index